EXCERPTS FROM LETTERS TO THE AUTHOR

"The Pro-Vita! book is excellent. After reading it, I changed many of the nutritional programs for my clients to your way of giving protein and vegetable breakfast and lunch with a light soup-grain-salad-vegetable dinner. I adopted it also for myself. I noticed that I can avoid in this way oncoming allergic reactions (sinus and burning, watery eyes) which usually showed up during the night."

— CL, *Physician, Germany, 9/14/90*

"I purchased the Pro-Vita! book and started on the Pro-Vita! diet. Never before have I experienced such a balanced awareness of how bodily dysfunctions can be corrected. It made more sense than anything I'd ever heard of and all the information was coming from one source. This was the culmination of my 20-year search for a plan to improve my health. The Pro-Vita! diet has completely changed my life. It has increased my vitality, my spirituality and my overall attitude towards life. To those who may read this letter, I would like to say without any reservations that they couldn't find a more effective life-style than following the Pro-Vita! diet."

— SMM, *Sepulveda, CA, 10/23/89*

"Before I had been following this food plan for even a week, I had lost seven pounds; so many of my friends are now very interested in your book! I feel so much better, and better about myself for following this diet! This is the first book I have found with such authoritative research backing up the claims being made. It really answers my

big question of how to know which foods to eat with which other foods without knowing what happens inside my body, chemically speaking. I have been waiting for just such a book for a long time—thank you, thank you, thank you!"

— SH, Houston, TX, 12/15/91

"After extensive blood work my diagnosis was as follows: Severe hypoglycemia, mononucleosis, Epstein-Barr virus and elevated serum cholesterol. My muscles were filled with pain and I looked like a huge balloon with two tiny beady eyes. I was unable to think and speak clearly. It was at this time that my colonic therapist handed me two books to read, *The Pro-Vita! Diet* and *The Liver Triad*. This is when you walked into my life, Mr. Tips. As I read *The Liver Triad*, I understood what had happened within my body. As I covered the pages in *The Pro-Vita! Diet* I decided, Do It Now! As unbelievable as this sounds, it is a true statement: After five days of being on the Pro-Vita! Diet I felt better than I had in eleven months. A happy ending. As of today I no longer have any hypoglycemia attacks, nor do I experience extreme fatigue, and my digestion has improved 80%, and my bowels are functioning! I am back to running my company—part time, but look forward to working full time in another month. My zest for living has returned."

— KWY, Orlando, FL, 9/14/90

"Recently I discovered at Whole Foods Market your books, including *The Pro-Vita! Diet*. Since your discussion made a lot of sense to me, I followed your dietary suggestions. To my great surprise, just three days of the Pro-Vita! diet cleared up my chronic GI tract problems.

Two weeks into your diet I noticed two additional benefits: A chronic post nasal drip and a perennial and seemingly undiagnosable vaginal drip had practically ceased. Most of all, a persistent pressure and dullness in my head had given way to clarity of thinking to my great delight. All of these events encouraged me to seek out further fine-tuning of my health at your clinic. What a lucky day for me to discover your books at Whole Foods!"

— *IHM, PhD, Austin, TX, 12/29/88*

"I met Stu Wheelwright here in Dallas some 20 years ago and took some courses from him on nutrition and sclerology. I never really understood his dietary recommendations—back then we were making green drinks from weeds—but he was successful in changing my diet in three major regards: 1) I stopped eating red meat and began eating low-stress proteins, 2) I began gardening and added vegetables back as a large part of my diet, 3) I stopped eating protein and carbohydrates in large quantities at the same meal. Thus I attribute to Stu the fact that I've lived in good health these last 20 years.... I'm 88 years old, and in excellent health for the shape I'm in. Reading the Pro-*Vita!* book, I can see where it was indeed a blessed day when Jack Tips came into Stu's life to organize his great research. It was a moment of destiny, and I am truly thankful. Now, for the first time, I see clearly the genius Stu was... we always knew that, but now I understand more...and what a fine thing it is to get his message out to others so they can live well. I've outlived all my family, but every day when I work in my garden, I think of Stu and how he touched my life. Thank you."

— *JL, Dallas, TX, 2/21/89*

THE PRO-VITA! PLAN
Your Foundation for Optimal Nutrition

FEATURING
THE WHEELWRIGHT 5 + 5
MEAL PLAN

Jack Tips ND, PhD

©1993 Edition edited by Rev. Bea Borden
Drawing of 5 + 5 meal on plate by Kathy Brown
Cover design and graphic art by Dale Wilkins
Book Design/Layout by Cath Polito
Indexing by Linda Webster
Proofreading by Janine Tips
Special thanks to Dr. Maesimund Panos and Jane Heimlich, and their
publisher St. Martin's Press, for permitting us to excerpt "What Is
Homeopathy?" from their book, *Homeopathic Medicine At Home.*

Copyright © 1987, 1989, 1992, 1993, 1995, 1996, 1999, 2004 by Jack Tips, ND, PhD.
All rights reserved. No part of this work may be reproduced in any form without
permission in writing from the publisher. New and expanded version.

Published by
APPLE-A-DAY PRESS
1500 Village West Dr., Suite 77
Austin, Texas 78733
Phone (512) 328-3996
Fax (512) 263-7787
website: www.apple-a-daypress.com

This information is provided in good will for informational and educational purposes only. All rights regarding the publishing of this material are owned by Life Resources, Austin, Texas.

LIBRARY OF CONGRESS CARD NUMBER 92-070715

Publisher's Cataloging in Publication (*Prepared by Quality Books, Inc.*)

Tips, Jack, 1950–

The pro-vita!plan: your foundation for optimal nutrition featuring the
wheelwright 5 + 5 meal plan / Jack Tips.
p.cm.
Includes bibliographical references and index.
ISBN 0-929167-05-8

1. Nutrition.   1. Title

RA784.75 1991   613

QB192-427

02   03   04   05   17   16

FOREWORD

We become what we think about.

We become what we eat during twenty-four hours a day.

What we choose to eat today will show up tomorrow in our health.

This is the eternal law of cause and effect with its implications.

We can set ourselves up to be sick, or we can choose to stay well.

It becomes more and more difficult to choose the right food since the progress of technology has shown a great influence on the production of our foods, causing considerable damage to our health. There are many environmental concerns. Vegetables and grains are grown on depleted soil, treated with pesticides, and gassed to preserve shelf life. Animals for human consumption are fed with antibiotics and hormones, and often treated inhumanely. Refined sugar and flour products, and many chemicals are added to foods.

We need a guide to help us find our way through this labyrinth to achieve our basic desire for optimal health. Dr. Jack Tips in this new book, *The Pro-Vita! Plan*, gives us far-reaching ideas of a new approach to our nutrition. He provides clear, precise answers and explanations to many important nutritional questions in general, while answering many questions about the Pro-Vita! Plan in particular. Moreover, he gives us an understanding of how disease originates as one of the effects of incorrect eating habits; and he shows us the way to heal ourselves. It is our responsibility to follow his guidelines.

Life manifests itself in the cell, which duplicates constantly, requiring the best nutrients for optimal functioning. How do we find the superfoods containing these nutrients? The author has the answer with his concept of "Bioenergetic Nutrition," found in the inherent life force of both plants and human beings, and their compatibility with each other. This perspective underlies the Pro-Vita! Plan and makes the most favorable nutrition at the cellular level possible.

The question arises, how much of this energy can be made available to the body? Does a specific food give the amount of energy our bodies need to sustain and enhance all faculties for the best state of health, or does what we eat take energy away from us by requiring excessive amounts of energy for the digestive process and waste disposal?

The author's answer is to distinguish between high, medium and low stress proteins. He points out that the digestion time a certain food needs is one parameter to measure the stress potential of that food. By this method it has been possible to develop charts of these high, medium and low stress foods. The stress level inherent in foods is one of the basic aspects of the Pro-Vita! Plan.

The author monitored two thousand patients about the results of this plan, and he assures us that it is highly effective. The Pro-Vita! Plan gives our body the right food at the right time in the right combination. With these and a positive attitude the body can better shift from imbalance, or disease, to balance and health, with the help of its inborn healing system.

It is not difficult to put the Pro-Vita! Plan into action. Once we get acquainted with real food as a living substance nurturing our body—another living substance—we will not desire to eat overcooked, dead food again, or foods to satisfy only our taste buds. We will not need to use food as a pacifier, when we find ourselves in a state of depression. Instead, we will enjoy the new adventure of choosing foods, which will make the difference between feeling tired, fatigued and sluggish, or feeling invigorated and happy. Each cell in our body is just waiting for the best support, not only concerning the right nutrition, but also in form of a positive and happy outlook for the best performance. All of our cells will rejoice with their inborn intelligence and capacity to remember, paying back with big dividends in the form of vibrant health and longevity.

The Pro-Vita! Plan gives us all the precise information and knowledge to initiate new health endeavor. The beauty of the plan is its great flexibility and the freedom we can feel from not being locked into a routine. We can get a taste of the significance of having a strong healthy body and mind. The desire to have a healthy body and mind will encourage us into action.

Here I can speak of my own experience, when I started to experience lower back pains, heart palpitations and unaccustomed tiredness. After I read the book, I kept completely to the plan. Two weeks later I noticed that the symptoms subsided, and soon they became just a memory. Also, I was able to eliminate all the little side-snacks I needed to maintain proper blood sugar and other temptations to indulge in non-foods. As a result, my way of thinking became clearer and more decisive. There is a certain discipline in this way of eating (not to be misunderstood with rigidity) which will mirror into your daily activities. Thank you, Dr. Jack Tips, the learning process never ends.

In finishing, I repeat what I stated before: It is not difficult to start the Pro-Vita! Plan if you have the desire to be as free as possible in your life's expression which encompasses the freedom and quality of the life you live. We might find treasures we never thought could be ours: health, happiness and longevity. We can choose to stay sick, or we can choose to become well. We also can choose to get this outstanding book to read and apply its principles to our daily life. It is our choice.

Congratulations!

Charlotte Lodi, *Doctor of Medicine, Germany*

PREFACE

The seed for this book was given to me by Stu Wheelwright in his "Rational Diet" lecture presented in 1985 in Austin, Texas. Afterwards it was announced I would be leading the next lecture just two days later. I was left with an audience of sixty people who wanted the lecture explained in greater detail and little did they know I was as familiar (or should I say unfamiliar) with the principles as they were. With the help of a chalkboard and some keen octogenarians who had encountered Wheelwright some ten years prior and were thriving on the diet, I outlined the rules and concepts to an audience eager for more information. Fortunately, teaching is one of the most excellent ways to learn.

During the next few months, I was able to experiment with Wheelwright's 1985 version of his life-long diet research called "The Lo-Stress, 5+5 Diet." I realized that some written material would be good support for people interested in trying the diet. Thus, I outlined Wheelwright's concepts in a four-page flyer and gave it to each attendee at his subsequent consultations and lectures. A year later, the written material had grown to a booklet.

In 1986, Wheelwright came back to Texas with the primary purpose to help me author his diet book and follow up with the herbal programs of his consultees. We isolated ourselves at my family's ranch and attempted to work. While writing I would challenge his ideas and ask for substantiation so I could explain it to the reader. However, even though Wheelwright was a veritable walking encyclopedia of nutritional and biochemical knowledge, he did not enjoy the writing process. Somehow, the laborious development of ideas for written communication was not in sync with his quick, creative mind.

Thus, I turned to cassette tape and interviewed him. This verbal interview technique worked best, leading to the discussion of many aspects of his diet and miles of tape.

Wheelwright was a great philosopher. We talked at length about how plants support human life on this planet and impart elemental vitality for our continued life processes. He spoke of his research with grasses and how he believed there was a grass to heal every ailment of humankind. He spoke of the herbs he found in the Amazon, of isolated peoples who eat instinctively, and of the wisdom of primitive peoples. He spoke of his work with Native Americans, and how he developed the ability to feel what an herb could heal before it was picked. And, very interestingly, he spoke of diluting his herbal combinations to free the energies so they could work deeper to nourish the spirit of human beings.

On one occasion, Wheelwright even outlined a model of a perfect living environment for a population of 144,000 people. I was absolutely amazed at his ingenious solutions to so many of our society's problems. No wonder it was hard to hold him to clarifying how amino acids were absorbed through the intestine. I was trying to write for the non-technical reader, when his level of thought was often expansive and global.

As the material evolved, more and more of my personal experience and clinical research with applying dietary principles became incorporated. With the first printing of the book, *The Pro-Vita! Diet*, the material was 50% Wheelwright's dietary insights and 50% of my own explaining of general dietary principles and philosophy which were not part of Wheelwright's teachings. I sought to help people understand Wheelwright's insights and correlate the information to current nutritional beliefs. Wheelwright recommended the book enthusiastically throughout his visits.

Wheelwright's dietary concepts were given *ex cathedra*, meaning that he would lay the law down and not give substantiation for his principles. For this reason I became the detective for finding substantiation for the principles of his ideas both as "devil's advocate" and proponent.

The Pro-Vita! Plan still retains the original Wheelwright seeds, and thus approximately 25% of it are the principles which he originally taught. The other information of this text derives from my research on, and my own clinical experience with, nutrition, health and natural cure. Throughout the book, I have made it as clear as possible which parts of the information come from Wheelwright's insights.

Wheelwright had a large following of health-conscious people who dearly loved him. In respect for his memory and the gift of improved health which he left to so many people, I differentiate his teachings from my own insights.

Over the years, my perspective has come to differ from Wheelwright's in several regards. First, as a classical homeopath, my foundation for understanding what health is, how to treat the whole person, and how the body heals itself, is based on the *Organon of Medicine*, 6th edition, by Dr. Samuel Hahnemann who was the originator of homeopathy. It is primarily through the matrix of Hahnemann's teachings that I synthesize the gems for better health which Wheelwright left us.

The second point where my approach differs is that Wheelwright felt that his dietary plan was ideal for everyone. In contrast, I am convinced that a nutrition plan must be tailored to the individual. Wheelwright would not allow people to tinker with his plan, yet I feel it fundamental to the success of the Pro-Vita! Plan that people adapt the diet to their particular circumstances. This is another reason for clearly identifying Wheelwright's principles in this book to help you differentiate the master's seeds of wisdom from the evolved application of these seeds.

It is my sincere wish to increase the quality of your life. As a person dedicated to the healing of the whole person, I am convinced that optimal nutrition plays a vital role in health, healing and the freedom we want to experience in our lives. It is my wish that the information contained in this book will be of good service to you.

Jack Tips, 1992

ACKNOWLEDGEMENTS

My heartfelt gratitude and deepest appreciation is hereby expressed

To **Dr. Stuart Wheelwright** who, with his provocative and iconoclastic insights, ignited the spark that launched my seven-year quest for understanding the role of nutrition in optimal health.

To **Dr. Samuel Hahnemann** for providing the foundational philosophy that diet (internal hygiene) and therapy (the correct remedy) constitute the most comprehensive and complete method for restoring the precious gift of health to the ailing human condition.

Thanks and gratitude to Janine Tips for her support in so many varied ways.

CONTENTS

CONTENTS (CONTD.)

CONTENTS (CONT D.)

CONTENTS (CONT D.)

PRO-VITA! KITCHEN AND RECIPES
PART IV: RECIPES

26 • Two-Week Pro-Vita! Menu

CONTENTS (CONT'D.)

VITALITY SCALE

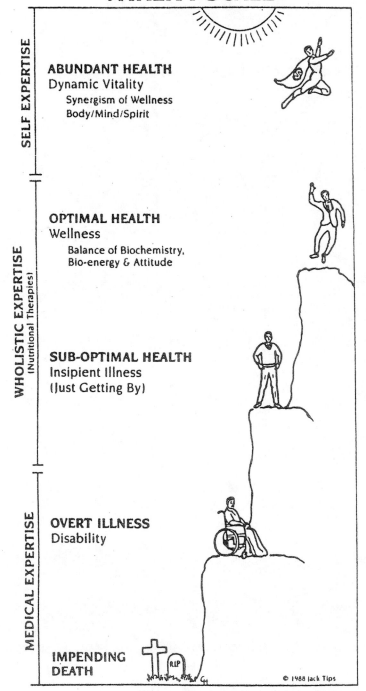

SELF EXPERTISE

ABUNDANT HEALTH
Dynamic Vitality
Synergism of Wellness
Body/Mind/Spirit

WHOLISTIC EXPERTISE
(Nutritional Therapies)

OPTIMAL HEALTH
Wellness
Balance of Biochemistry,
Bio-energy & Attitude

SUB-OPTIMAL HEALTH
Insipient Illness
(Just Getting By)

MEDICAL EXPERTISE

OVERT ILLNESS
Disability

**IMPENDING
DEATH**

R.I.P.

© 1988 Jack Tips

PART I

THE FOUNDATION OF THE PRO-VITA! PLAN

This section provides a discussion of various nutritional tenets and philosophies, as well as the key components of human biochemistry, bioenergy and health. This part is our foundation for understanding nutrition, health and the Pro-Vita! Plan.

THE ROLE OF NUTRITION
IN HEALTH AND DISEASE

NUTRITIONAL PATHWAYS

Over the past 30 years, a confusing array of nutritional pathways has crisscrossed the health field, giving promise of greater health. Some of these nutritional plans help people, others hurt people, and some plans merely substitute one nutritional imbalance for another.

How do you know which nutritional pathway is the right one for you? The confusion and controversy about diet plans are symptoms of working with the isolated parts of human health instead of working with the whole nutritional picture. A diet promoting health, well-being and longevity does not have to be confusing and controversial. Simplicity and ease can replace confusion; clear overview and balance can transcend controversy. The result is a rational way of eating for optimum health and the associated benefits of mental clarity, creativity, longevity and vitality.

As people of the twentieth century, we have a unique dilemma: We are constantly bombarded with a barrage of time-saving, instant, sense-stimulating, but inappropriate foods in our stores. At the same time, we are confronted with a medical philosophy which suppresses or palliates symptoms of illness rather than curing according to Natural Law. When we learn that we do not have to trick or cheat nature to enjoy our innate vitality, then we find the reward of optimal health for understanding and cooperating with Natural Law.

This book provides the information for you to determine your nutritional pathway. Once you find and understand this pathway, you will move with ease on the road to dynamic health.

The Pro-Vita! Plan is not a new nutritional plan, because the Natural Law has been with us since time immemorial. But unlike many methods for eating for health, it has withstood the shifting opinions and advancements of nutritional science over the past few years. In fact, the newest discoveries verify the completeness and adaptability of this plan. Thus, we find that the Pro Vita! Plan is not so much a nutritional pathway as it is the nutritional hub from which a personal plan for healthy eating is derived. For this reason, the Pro-Vita! Plan is compatible with many life-styles and beliefs.

DIET VERSUS NUTRITION

In its simplest definition, diet is what you eat and drink over a period of time. This has an effect on your well-being. The term diet does not refer to temporary diet plans for various goals, such as cleansing, healing, weight loss, candida control, blood sugar balance, or ulcer relief, for example. Such diets are specific therapeutic treatments rather than a nutritional plan for building and maintaining optimal health.

Nutrition, for our purposes, is a PLAN to supply the body with the raw materials it needs for growth, maintenance and vital processing. A plan implies maximizing beneficial nutrients while minimizing detrimental intake of substances. Throughout this book we will examine nutrition in terms of its quality, bioenergy, biochemistry, quantity, composition, stress-level and overall effect on health.

In the context of a nutritional pathway, where is your present diet leading you? Is it leading, like most people's, to heart disease, cancer, osteoporosis, diabetes, Alzheimer's, an early grave; or is your nutritional path leading to vitality, joy, self-discovery, creativity and longevity?

For an honest answer, you need to know that health is built in layers. For example, what we do in our teens predisposes our health in our twenties. If in our twenties we correct past mistakes and heal tendencies to disease portrayed as symptoms, then our thirties will be more healthful, vital and creative.

Disease is built in layers, too. For example, high intake of sugar in the teens predisposes some people to hypoglycemia in their twenties.

If, in the twenties, this tendency is not corrected, but is covered over by using even more sugar and perhaps stimulants such as coffee, or if it is suppressed by drugs such as antidepressants, then is it really any wonder that diabetes could occur in the thirties or forties?

Every day we are given a choice to build and support health through nutrition. At the same time, we can correct symptoms which are the body's way of telling us that a disease trend is possible. Or we can ignore the incredible workings of our vitality and continue the disease process until we are seriously stressed in our health.

Each day we have the opportunity to take charge of our lives and build health into our future. Or we can buy into the great deception that medicine will find a cure for cancer, heart disease, arthritis or allergies which we are creating day by day through our unhealthy life-style.

We need to understand right here at the start that when I refer to "medicine," I am referring to the whole medical industrial complex, not to the individual doctors. I am often critical of "medicine" for its ignorance of natural law and nutrition; its suppressive drugs that always have side effects; its philosophy of suppressing symptoms instead of curing; its history of persecuting alternative treatments and cures to illness; its excessively high costs; and its misguided fundings of research. But I am not being critical of the dedicated, though possibly misled, men and women who are dedicated to the practice of medicine. Doctors are individuals and their personal beliefs and ethics are a personal matter. There are many fine doctors dedicated to a complementary approach to healing who encourage nutrition, herbal therapies, food supplements and homeopathy. I have personal respect for many men and women degreed in medicine.

Here's a quick example. The medical industrial complex knows by their statistics that 35% of all cancers are caused by dietary factors. Yet, only 2% of their financial allocations have anything to do with nutritional research. The bulk of the research and the research dollars is geared toward methods of early detection. Early detection sounds honorable until it is realized that the bottom line motivation is that there will be more time to put people on more drug therapies, give more tests, and have more doctor visits. Thus, more money can be paid to medicine before the patient dies.

Since nutrition does not yield dollars for the medical industrial complex, money is withheld from nutritional research. In fact, nutrition can prevent a large portion of diseases, both chronic and acute. But improving nutrition threatens the financial basis of medicine because with proper nutrition there would be much less illness. Medicine is big, big business; and the organization thinks only to protect its own interests.

In our society, billions of dollars are spent each year for products to hide our symptoms brought on by inferior diet. A healthy body has pleasant breath; a pleasant scent; a strong gastrointestinal tract; and healthy skin. So what does the need for aisles of mouthwash, harsh toothpastes, breath mints and breath sprays tell us? What does the need for aisles of deodorants, antiperspirants, perfumes, deodorant soaps tell us? What about the aisles of antacids, laxatives, stool softeners, and scented toilet paper? And what do aisles of acne preparations, cosmetic cover ups, steroid creams, ointments, and powders tell us? The array of such products tells us we are a society adept in hiding our sickness. We prefer to do that which is wrong for our health, cover it up, suppress it, and then hope our doctors can cure us when whatever is wrong degenerates into something life-threatening.

I once heard my high-school English teacher, an elderly gentleman, say that he wished he had the wisdom of age when he was a young man, because now, when he had wisdom, he had such little time left to apply it. When he was young and had the energy to succeed, he had no interest in the things that he now felt were important. Since my English teacher's situation is a common fact of life, one solution is to eat and live so that middle age and old age can be a dynamic, productive time free from the limitations of inhibiting illness.

If you share this goal, this book will provide you with the tools to build good health for your future. This book teaches Natural Laws that govern health to help you find a simple, enjoyable, healthful way of eating tailored to your body and life-style.

THE IMPORTANCE OF A NUTRITIONAL PLAN

Currently, there is much emphasis on therapeutic diets: weight-loss schemes, so-called "immune power plans," candida diets, "Fit For" and "Eat To" plans, and athletic regimens. Therefore, it is necessary to affirm that a food plan along with exercise and a proper, loving attitude is more than a crash therapy or a quick means to an end. In effect, a food plan is a major foundation upon which to build health, well-being and longevity.

People often mistakenly make therapies their food plans. They constantly cleanse without taking time to rebuild. They rely on vitamin pills to supply factors their diets lack. They rely on stimulants such as coffee, sodas, tobacco, sugar and drugs to produce metabolic and physical activity as discussed in the book, *The Next Step to Greater Energy*, Tips (1990). But such diets simply will not promote health, though it may take years to discover this fact. Good health will remain only an empty hope until the nutritional plan is more in accord with Natural Law.

The human body was originally designed to prosper on the "fruits of the earth." Fruits translates to what the earth bears forth and may include plants, sea food, animals and rocks for that matter, depending on your interpretation. However, the most logical place to start is with fruits and vegetables in their raw state. Non-life source chemicals are excluded. Yet, the average person is exposed to more than 200 non-life-supporting toxic chemicals every day if tap water is used, the air is breathed and commercially grown produce is consumed.

The idea of eating natural foods is based on the fact that nature provides the necessary ingredients for health through diet. This is the natural law and defines the covenant between human beings and earth. If we neglect this fundamental law, we will remain out of sorts with our health and life. Thus, the importance of a well-designed nutrition plan grows each day because we want to maintain our bodies in good health. To achieve this, we have to provide our bodies with foods that are compatible with health and avoid the substances that destroy health.

A food plan should offer full and varied food selections so that there is a broad base of nutrient sources. Because restrictive diets are reflections of restrictive attitudes, a nutrition plan should be varied and flexible. Flexibility and adaptability are keynotes of a successful plan for eating and a life free of concerns about health.

Life begets life. Foods for health are whole, vital, fresh, delicious and ALIVE! Primitive peoples are guided to foods by an intuitive use of taste, a faculty lost to civilized people who live on processed chemical foods. However, the faculty for wholesome foods and the intuitive sense of what is needed when, can be regained.

HOW DIET AFFECTS HEALTH AND DISEASE

It is important to understand the role of foods in health and disease to know what nutritional health we can accomplish with the proper diet. If we correctly understand the role of diet, we do not have false expectations for trying to accomplish things with our nutritional plan that it cannot provide or correct.

To establish the parameters for a nutritional plan, here is a yes/no game to see which answer is correct.

1. Can an optimal diet alone provide optimal health?

NO! A human being is much more than the food eaten. Several distinct, but interwoven dimensions affect a person's optimal level of health including thoughts (purpose in life and expectations); emotions (love and hate, for example); heredity (constitutional predispositions); free flow of life-force energy around and through the body; and how the body assimilates its foods. Most importantly, a person's spiritual life affects health. Consequently, diet is only a small, but important piece of the puzzle of health.

2. Can just any diet work if a person has a beneficial spiritual life, good mental health and emotional stability?

NO! Many spiritual giants who have given evidence of their wise, peaceful and loving attitudes, have suffered poor physical health. Spiritual law does not exclude a person from the dynamics associated with proper maintenance of the physical body. Ignorance of how to maintain physical health properly is no excuse. Nature is dispassionate.

3. Some people seem to be so healthy, yet they eat commercial beef hamburgers, containing antibiotics and hormones, and chocolate ice cream which is usually laced with chemical toxins in addition to the antibiotics and hormones contained in milk. Can some people get away with this way of eating?

NO! At the present time, the vitality of these people is able to adapt to their poor choices of food. Therefore, these people maintain the appearance of getting away with this way of eating. Furthermore, a person may be biochemically predisposed, pH-wise, to benefit from such foods as they normalize the acid/alkaline balance, but better food choices could do the same thing without the detrimental side effects. Eventually, such eating practices, if repeated often enough, will result in a lower quality of health. For example, the high fat contained in such food choices may later result in early menarche and menstrual difficulties, gall bladder disease and coronary disease.

4. Some people eat so well with raw foods, sprouts, properly combined foods and special supplements, yet they have so much trouble with environmental sensitivity and health. Is their diet failing to restore their health?

NO! At the present time, the vitality of these persons is deranged and foods do not have the power to affect a cure. Everything is a stress to the system of these persons. But their healthy foods are not failing such people, because the restoration of health is not within the scope of the foods' healing abilities in these cases. Instead, a healing therapy such as homeopathy is required to restore health. However, the good quality foods are helping such persons to avoid the additional aggravations which would occur with poor food choices. Thus, these good foods provide the type of supportive nutrition the body will use to repair itself in conjunction with the healing therapy.

5. Can diet cause disease?

YES! No doubt! Most diseases are, in fact, caused by poor diet. What we eat is a major factor in determining our biochemical terrain. Dietary stress weakens the gastrointestinal mucosa, inhibits the liver's function, taxes the kidneys and damages the heart and brain. The by-products of inappropriate dietary intake weaken the immune system. When this occurs every day, the body becomes prey to pathological organisms such as yeasts, fungus, bacteria and virus which can flourish in a hospitable terrain. Other dietary indiscretions damage tissues as in the case of low density cholesterol and free radicals, such as nitrates, nitrites and food colors found in red meat products. Because diet plays a key role in the cause of disease, it also plays a key role in the prevention of both acute and chronic illness.

6. Can diet cure some diseases?

NO! Only the body's inherent vitality cures, but YES, diet can help to correct many diseases. However, diet cannot correct all diseases. It would be better to say that diet can cure those diseases caused by misuse of foods, provided that such diseases have not yet deteriorated into "beyond repair" states such as abnormal cell proliferation. If the etiology of the disease is dietary indiscretion, then changing the diet to a more natural nutrition can stop the disease and restore health. For example, diseases such as high cholesterol, fatty liver, gall stones, kidney stones, colitis, constipation, high blood pressure, premenstrual syndrome and hypoglycemia may well be caused by diet and thus cured when nutritional changes are made. The return to a natural life style will allow the body's innate healing power to apply itself to many diseases including cancer and multiple sclerosis in some instances.

We need to keep in mind that the cause of disease is most often the result of one or more causations and a host of contributors. Thus, seldom is diet the SOLE etiology, or cause, of illness. When nutrition is only one factor in the etiology of disease, diet alone probably will not cure, and a therapy is required. As an example, we look at all of the factors that may add up to a case of emphysema taken from our clinical records. The person suffering from this disease of the lungs exhibiting shortness of breath, may have the following background factors resulting in this chronic, degenerative illness:

- Grandfather had tuberculosis.

- Allergy to dairy products as a child. Allergy shots suppressed the symptoms and allowed the continuance of the dairy products to unnaturally be included in the diet.

- Asthma at age 5-7. Treated with drugs, including steroids.

- Smoked, age 16-24.

- Pneumonia twice, treated with antibiotics.

The question is, can dietary changes alone affect gentle, rapid and permanent cure in this case? Probably not, but improving nutrition will help. Why will diet alone not effect a cure?

- Because there exists a constitutional predisposition to respiratory problems.

- The body's vitality has been significantly altered by drug therapy which suppressed the symptoms and allowed dietary indiscretions to continue.

- Tissues have been significantly changed by smoking and drug therapy.

- The illness was not created by an imbalanced diet.

So perhaps our question in this case should be, "Does good nutrition have an important role in effecting cure of this chronic condition?" It certainly does! By all means, the intake of dairy and red meat must be stopped. Instead, the focus should be on light foods, raw foods, soups and whole foods. This nutrition helps to relieve the stress which the bowel puts on the lung via toxins and gas in the blood stream. Consequently, diet becomes the foundation for the natural therapy employed to restore health. That health can be restored in such cases of emphysema is shown by many natural practitioners' clinical records. The turn of the century homeopathic journals show effective cure of many diseases. Both a good nutritional plan and natural therapies were needed to overcome the degenerative process at work in this case of emphysema.

NUTRITION AND THE CHINESE FIVE ELEMENT PHILOSOPHY

To further define the role of diet in life let's look at Chinese principles relating to nutrition. The well-known Chinese Five Element Theory provides a model for understanding the basic life processes and a perspective on the role of nutrition in overall health. Forming the basis of the oriental view of health and disease, this ancient philosophy explains the interrelatedness of the five different, yet interrelated, aspects of health.

The five elements are substances the body must have to live. Another way of looking at this is that lacking any one of these five elements, the body will die. The five elements are:

Earth — Food to eat

Air — Oxygen to breathe

Fire — Heat from the sun

Water — Water to drink

Ether — Vitality, Life Force

In the Five Element Theory, each element governs certain organs and body processes. Acupuncture, the oriental science of restoring health via the meridian-energy flow, is based on helping the body to regain balance in the five elements.

For our purposes of examining the role of nutrition in health, we are most interested in the Earth and Water elements, because we are concerned here with food and drink. We learn from the Chinese theory that diet represents two-fifths of the team of elements responsible for life maintenance. Thus, diet plays a vital role in health which is viewed as balanced, free-flowing participation in the whole five element dynamic. In turn, diet is also important in disease when viewed as an imbalance in the five element dynamic.

How do the other elements affect health? Without Ether, the body quickly dies. Solomon wrote in *The Song of Solomon*, "When the silver cord is broken, I will die." The silver cord represents the body's connection with the Etheric element, a covenant with the Life Force which animates the human body. The Ether element is the sparkle in our eyes and the light of our personalities. It is self-awareness or the ability to discriminate ourselves as individuals. More specifically and less esoterically, the Ether element is the bioenergetic, or magnetic, field of the human body.

Without the element Air, the body also dies quickly. Consequently, oxygen is quite precious for the life processes at the cellular level. Oxygen facilitates combustion of our cellular life-fires. So biochemically, oxygen plays a critical role in maintaining our metabolic rates and all our life activities. A chronic shortage of oxygen often results in cancer. For this reason numerous natural cancer therapies focus on oxygenating the body.

In our bodies, air is transformed and combined with our dietary nutrients to become liquid blood and solid molecules of tissue. Air is rich in the etheric element Ch'i which is the Chinese word for "breath," and thus air imparts invisible energy to the body. It is Ch'i, electrical energy, that flows through the body's meridians and is the dynamic for the adjustments to health accomplished by acupuncture. So the Air element interfaces with the Etheric element and brings life with each breath.

Without the element of Fire, or heat and energy from the sun, the body's environment would turn to ice, and life would be lost in a matter of hours. The sun, too, imparts an invisible energy for the balance of our planet and our bodies. But the sun alone is not utilized by our bodies for food. We lack the ability to transform its energy, as a plant can do via photosynthesis, into food. Thus plants, such as the oils in seeds, become the mediary, or converter, for sun energy into food energy that we as human beings can then assimilate and convert to our body processes. It is impractical to sit in the sun and try to absorb and convert its energy for the body's life processes. It is much easier to have a salad and some enchiladas. It is in this relationship between human being and plant that the foundation for human nutrition is established.

Without the element of Water the body can live for a few days, but then life ceases. Water provides the fluid, or medium, for the body's chemical reactions. The crystalline structure of water holds energy just like a video tape holds the light and sound patterns of a movie. Water is the reducing agent for strong elements and the medium for chemical movement of energies within the body.

Without the Earth element, or food, the body can survive for quite a while depending on the individual's mind set. Some people have starved to death in just three days, while others have fasted on water alone for 90 days before taking food. It is important here at the onset to establish that food provides the body with the chemical raw materials or nutrients for health, and it also contributes to the circulating Ch'i energy for nourishment of the bioenergetic processes.

To truly understand diet and nutrition, we must account for both the biochemical and bioenergetic processes of health.

Although food is the least important element for keeping the body from dying, it is nevertheless very important for the quality of life because of it stabilizing effect on body processes. Since food is not as critical to maintaining life in the way Ether or Air are, it works foundationally in body processes.

Minor dietary indiscretions often pass unnoticed, because they do not rock the broad biochemistry or bioenergy of the body's homeostasis, it equilibrium. In the same manner, a small amount of truly great food has little impact in the entire dietary balance. Ultimately, food and diet function in an arena of constancy and quality. Repeated dietary indiscretions (eating foods detrimental to health), or repeated dietary enhancers (eating foods that build the life processes), affect the whole person by their impact on the biochemical or bioenergetic balance of the body.

We are making the important point that causing changes in health through nutrition is usually a slower process than reviving a thirsty person with water or warming a cold person with heat. In essence, nutrition functions in a fundamental way in the grand scheme of life.

A consistently poor or detrimental diet reduces health and the quality of life. Over time, such a pattern will lead to disease and death. On the other hand, a consistently good diet will promote and maintain health, providing a good quality to life. Over time, good nutrition will lead to a strong foundation for health and form the basis for a person to live a full, vital and creative life.

The Pro Vita! Plan demonstrates how to build your health on a solid foundation that is free from the flaws of nutrient deficiencies as well as nutrient excesses. And just as importantly, it helps protect your health from the toxic effects of pesticides, additives and preservatives. The Pro Vita! Plan is packed with life-supporting nutrients that enhance the quality of life.

THE PRO-VITA! PLAN

DISCUSSIONS WITH WHEELWRIGHT:
THE LOW-STRESS PLAN

My own nutritional philosophy was significantly influenced by Stu Wheelwright's insights into food planning. Wheelwright toured Texas in 1985 and 1986, teaching his dietary philosophy, ideas and practical experiences. In 1985, in Dallas, after a busy day consulting and teaching the principles of the low-stress diet, I questioned Wheelwright about several of his ideas.

I asked: "Stu, for food planning you're teaching principally a meal consisting of vegetables combined with some low-stress proteins. This suggestion for eating is in direct contrast to the currently advocated diet emphasizing complex carbohydrates. What about the research supporting this kind of a diet, such as beans and rice combinations, as the perfect fuel system for the body?"

Wheelwright leaned back in his chair, his head nodding a bit as if falling asleep—he was after all elderly and had just consulted with 32 people and lectured for two hours—but then with startling clarity he answered: "Jack, you are not a dough boy. What's your body made of?" His bright eyes stared at me unblinking, as I replied: "Mostly water, then amino acids, then some minerals...." His hand turned palm up over his bowl of Chinese vegetable and chicken broth soup, and he commented: "Well...." Which was all he would say in answer to my question.

Six months later in Houston, Wheelwright gave another lecture on nutrition and then prepared a meal for his audience. Later that day, we stopped to eat tortilla soup in a Mexican restaurant. Again I had the chance to question some of his dietary principles.

"Stu," I said, "Are you aware of all the research suggesting that complex carbohydrates are the perfect fuel for our bodies? How does the body gets its fuel from the meal which you prepared for us?" That I was returning to this topic was an obvious irritation for Wheelwright, particularly since it interrupted his discourse on his world travels.

He answered me with another question: "Are you aware of all the research that Exxon is doing to perfect gasoline?" When I replied vaguely that I was, he said: "Gasoline alone will not keep your car out of the shop and on the road. Now, when I was in the Philippines...."

I understood Wheelwright's analogy of gasoline with food quite well, but it was not enough to offset my earlier nutritional education derived from my biochemical research about complex carbohydrate diets influenced by several respected nutritional authorities. When Wheelwright came to Texas again for our next statewide tour, I planned to approach him again about his principle dietary idea, perhaps to get a better explanation. By the time he gave his final lecture in Austin, I had already collapsed from exhaustion and my friend, Timothy Kuss from California, had to substitute for me to introduce Stu at the lecture. The "old man" had clearly outpaced the young nutritionist and made it to the finish line of a non-stop, action-packed month. When I took Stu to the airport two days later, I had my chance to again challenge his diet of vegetables and low-stress protein, his "low-stress diet," as he called it.

We were discussing writing down all of his valuable information, and he encouraged me to write a small book about the low-stress diet. He thought that the name "The Biogenic Diet" would be a good title. To approach once again the subject of complex carbohydrates as a diet, I said: "Stu, to write the book we are talking about, I need to examine the current nutritional philosophies and then explain why they are not the answer to good human health. Then I need to explain in sound biochemical terms how the low-stress plan works differently and better. Now, the experts on the complex carbohydrate diet claim...."

"The experts!" Stu exclaimed. "What do they know? They read books that somebody else wrote by copying down what somebody else wrote previously. We are a nation of copy cats. Think for yourself! First try the low-stress diet for yourself for two months. Then talk to me." With that he penned down his private telephone number. "And learn your biochemistry!"

Thus rebuked by Wheelwright, I replied, "All right, Stu, I will. You can count on it." And delivered him to the airport.

In this way, I began a diet of vegetables, seeds, fish soup and all the new and exotic foods that Stu loved and had taught me about. After just three weeks I really did have more energy and a clearer head, but I had to phone Stu with one problem: "Stu, I have a low-stress breakfast of vegetables and low-stress protein at 7:00 am. But by 10:00 am I am starving for something sweet like a cookie."

To this he replied: "Eat some Swiss chard or other greens such as kale with your breakfast, and your 10 o'clock hunger will stop in about a week. Also work on your liver with the liver triad formulas." Sure enough, that's what happened! And this is how we started our dialog to perfect the low-stress diet. I would advocate for humanity and the practical concerns, while he would discuss the solutions and refinements of the food plan with me.

After three months on the low-stress diet, I was much improved healthwise. But I never did learn exactly why the kale helped with the transition away from cookies. Then I started taking liberties with the diet by eating pizza, ice cream, and by eating late at night. The consequences are not hard to guess!

I also followed Stu's advice to continue further studies in bio-chemistry. I reread my college textbooks and numerous other books and research studies on a wide range of nutritional and biochemical topics. During 1986, Wheelwright visited Texas several times for lectures and discussions. By 1987 I had understood his nutritional approach well enough to write a slender book explaining the diet's basic principles.

More important than understanding Wheelwright's low-stress diet cognitively, were my experiences to observe and talk with people who used Stu's dietary suggestions to overcame fatigue and illness. People who were fatigued, bent-over, ill, unhappy in 1986 before knowing Wheelwright's nutritional plan, were bright, more youthful and well in 1987. When I interviewed a number of these persons, I confirmed that they followed Wheelwright's food plan and took his herb formulas. Amazingly, these people followed the low-stress diet 80% of the time! Clearly, it was quite simple to switch from a traditional American diet to Wheelwright's healthful low-stress diet consisting mainly of vegetables and small amounts of low-stress protein.

Previously, I had studied with several great nutritionists who operated health ranches and fasting clinics. But I never saw the consistent health improvements in the dietary arena as I did by Wheelwright's nutritional program.

THE NEW PRO-VITA! PLAN

Early in 1986, the Wheelwright diet became a fundamental part of my clinical practice. Initially, Wheelwright had called his nutritional regimen "The Lo-Stress Diet", "The Rational Diet", or "The 5+5 Diet." I performed much clinical research revolving around the diet: Blood tests, electro-acupuncture analysis, urinalysis, hair analysis and careful tailoring of the dietary principles for individuals over a period of five years. Subsequently, Wheelwright's son, Stuart, and his friend, Will Thompson, called this remarkable nutritional plan the "ProVita Diet".

Pro-Vita! means FOR LIFE! Experts in nutritional circles often say that we live and die at the cellular level. The Pro-Vita! Diet addresses the fundamental needs of the cell as the basic unit of life.

Realizing that the word "diet" implied too many negative connotations of strict adherence to a weight loss plan, I changed the name in 1991 to "Pro-Vita! Plan." I made this change also, because we now present a plan for cooperating with a person's inherent vitality, or life force, to bring out the best possible state of health through food and nutrient intake.

Since I began to implement the Pro-Vita! Plan in my clinical work, hardly a week goes by without a letter or two from a client who is benefiting from this fine nutritional program. A few of these letters are included in the back of this book. I have observed clinically how the diet helps to balance blood chemistry, builds energy, halts the disease process, rebuilds weak tissues and provides mental clarity in children and adults.

I have added my own refinements in the form of individualizations of the diet. Stu would tell people to eat the 5+5 meals (that is, 5 vegetables and 5 low-stress proteins) and no straying from the plan was allowed. He probably felt that individualized plans would allow too much room for harmful personal deviations. However, by working clinically with more than two thousand people and monitoring the Plan's results over the years, I have observed how the principles of the Pro-Vita! Plan must be tailored to the individual's needs.

Where Wheelwright would say dogmatically, "Eat like I tell you," I say, "Learn the principles of the Pro-Vita! Plan and apply them to your individual life-style with your specific needs and to suit specific times of your life." This way, the individual also learns more about the program's fundamental features and takes more personal responsibility for the nutritional planning.

For our discussion of nutrition it is important to realize that according to the fundamental naturopathic premise, the original design of the body—its archetypal blueprint—is considered perfect. This premise is a vital point for our discussion about nutrition. If the body's blueprint is perfect, then as ailing human beings we are not realizing our full level of health. Another important point is that the body has the innate wisdom and power to heal itself. The sciences of homeopathy, naturopathy, acupuncture and a few others are the study of, and cooperation with, the healing force within each individual. Thus, we can say that the body knows best how to heal itself. The treatment, remedy or therapy recommended by the natural health practitioner helps the body to adjust its vibratory rates. The healing occurs according to the body's inherent wisdom, provided that the body receives the right information to initiate healing. In homeopathy, and to a large extent in systemic herbology (particularly the way Wheelwright applied herbology), the right information is known as "similibus similia curantur" or "likes are cured by likes." This critical law of similiars is explained in the essay, "What is Homeopathy?" in Appendix A.

Proper nourishment is also a treatment for the body. Nutritional researchers estimate that 90% of our illnesses and diseases are caused or exacerbated by: 1) improper food consumption, causing nutritional deficiencies and excesses; 2) autointoxication or low oxygen, fermentation in the bowel which poisons the blood and lymph; and 3) poor elimination of toxins and metabolic wastes. All three of these physical causes of illness are nutritional issues. Proper nutrition can, in effect, help the body to heal itself!

Improper internal hygiene, or nutrition, sets the stage for opportunistic pathogens, such as virus, bacteria, yeast and fungi to flourish and disrupt health. Other causes of poor health include genetics, birth defects, miasmatic taints (bioenergetic tendencies towards diseases inherited from ancestors), poor attitudes, injuries and incomplete adaptation to the environment.

Wheelwright took upon himself the mission to discover what he believed to be the optimal diet for humanity. For my part, the task is to advance, apply, explain and amplify his nutritional tenets so more people may benefit. The information contained in this book explains the basic as well as the more esoteric features of the Pro-Vita! Plan in such a way that you can apply them easily to obtain maximum health.

WHEELWRIGHT'S CONCEPT OF PLANT BIOENERGY

An important and far-reaching dimension of Wheelwright's plan is the concept of the bioforce, or bioenergy, of plants. This bioforce is not the metabolic energy derived from food. Instead, it is the bioenergetic compatibility of the food's energy pattern with the individual's proper, vital energy pattern. The food's energy pattern is based on how the plant manifests the vital force into configurations of minerals and other nutritive factors. The energy pattern is the synergism of the plant's organization. Wheelwright's concept of bioenergetic nutrition has profound consequences.

The concept of bioenergy has traditionally been the domain of homeopathy, acupuncture, electro-acupuncture, bioenergetic medicine, anthroposophical medicine and systemic herbology. These healing systems all affect, to a greater or lesser extent, the patient's bioenergetic fields to initiate a healing process.

From the perspective of bioenergy, nutrition takes on a more profound significance, because it plays a vital role in the synergy of life. Synergy of life means that the individual elements add up to something greater than the sum total of the parts. For this reason, diet can enhance or hinder the quality of a person's life. Finally, the importance of how well a person feels has a profound impact upon happiness and success.

If we look at the biochemical aspect of nutrition we find that the body's processing of food is based on two fundamental factors. First, there has to be proper intake and assimilation of nutrition, and the liver has to have the ability to process the food. Second, the metabolic wastes of the food have to have proper elimination. Linked with these two processes are the availability of enzymes and proper amino acids.

It is of interest to note that from the perspective of bioenergy, a person's attitude is a predisposing factor in how food is used by the body. A person with a positive, enthusiastic attitude can eat a mediocre diet and still have better health than a person with a poor attitude eating a perfectly healthy diet.

As I delved deeper into the biochemical and bioenergetic processes of health, I discovered that the fundamental features of Wheelwright's diet form the core for optimal nutrition. His nutritional philosophy becomes the basis for the perfect prenatal, cardiovascular, athletic, school, allergy-avoidance, weight loss/gain, anti-arthritis and health maintenance diet.

Ultimately, Wheelwright's dietary insights represent a sophisticated, upgraded bioenergetic version of the earlier models of food combining. Advancing the general dietary research, Stu placed new emphasis on bioenergy concepts as they relate to the biological and biochemical processes. Looking at foods, nutrition and health from this new overview allowed Wheelwright to advance beyond the prevailing limitations of each science and examine human nutrition in a new light.

Wheelwright was internationally known for his work with the body's electrical energy called "bioforce." The application of his work regarding nutritional biochemistry is currently named "quantum chemistry." Rather than placing his dietary insights on philosophies and theories, he founded it on biochemistry and bioenergy. His simple question about nutrition was, "Does what you eat, and how you eat it, give you more physical and essential energy than you had before eating?" Included in this question is the whole spectrum of nutrients as well as the energetic factor "Ch'i." A result of winning on the dietary energetic scale results in food providing the bioenergetic qualities of health, calmness and well-being. Conversely, does what you eat take more energy to digest and dispose of its wastes than it gives you? In order to stay on the plus side of energy, a bioenergetic perspective on nutrition is important.

Wheelwright's bioenergetic approach to nutrition together with other commensurate dietary factors are the foundation for the Pro-Vita! Plan. The plan is built on basic food combining to optimize digestion and enzyme function; fresh, whole and organic (whenever possible) foods for a basic life support system; the understanding of how the body uses its nutrients; the effects of nutrients (biochemistry); and deriving the vital energy to support vibrant health.

To provide you an easier way to understand the concept of "Ch'i," or the body's electrical field, we include a brief excerpt by K. C. Cole from *Discover Magazine* (February, 1984).

Electricity is almost certainly the most elusive of everyday things: It lives in the walls of our houses, and regulates the lives of our cells. It bolts from the sky as lightning, and sparks from your finger if you touch a metal doorknob after shuffling across the rug. It shapes the structure of matter—making plastic pliable, oil slick, and glue sticky. It runs electric trains and human brains . . . Light is electromagnetic radiation—and that includes everything from visible light to x-rays, microwaves, and radio waves. The magnetism in iron magnets is caused by the spinning of countless electrons twirling in unison, just as the magnetic field of the earth is most probably created by the swirling of electric currents in its molten metal core.

Your entire body is a giant electric machine: body chemistry (like all chemistry) is based on electrical bonds. It even runs on electricity. The energy you need to see these words comes from the egg you ate for breakfast; the egg got its energy from the corn consumed by the hen, the corn extracted that energy directly from the electromagnetic light of the sun through photosynthesis.

When you think about it, the universe is positively (and negatively) electrifying. But because of the usually perfect balance between positive and negative forces, most of the electrical power around you is neutralized—and therefore unnervingly invisible, at least in the normal sense...Essentially, everything around us is elec-trically charged empty space.

The important perspective of bioenergy brings new insights to nutrition which surpass those provided by a biochemical perspective alone. To illustrate this point more precisely the soybean story provides insights into the many nutritional considerations of a single food.

BIOENERGY AND BIOCHEMISTRY OF FOODS: THE SOYBEAN STORY

Research about soybeans provides fascinating information into a food's bioenergetic and biochemical properties. From its biochemistry we know that the soybean has a high content of protein. But biochemistry also makes it clear that the soybean's energy is not particularly suitable for human health unless the soybean is first predigested, most often done by natural fermentation.

From a bioenergetic perspective, the plain soybean does not test particularly well for nutrition either. However, once it is fermented, or predigested, as tofu or miso, the soybean's energy pattern improves. This fact has been documented by Kirlian photography, a method of imprinting the bioenergetic pattern of a life form on a piece of film.

When soybeans are fermented, as in tofu, the digestive system gets a headstart on breaking down their complex protein structures. From a bioenergetic perspective, a 600-molecule amino acid chain that cannot be broken down mathematically by enzymes into two or three molecule chains, will test incompatible. In contrast, a 16 molecule chain that can be reduced to two and three-molecule chains, will test compatible. All of this simply means that the human enzymes can split the latter short amino acid chains better and have the optimal, nucleo-proteins available for the cells. Fermentation produces shorter molecule chains and alters the energetic pattern of the food.

We have discussed how plants convert, or transform, sunlight into useable chemistry and bioenergy for our bodies. The additional process of fermentation accomplishes this transformation for the soy bean. Fermentation transforms the coarse nutrients into more useable nutrients.

Consequently, the facts from biochemistry about the soybean protein need further clarification. It is not as important to know how much protein is in soybeans as it is to know how much of this protein is available to the body's cells. It is also important to know how much energy it will cost the body to process the soybean protein. In effect, this is the well-known issue of quality versus quantity. But in this case, the bioenergetic approach tells us about quality, while biochemistry addresses the issue of quantity.

By looking at the soybean story a bit further, we understand that health is not based on biochemistry or orthomolecular nutrition alone. Soybean protein will not break down sufficiently into nucleoproteins—the short amino acid chains—which the cells use for nourishment and energy unless it is first hydrolyzed, or predigested, or fermented.

A simple observation of the Oriental use of soybeans reveals that the Chinese and Japanese seldom use them until they are fermented, as in miso, tofu and tempeh, or cooked as sprouts in eggrolls. The Orientals do not eat soybeans as simply cooked beans the way we eat pinto beans or black beans.

Recently, many soy protein products have appeared in our markets. Such products as soy protein powders and textured vegetable protein (TVP) patties are indeed high in protein, as advertised. But these products were invented by biochemists who paid no attention to the fact that these proteins are not very biologically available to the body's cells. Therefore, these products are high-stress foods that take more energy from the body than they supply. The same is true of cotton, a plant high in protein but so complex that it does not work well as fodder or food.

The following explains why unfermented soy protein is difficult for the cells to use. Soy protein is complex with long chain molecules. The adult body lacks the digestive strength to break down its long structures into chains of less than 16 molecules which are still too large for cells to use effectively. Instead, cells require 1, 2, and 3-molecule chain amino acids which are called "nucleo-proteins." In fact, 16 molecule chains can tax the kidneys, clog the lymphatic system and stress the liver. This is what many nutritionists write about as "large molecule proteins."

Furthermore, raw soybeans contain an anti-proteolytic enzyme that interferes with protein digestion. For this reason, in Chinese cooking the bean is separated from the sprout. The sprout is then cooked in an eggroll or is stir-fried. When the soybean sprout is lightly cooked, the anti-proteolytic factor is broken down, making the protein structures more easily available. This is one of the few instances when light cooking or fermenting improves the nutritional value of a food as compared to the value of the raw food.

The information about protein availability in soy beans is of vital importance for VEGETARIANS. Such persons often lack understanding about the biological availability of the vegetable protein. As a consequence, they exhibit symptoms of protein deficiency at the cellular level. Frequently they also demonstrate weakened tissue integrity. The bodies of vegetarians often must labor with unusable and difficult-to-use, large molecule protein chains. Under these circumstances, the body's tissues have to give up their proteins to perform basic metabolic functions and are thus weakened.

Over a period of years—usually three to seven—as more carbohydrates are brought into the diet to compensate for the lack of energy, the body learns to make do with inferior materials, thus weakening the quality of tissues. Complex carbohydrates do not contain the proper enzymes or protein structures to build quality tissue. Adopting the principles of the Pro-Vita! Plan helps vegetarians maintain their health and tissue integrity. By using soy ferments with seeds and raw sprouts (sunflower, chia, alfalfa, mung, and others), vegetarians can introduce biologically available, complete proteins to their bodies. Thus, they can avoid the use of animal flesh, provided they maintain a strong digestive system.

Dr. Royal B. Lee, the twentieth century's premier nutritional researcher, investigated the nutritional problems of vegetarians. He found that a child would not be able to effectively process soybeans as an adult, unless fed considerable quantities of soybeans and other complex vegetable proteins prior to age eight. Evidently, the digestive system can be trained in the early years to accommodate complex vegetable protein. But, as Dr. Lee found, unless this occurs during early childhood, a person will not likely be able to fully develop the ability later on. Although there is a way to strengthen the digestive system of an adult desiring to live on plant proteins through homeopathy and breathing exercises, it takes a strong commitment and some focused effort. In general, Lee's research is quite valid, as such health-committed adults are rare to find.

Dr. Lee discovered another prerequisite. He found that a child must not eat meat during these early years so that the training of the body's digestion of complex vegetable proteins is not interrupted. Moreover, Dr. Lee discovered that ancestry is a factor. A history of vegetarianism in the family predisposed a child to be able to process complex vegetable protein.

This digestive factor which converts niacin to niacinamide by attaching an amino acid and synthesizes Vitamin B-12 from amino acids, is inherent in some persons via vegetarian lineage. It is called the "intrinsic factor." Herbaceous animals like cows have this factor to convert grass into protein. Many varieties of fish also possess this intrinsic factor to convert sea vegetation into protein. However, many occidental people, unless they have East Indian or oriental ancestry, do not have the intrinsic factor. If they do have this factor, then they can support their bodies adequately on a vegetarian diet, relying on vegetables, seeds, fermented soy products, beans, sprouts, and a few nuts properly prepared, combined and digested to provide the proteins.

If, however, the intrinsic factor is lacking, a person will not be able to adequately support the body without at least some fish protein, according to the Lee research and subsequently researched and substantiated by Wheelwright. The proteins in fish—as well as in fowl and other meats—supply the necessary intrinsic factor, because the protein structures are already converted, that is, the fish has converted sea vegetation into tissue. Even as little as two cubic inches of fish per week will provide enough intrinsically factored protein for a person to be healthy on a vegetarian diet, provided that carbohydrates are kept to a minimum when the protein is eaten.

It is interesting to note that *Webster's New World Dictionary* defines the intrinsic factor as "a substance secreted by the stomach which permits the absorption of vitamin B12 in the intestines...." Dr. Lee had found that the B-vitamin niacin could help determine, in the following manner, whether a person has the intrinsic factor. Niacin must be converted to niacinamide—a proteinated form of niacin—by the intrinsic factor in the stomach, otherwise a phenomenon known as "niacin flush" occurs. Such a niacin flush causes a person's face to turn red as if it were sunburned. The back of the arms can itch from the release of histamine and the skin can feel warm. No harm is done by the niacin flush because it is simply a dilation of the blood vessels near the skin. In fact, some people deliberately take niacin in high potencies (more than 100 mg.) to bring blood to the skin to promote better skin health and a clearer complexion. The flushing seldom lasts longer than 20 minutes, although it can last as long as two hours.

According to Dr. Lee, the niacin flush can be used to determine if a person can physiologically be a vegetarian. The test is to take between 100 and 200 mg. of natural niacin—but not niacinamide which is often sold as supplemental niacin—on an empty stomach. If a person flushes, the niacin was not converted by the stomach to niacinamide because the person lacked enough of the intrinsic factor. Thus, a niacin flush at 100 mg. indicates the person's inability to prosper on a strictly vegetarian diet, or that very special attention to diet and health will be required to make the transition to vegetarianism. Note, if higher amounts of niacin are used, such as 500 mg., anyone can flush. When there is more niacin than can be converted to niacinamide, a flush will occur. The test is to detect low levels of intrinsic factor which will make vegetarianism a detrimental diet to follow until the digestion can be strengthened.

Homeopathy has helped people to improve the vitality of their digestion so that they can make the transition from eating meat to a vegetarian diet. By strengthening the vital force via the appropriate, fundamental remedy and by following the tenets of the

Pro-Vita! Plan, a person can endeavor to become vegetarian without sacrifice of health.

While on the subject of vegetarianism, I would like to share an observation from my clinical practice. I have never seen a true vegetarian among all of the people who claim to be vegetarian, with the exception of perhaps one person. I find that most vegetarians, instead of eating green, leafy VEGETABLES, subsist on carbohydrates like bread, fruits, rice, potatoes, pasta or cookies. Thus, a better name for them would be "carbotarians." After a few years, carbotarians often get a little pudgy, a little water-retentive, a little tired and washed out, and quite deficient in protein at the cellular level. If these persons had focused on vegetables and good quality proteins, they would have fared much better.

Of course, the case against heavy eating of meat is well-founded, because of its toxic effect on the body and its detrimental ecological effects as well. On a global scale, animal foods take more resources from the planet than they return nutritionally. The acreage used to maintain cattle can provide more food per-capita with other agricultural endeavors. The dire consequences of the cattle industry have been explored eloquently by Frances Lappe in her book *Diet for a Small Planet* (1971).

For most people, once they are biochemically stable and have adequate protein at the cellular level, a diet of vegetables together with low-stress proteins will provide a much better level of health than a diet focused on complex carbohydrates. We repeat this because the current dietary trend is towards grains and complex carbohydrates. While this trend is indeed an improvement over a diet heavy with meat, it still does not work to build the maximum dimension of health. We will continue throughout this book to look at these important issues.

Our discussion of soybeans has shown that just because a food is high in a nutrient, this does not mean that it is more nutritious. Nutrients have to be ASSIMILATED and used, a factor which is called the food's bioavailability. If we look at nutrition from the perspective of bioforce and bioavailability, we will not be misled by information brought forth from a more limited view used to market a product or from a rigid diet philosophy.

Although many people adhere to the tenets of the Pro-Vita! Plan, they are in fact a diverse group, including meat and potato people, vegetarians, macrobiotic-based persons and many others. Such multiple adaptations of the Pro-Vita! Plan are possible because it will teach you how to optimize the foods you choose for your individual program. The Pro-Vita! Plan does not lock you into a philosophy or rigid nutritional pattern. Use it to build both health and freedom in your life.

Let's return to our new bioenergetic perspective gained from the soybean story and apply it to other areas of nutrition. A high-potency vitamin supplement may not be better than a low-potency one. In fact, it usually is detrimental to the body. To determine which potency is maximal for the body, kinesiology (muscle testing) and electro-acupuncture (electric measurement of the meridians) can be used. Although there is a considerable margin of error in such testing, in the hands of a gifted practitioner these techniques can be quite revealing and helpful. Both of these methods are based on an energy perspective and provide insights into what works best.

Wheelwright, in creating his famous nutritional formulas, endeavored to provide nutrition for the body to use as it directs, rather than the supplement directing the body to react. High potency supplements act like drugs and force the body to react. But Wheelwright's goal for most of his formulas was to gently nourish and encourage balance to specific body systems.

Applying the bioenergetic view to your present diet: If your current plan is taking away more energy than it provides, you are munching your way, bite by bite, to ill health and an early grave. Since we know that foods inherently contain healing power, it follows that the misuse of them has the power to kill. Although a slow process, since the body has many safeguards, this power of foods affects all of us.

If, on the other hand, your diet is providing more energy than it takes for processing the foods, then you have energy to make repairs in your body, to maintain a strong extra-cellular matrix of collagen and elastin, to support immunity and adaptability, and to possibly experience that dynamic state of being called "abundant health." Not running on energy deficit, or using a nutritional plan that makes demands on the body's vitality to adjust, means that energy is available to promote well-being and refreshment of spirit.

However, proper diet is only one part of optimal health. Exercise is also vitally important to mobilize the waste-disposal system. The most crucial aspect of vibrant health is attitude and right thinking. The Pro-Vita! Plan can provide the nutritional foundation upon which to build your own fountain of youth! Learn the basic features of the program and you will be able to tailor your individual dietary pattern suited for your life-style. Try the Pro-Vita! Plan for a few weeks to see if this rational and inspirational plan for a greater life provides the nutritional freedom and health you are seeking.

The important aspects of the Pro-Vita! Plan are displayed in the following graphic.

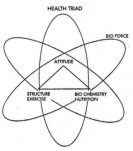

In this book you are invited to take a new look at both the science of nutrition and YOUR PERSONAL NUTRITIONAL PATHWAY. By reading this information you can cultivate a nutritional overview to guide your journey through the controversies of multiple dietary theories so prevalent on the present nutritional scene. From our information you can formulate for yourself a simple, flexible and balanced plan which works well for you to attain optimal health.

If you are reading this book for possible answers to conditions of failing health, you will find answers. But they are not listed as specific remedies in these pages. Instead, you will derive your own answers by applying your newly discovered nutritional principles and seeking the advice of your natural healthcare provider. A cure to an ailment may or may not be nutritionally based, but an overview of dietary facts is often the key to finding answers. Consequently, by acquiring a valid nutritional overview, you also develop an overview of health or healing concurrently.

If you are studying this book to verify your current nutritional beliefs or to explore new areas of diet, you will find a matrix that provides new insights into what is working for you nutritionally. And the matrix will also point out possible means for enhancing your food plan.

This book may challenge you, put your nutritional theory to a test and evaluate it for its validity. But you are the person who decides what is beneficial for you. Our information provides the necessary tools for you to know what food plan is good for you. Ultimately, this book imparts a rational, balanced plan from which you can develop your personal nutritional pathway. And that is the purpose of this book!

To summarize this discussion: Our energy has a physical, biochemical side and an etheric, bioenergetic side. These two aspects are thoroughly interwoven; each supports the other, and each affects the other. The major shortcoming of nutrition as a science is the lack of understanding of nutrition's bioenergetic side. The Pro-Vita! Plan is founded on the principles of both biochemistry and bioenergy.

THE PRO-VITA! NUTRITION PYRAMID

In the next four chapters we examine the four Pro-Vita! food groups in detail: Vegetables, Proteins, Oils and Carbohydrates. These food categories make up the essential nutrient requirements of the body. The key issues are what to base human nutrition on, what proportions of each food group are optimal, and what roles each food group plays in maintaining health.

The Pro-Vita! Nutrition Pyramid is portrayed here to depict both the QUALITY (order of importance to health) and the QUANTITY of the foods as they make up an optimal diet.

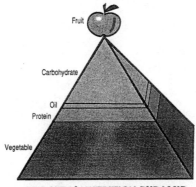

PRO-VITA! NUTRITION PYRAMID

The nutrition pyramid is unique to the Pro-Vita! Plan. It is based on years of applying the insights that Dr. Wheelwright shared with me, and my clinical observations that people's vitality and body chemistry improve when applying its principles.

As you can see in the pyramid, VEGETABLES form the foundation for human nutritional health. By volume, 65-75% of a Pro-Vita! protein meal will be vegetables. This means a generous bowl of salad as well as one or two lightly steamed vegetables, plus the protein foods. A carbohydrate-based meal—different from the Pro-Vita! protein meal—will most likely be 95-100% from the plant kingdom.

The next food group represented in the pyramid is PROTEIN. The smaller layer it occupies in the pyramid is representative of the small amount of protein recommended in the Pro-Vita! Plan. This book focuses extensively on low-stress protein use as the determining factor in health. If a person eats plenty of vegetables and the recommended Pro-Vita! proteins, health and vitality will increase.

High quality OILS are also vitally important because they build health and prevent cancer. The chapter on oils presents vitally important information about how to work with this essential nutrient.

And lastly, CARBOHYDRATES. Important for day-to-day energy and very easy to come by, complex carbohydrates serve a less critical, but necessary role in human nutrition. As the top section of the pyramid, carbohydrates are the least important nutrient, but only because they are so readily available, and there is less risk in their misuse than there is in using proteins and oils.

On the top of the pyramid is an apple, the symbol of health and freedom from disease. It also represents the FRUIT category of foods which, in the Pro-Vita! plan, are used for recreation and enjoyment, and of course, for their valuable enzymes and minerals.

Currently, the United States Department of Agriculture is considering creating its own pyramid of the basic food groups. They are now admitting that the four basic food groups that dieticians and medicine have been pushing on the American public for decades are not designed to produce good health. The current four basic food groups are simply representations of the four basic food lobbies in Washington.

The Department of Agriculture has the data that clearly states that red meat and dairy are endangering human health, so they want to reconstruct the four basic food groups and not give equal proportions to each group. Their new pyramid is certainly a move in the right direction.

However, we'll not likely see an honest portrayal of human health in the Department of Agriculture's work, because they are not looking at the individual people. Instead, they must compromise among the powerful food lobbies and the medical-industrial complex. Each of these powerful organizations want to ensure that their vested, financial interests are protected and generously represented, whether or not they are in the public's best interest.

The model currently under consideration by the Department of Agriculture places primary importance on complex carbohydrates (starches). While this is not the optimal foundation for human health, it is a large step in the right direction because it changes the focus of the American diet away from red meat and excessive use of dairy products, to a plant-based food group.

Keep in mind that large governmental organizations seldom care about the individual. It's just not their role. Their job is to evaluate national trends and broad-scale concerns. They must consider the agricultural ability to provide food for the masses so there is no shortage or famine. Thus, the Department of Agriculture will tell us a food like carbohydrate is the most important for reasons other than studies of human health. Their reasons include such facts that the farmers can grow carbohydrates more economically and more massively than meat; carbohydrates store better and can be more easily transported; carbohydrates fill more tummies at a cheaper price, so low income families will not become malnutrition statistics and make the country look bad statistically. With a few facts about lower cholesterol and lower cancer rates, the government will most likely compromise with a less than optimal plan as their official position. From a governmental perspective, the official plan will have to be a compromise between the known nutritional facts and all the lobbies and vested interests that want to be represented in the foods we buy. Once their official position is established and agreed upon, medicine and dieticians will promote that position to the American public, and it will become a "fact."

The Pro-Vita! plan only addresses what is optimal for your health and explains how you can eat, each day, for greater vitality and freedom from disease. So for you, the individual, here is the way to better nutritional health.

Now you are ready to delve into the four Pro-Vita! food groups and become well-versed in how to make your foods work for your health!

GLORIOUS VEGETABLES: THE FOUNDATION OF HUMAN NUTRITION

VEGETABLES ARE ESSENTIAL FOR A HEALTHY LIFE

Unlike a mystery novel that leads the reader to a startling conclusion, we start this chapter with its conclusion: VEG-ETABLES—MOSTLY RAW, SOME COOKED—FORM THE FOUNDATION FOR HEALTH THROUGH NUTRITION. We'll now discuss this issue from a variety of perspectives, but you should know here at the start that we're not going to advocate a raw foods diet. Yet, vegetables are so important, and so often neglected, that we must emphasize their fundamental and essential place in human nutrition as the foundation upon which to build our nutritional values with other food categories.

Stop and think for a moment. When you prepare a meal, do you first plan its meat or starch portion? Is it like, "Let's see, I have a lamb roast. What do I have to go with it?" Or do you proceed in this way, "Let's have spaghetti. Let's see if I have some garlic bread and olives to go with it." If these are your natural thought processes, then your food plan is NOT prioritized to focus on health.

On the other hand, if your focus on food is, "I have beautiful fresh salad makings. I think that some spaghetti on the side would be fun." Or, "Look at this fine organic broccoli. I think I'll make a sesame-miso sauce and have it with a bit of fish." With these approaches your orientation is geared towards vegetables and health.

Unless we first focus on vegetables, we run the risk of compromising our health. By vegetables we mean fresh green, red, white, yellow, or orange vegetables, the kind that grow in the garden, often called "pot-herbs", not grains, fruit, nuts or tubers.

Don't be alarmed—this is as radical as the Pro-Vita! nutritional information gets! We are simply stressing two points. First, vegetables are a vitally important part of human nutrition and are sorely lacking in the diet of most people. But then, most people also have nutritionally related health problems. The focus on vegetables will greatly reduce many health problems. Second, we are talking about vegetables, not boiled or cooked grains which are carbohydrates. Altogether, we want to build up the importance of vegetables in overall nutritional health.

Many people say that they don't particularly like vegetables and instead much prefer smoked meats, spicy sauces, tangy cheeses or sweet deserts to the common and ordinary vegetable. In Natural Health we understand that vegetables can taste bland and boring to people whose taste faculties have been titillated by salt, spices, chemical flavors, sugar and smoke. Like an addiction, constant stimulation of the taste buds with strong impulses can alter the sense of taste and establish a need for strong taste sensations. Some people can become mildly addicted to hot peppers as the pain of eating them causes the release of endorphins in the brain and thus imparts a feeling of well being. When the natural ability to taste fresh and subtle flavors becomes jaded, or warped, due to the onslaught of dead foods doctored with additives to make them palatable, then people find the basic, wholesome foods less palatable. Please do not interpret this as a hint for a bland diet. Peppers, herbs and spices can enhance foods tastefully and nutritionally.

We have an unequivocal guarantee for you, if you are a person who currently shuns vegetables. As you reintroduce a variety of fresh vegetables into your diet and decrease the overstimulation of your taste buds, the vegetables will taste better and better every day. In their natural state, organic foods are vibrant with delicious and subtle flavors so that the body naturally desires them. Please let me underscore that we don't advocate a bland, lackluster diet. In fact, nutrition should be exciting, flavorful and satisfying to all of our senses: sight, smell, taste, feel and even sound!

In the natural health field, it is common knowledge that the flavors of fresh, organically grown vegetables are exquisite for a person in a healthy state. Imagine the wonderful, fresh crunch of sweet celery; the tang and flavor explosion of a slice of red bell pepper; the touch of tart lemon juice; the sweet, smooth taste of jicama; the pungent essence of fresh basil; the surprising bite of a piece of radish; the prickly aroma of parsley; and the crisp coolness of green leafy lettuce. All of these vegetables impart their precious fluids, enzymes and minerals for the cells of our body to thrive on!

Sadly, most people today have lost the ability to enjoy a bite of crisp carrot, sweet juicy corn, earthy sprouts and chewy cabbage. Some people have even lost the desire and ability to enjoy fresh fruits, and thus miss the sour, but luscious, sensation of biting into a ripe plum or the aromatic explosion of chomping down on a crunchy apple.

More than one reason exists for the misplacement of this sensory ability. One reason is the overstimulation by chemicals and additives which leave a person unable to experience the flavorful subtleties of basic healthy foods. Another cause is the use of alcohol, tobacco or coffee which dull the taste faculty.

The following is an example of common overstimulation. While at the beach recently, I saw a teenager running around with a big radio held to his ear blasting out heavy metal tunes. The teenager was certainly stimulated in an auditory way and enjoying himself, but he was no longer in tune with the surge and rhythm of the waves breaking and washing over the sand, the mournful cries of the gulls as they glided on the breeze, or the rustle of the grasses and reeds as the wind whispered across the dunes. We must remember that where we place our attention, or on what we place our attention, often determines the extent of our experience. If our focus is on enjoying the rich and subtle flavors of plants, then we enjoy the flavors.

Another reason for not being able to enjoy the subtle flavors of many vegetables and fruits is that commercial farming and synthetic fertilizers have given us an object that merely looks like a carrot or a peach. It may be jumbo in size, but it's hollow in nutrients. The commercial vegetables and fruit do not contain their full flavor due to the absence of important trace minerals and the plant's full, natural vitality. Because commercially grown foods often taste and look less than appetizing, the food industry adds synthetic colors and waxes to trick our eyes. Then we add sugar and spices to provide the taste sensation we inherently know the food should have.

However, the lost taste faculty will readily return when a person follows a more natural food plan. If you can just get through the transition period as a person must with any addictive process before coming clean, you will get the reward of rediscovering wonderful "new" taste sensations.

HOW TO IMPROVE THE VEGETARIAN DIET

Many people who call themselves "vegetarians" are actually living on a less than optimal diet because they overuse cooked grains at the expense of vegetables. Many health authorities have examined various physiological factors to draw conclusions about what is suitable for humans to eat. Although such research often goes to extremes or forces conclusions to prove a point, we endeavor to keep an open perspective about these issues.

For example, some proponents build their philosophy of vegetarianism on such facts that gorillas are very strong and live on a diet consisting mostly of vegetables and fruits. As a consequence, these researchers maintain that humans also can be very strong as vegetarians. While this statement is 75% correct, its logic is however specious. The analogy with the gorilla does not take into consideration several facts: Gorillas eat insects; they have a different blood chemistry and physiology; they have a shorter life span; they have obvious intellectual differences—which in some ways make them smarter than humans!

The view of many proponents of vegetarianism is essentially correct that vegetables are the basis of the human diet. But they have extracted the right conclusion from faulty, or stretched reasoning, particularly if their conclusions exclude other food groups as is done, for example, in fruitarianism, where only raw fruit is eaten.

A similar type of logic is often used when researchers evaluate the human teeth to determine what foods we are suited to eat. Our flat, grinding teeth show that we are best suited to eat an herbaceous (vegetable) diet. Yet, our teeth are not completely herbaceously oriented because we have canine teeth more suited for tearing food. An honest appraisal of the function of human teeth is that we are 90% herbaceous. Vegetarians will take this 90% of fact and make the assumption that people should be 100% vegetarian.

In contrast, people who advocate eating of meat pretty much ignore the facts that humans are not well-suited to subsist on meat. If we consider the fact that human teeth are not 100% suited to vegetable foods, we have only a small margin to consider other foods as well.

Another popular fact used to judge optimal nutrition is the length of the intestinal tract. Herbaceous animals have very long intestinal tracts so that their digestive systems have time to process the grasses and leaves they eat. In contrast, carnivorous (meat-eating) animals have very short digestive tracts to quickly digest meat and excrete it before it can putrefy in their intestines. These animals also have a special digestive enzyme, uricase, to break down uric acids which are so abundant in meat.

Interestingly enough, we find that humans have a lengthy intestinal tract which means that we are indeed suited for an herbaceous diet. However, our intestinal tracts are not quite as long as they should be for an exclusive diet of grass and leaves. Yet, the intestinal tract is definitely too long for a heavy diet consisting of meat. Again, we are looking at a fact which tallies only 90% towards vegetarianism. Clearly, the facts weigh very heavily, but not 100%, towards a vegetarian diet.

The following chart displays the conclusions about our digestive abilities.

	Vegetables/plants	Meat/other
Teeth best suited for	90%	10%
Length of intestinal tract	90%	10%
Enzyme capabilities	90%	10%
Ability to process by-products	90%	10%

From this chart we readily see that the score weighs heavily in favor of an herbaceous diet, but not 100%. The teeth are mostly, but not completely, geared to herbaceous food. The intestinal tract is well suited for an herbaceous diet but could be more so than it is, since humans do not have a four-chambered stomach like a cow or camel, for example. The length of the intestinal tract could be longer to better process the complex nutrients in grasses and leaves. Altogether, the intestinal tract is too long for digesting meat and too short for digesting grasses.

If we consider the presence of enzymes, we find that humans do not have the high levels of hydrochloric acid and uricase suited to heavy eating of meat. But humans do produce hydrochloric acid, trypsin, chymotrypsin and several protease enzymes to digest foods high in protein. In addition, the human body has the ability to process some, but not a lot of, toxins from foods high in protein.

Summarizing our discussion about a vegetarian diet, we find seemingly conflictive facts. First, the human body is particularly well suited for an herbaceous diet. At the present time we do not yet know precisely which amount of such a diet is purely vegetable and which part is vegetable protein, or carbohydrate, or non-herbaceous foods. Second, it is not certain that the human body is exclusively herbaceous. If it were, there would not be so many exceptions to people being able to be vegetarians. Nature is exacting in the adaptation of organisms to their ecological niche and place in the food chain. Also, if the body were attuned exclusively to one food source, humans would be less fit to survive. The ability to maintain life on a variety of food sources increases the chances of survival of the species.

Currently, it is accepted and common knowledge that the bulk of the human diet should be from the plant kingdom, such as vegetables known as pot herbs, sea vegetables, grains, seeds, nuts, sprouts, legumes and fruit. According to the statistics we have discussed, 90% of our diet should be from plant sources. In turn, a mere 10% of our nutrition could be from dairy, meat and various processed-food items that inevitably get ingested.

There is, however, much controversy and speculation about the 90%, the vast majority of our food. This controversy is about how much of a person's diet should be vegetables, how much carbohydrates like grain and potatoes, and how much protein such as seeds, nuts and properly cooked beans.

The current trend in nutrition is based on the body's energy system and emphasizes that the bulk of a person's diet should be grains. The Pro-Vita! philosophy does not agree with this perspective. Instead, the Pro-Vita! Plan suggests that the bulk of the nutrition must be vegetables, especially raw green, leafy vegetables. Certainly, the organically grown, raw vegetables and fruit are the only food which can provide its own enzymes for ease of digestion, organic minerals and vitamins, as well as the important fiber for the health of the gastro-intestinal tract.

However, we won't get too carried away and advocate a diet of only raw food! Wheelwright was decidedly against this kind of food plan. And I myself have observed clinically that people who eat a high level of, or exclusively, raw foods are not experiencing the abundant level of health their body is capable of. We will discover why a diet consisting exclusively of raw foods does not work optimally for the body as we continue to build the Pro-Vita! viewpoint on nutrition.

To be healthy, we must have reverence for the wonderful, fresh, natural, organic fruits and vegetables the earth brings forth for our sustenance and well-being. Living foods must be a part of our diet at EVERY MEAL! A basic part of health is that life begets life. Thus, we need to eat living foods for our bodies to maintain health. If a person does not desire luscious fruit and tangy fresh vegetables, then the innate sense of taste has been perverted by unnatural foods. Excessive use of sugared, smoked and chemically treated food items estrange people from their basic foundation of health.

In most people's diets, grains are not well prepared. Such grain products as rice, bread, pasta, chips have been cooked to a carbohydrate mush at the expense of their valuable enzymes and beneficial fiber. Such grains are not in the same life-vitalizing category as the glorious vegetables which provide such great nutritional value. Therefore, a vegetarian who says," Let's have brown rice and maybe a few veggies to go with it," is still missing the nutritional boat, so to speak. What's really needed is to have lots of different vegetables with a little bit of rice to open up a new dimension of nutrition and health.

The Pro-Vita! plan indicates that there is a place for fruit, raw vegetables and cooked vegetables, for carbohydrates (potatoes, grains) and protein foods as well.

Wheelwright advocated to have 1 cooked and 4 raw vegetables with every meal. However, he did not advocate protein or carbohydrates with every meal. But he did suggest vegetables with EVERY meal which means vegetables with breakfast, lunch and supper. As strange as it may seem to you at this point, there are very easy and tasty meals for this plan, as we will discuss.

The important point is that vegetables give us major nutrients for our health:

- natural vitamins to make the body chemistry work effectively;

- organic minerals to provide stamina and vitality;

- living enzymes, the key to staying youthful;

- water to purify the body;

- fiber to optimize digestion and elimination, and to prevent cancer.

No other food category can offer the body the foundation for health as fresh, raw, organically grown vegetables and fruit. Only in vegetables and fruit do we find the energy of the sun and the minerals of the earth joined together in water for nature's most complete nutrition package for our health, vibrancy and longevity.

GENETIC ENGINEERING OF VEGETABLES

The current controversy about the genetic altering of produce concerns us enough to include a short section here on this topic. Genetic engineering is the alteration of the qualities of a plant through changing the DNA codes in the genes or by adding new genes. As with any change, this genetic altering can be for better or for worse. Better changes are those that increase the nutritional value and vitality of a food. Worse changes are those that increase allergenic properties or weaken the nutritional value of a food.

The allure of better changes is to increase the anti-cancer properties, improve the flavor or enhance the healing factors in a food. Dr. Wheelwright worked in his own garden genetically engineering foods. To improve nutritional content and flavor, he removed generations of degenerations in the plant caused by hybridization. Wheelwright's garden grew in a magnetic field that harnessed the natural energies of the earth and repelled insects.

Wheelwright would often bring the results of his work to Texas to share with his gardener friends. From his garden, I sampled a potato that tasted like a strawberry, a tomato with the texture of an apple, and a cucumber with three times the flavor and refreshment. His produce was always delicious, energizing and vital.

However, the current goal of genetically altering plant foods is to extend their shelf life, not to improve human nutrition. And in the case of the altered tomato introduced to the marketplace right now, this food is nutritionally inferior because science has genetically deprogrammed the pectin that contributes to its spoilage. In fact, pectin is the best part of the tomato because it is the anti-bowel cancer fiber. Consequently, the engineered tomato has lost a major nutritional value in exchange for longer shelf life.

We cannot trust scientists who are ignorant about the nutritional relationship between plants and the human body, and who know nothing about the vital force, to genetically engineer foods that remain valuable for human consumption. Historically, genetically altered foods have become increasingly inferior.

An example of inferior altered foods is wheat which now contains an inbred anti-smut factor that causes wheat to be highly allergenic to so many people. The genetically engineered wheat is a prime example why we need to return to ancient grains such as spelt for our nutrition. Another example of poorly conceived food alteration is the cross-breeding of iceberg lettuce. This genetic alteration resulted in longer shelf life, the nutritional value of a sheet of notebook paper and the addition of bowel-retarding opiates.

In the present case of the engineered tomato, the scientists never asked what makes the perfect tomato for human nutrition, otherwise its pectin would have been increased! Instead, scientists prolong the tomato's shelf life by inhibiting the natural process of spoilage for only one reason—monetary gains. If a tomato can be grown that does not have to be picked prematurely green and artificially gassed into ripeness as happens now, then the producers do not have to spend money on that process. And the altered tomato's longer shelf life means that the grocer will pay more for the tomato because more can be sold and not so many are thrown away.

Although basically nothing is wrong with the technology of genetic engineering, the present controversy is about technology's misuse of the genetic alteration process. Also controversial is the motivation of the scientists who are not concerned whether such genetic alterations produce higher nutritional values in the altered produce.

The frightening aspect of the present controversy is that the U. S. government claims that the consumers do not need to know if a food has been genetically engineered. The FDA is willing to allow such foods to be slipped into the grocer's food bins without warning us about their altered nature. The same governmental agency, that is, the FDA, which wants to take vitamins off the food shelves and make them available by prescription only, now wants to put nutritionally inferior foods on our tables without warning on the labels that these foods have been genetically engineered.

Fortunately, several consumer groups are protesting the FDA's position. Jeremy Rifkin, president of the Foundation on Economic Trends, opposes genetically altered foods. As quoted in the *Austin American Statesman* (June 1, 1992), Rifkin demands that all genetically engineered food be tested and labeled "so the consumer can make the ultimate decision."

Rifkin further states, "You [the FDA] are playing ecological roulette with our food supplements. If a pear has a mouse gene, then it should say so on the pear. If there is a human growth hormone in my hamburger, then I want to know it. I think the American public is going to be very opposed to these foods. . . .To say industry will police itself is a joke."

For your and your family's sake, start a small garden, buy organically-raised produce and follow the Pro-Vita! Plan. Please remember the words of Dr. Wheelwright that I heard him say a hundred times, "Unless you have your own garden, even on a balcony, you will not be able to experience good health."

Ultimately, the concern for our food becomes a consumer issue. We must demand organically raised produce and let our dollars make nutrition the primary issue in foods. And we must vote people out of public office who do not work to protect our innate right to natural health.

NUCLEO-PROTEINS:
THE KEY TO DYNAMIC HEALTH

THE PROTEIN CONTROVERSY

The Pro-Vita! Plan has its roots in several traditional areas of nutrition: Food combining, biochemistry, pH (acid-alkaline balance), enzymes, digestion/elimination and, of course, the non-traditional area of bioenergy. Each of these roots nourishes the tree of greater health and well-being, but combined and reconciled by the bioenergy perspective, these traditional roots go deeper than ever before in a simple way each of us can master and experience individually.

There are many angles from which to explain how this nutrition plan works. This section of the Pro-Vita! Plan is based on one of the most controversial areas of nutrition, the proper use of PROTEIN. But proteins are only controversial because their PROPER USE is not understood. Wheelwright gave us this perspective on protein because he preferred to confront the difficult, most important area first, and let other nutritional considerations fall into place.

Proteins are vitally important. The word "protein" is derived from the Greek language and means "of primary importance." Amino acids, the organized components of proteins, are the biochemical basis for life itself and are required by every cell. The immune system's antibodies are protein. Endocrine hormones are protein. The extra-cellular matrix, or material between the cells, is protein. Nucleo-proteins make up a vital part of the body's energy system. They are used for daily activities and must be replenished.

Collagen, the "cement" that holds the cells together, is also based on protein. Cellular immunity depends on protein. All of the thousands of known enzymes are made with amino acids from protein. Bones and teeth are also made of a matrix of protein over which the minerals such as calcium and phosphorus are laid. And the brain's neurotransmitters, regulators of everything from sleep to feelings of joy, are protein, too.

Science has discovered 22 amino acids (and possibly another two or so) that make up the known components in the protein chain alphabet. Of these 22 amino acids, nine are classified ESSENTIAL because the body cannot manufacture them, but must rely on diet to provide them. (Some people speculate that an evolutionary or spiritual step is needed for the body to learn to manufacture the essential amino acids as well, so human beings can rely strictly on fruits and vegetables as foods.) The other 14 amino acids can be assembled or disassembled by the body in the liver as it sees fit, provided that the liver is in good working order.

From the 22 recognized amino acids, the body produces what science has identified as 50,000 amino acid structures necessary for body function. Out of billions of possible combinations which amino acids could form, approximately 50,000 are known to support life. This means that there are billions of combinations that have unknown potentials ranging from healing to killing.

That some combinations of amino acids are not healthy is one reason why some nutritional researchers are concerned about the use of NutraSweet (aspartame). Although this product is a combination of two natural proteins, it actually is a new form of protein, not found in nature, and it breaks down into alcohol.

For this reason, many nutritional researchers are concerned about the known and unknown side effects of NutraSweet. Side effects of NutraSweet intake are suspected to be hyperactivity, anxiety attacks and allergies. Unfortunately, the extensive brainwashing of the public by NutraSweet's TV advertising is at work to sell us this product. The fact that such a hard-sell campaign is thought to be necessary, is testimony that there is something wrong with NutraSweet. At this time, more than 4,000 food products contain this unnatural amino acid chain in addition to other chemical additives, thus contributing to the overall toxic burden being placed on the body.

Perhaps, to find a sugar substitute science should look to nature. For example, the Brazilian herb, stevia, is much sweeter than sugar, metabolizes slowly, does not deplete nutrients and is designed by nature. Some healthfood markets carry this natural sugar substitute.

The body's vital amino acids derive primarily from diet. The body digests the dietary proteins into amino acids. The liver re-forms these into usable protein structures, the nucleo-proteins. This process of changing dietary proteins into usable amino acids is called "humanizing" the proteins. During the humanizing process, a molecule of fat is added and the individual's biological warp to the electron shell "personalizes" the molecule. The biological warp, a bioenergetic term, means that the nutrients accepted by the body become a recognizable part of that body. This process is important immunologically because the immune system is supposed to attack "non-self" molecules, and not attack "self" molecules. A non-humanized amino acid chain, whether it be Lima bean, cedar pollen, or dust, is known as an "allergen" if the immune system overreacts to it.

Many people are aware of the expression, "You are what you eat." This statement is true if the liver can process the food. As a result of the liver's work, amino acids bear a unique molecular signature which identifies them as "self" rather than "non-self." The biological warp makes the nutritional protein part of that particular body's ecosystem. Without this vital liver function, the proteins would remain foreign, unusable, toxic and allergenic for the body.

The problem with many people's allergies is their body's excessive reaction to proteins in the blood stream which have not been, or cannot be, humanized. For example, pollens enter the body through the lungs; foods and non-foods such as NutraSweet enter through the stomach and the intestines. As consequence, the immune system in hypersensitive individuals can have violent reactions.

In the 1970s, many health authorities promoted "Hi-Protein" diets, such as 200-grams-a-day protein powders. These products made many people sick because too many poor quality proteins flooded their bodies and had to be processed. This caused acidosis, or an overly acid condition, leading to osteoporosis and other diseases, and congested the lymphatics with large-molecule proteins thus further inhibiting removal of toxins from the body. As a backlash to this excessive use of protein, many health authorities, in turn, promoted an extremely low protein intake. However, eventually people became sick from a lack of available amino acids and exhibited weakened tissue integrity and immune systems.

In the 1980s, the dietary push toward high complex carbohydrate (grain) intake began. Already there are trends showing that this is not the dietary answer, because a carbohydrate food plan does not build the quality tissues required for optimal health. Also, carbohydrates such as grains often become allergenic if used excessively. This may be caused by modern hybridization and agricultural methods rather than the natural grain. They are survival food and will do if no other food is available. Yet, most people want more than "make-do" with foods since foods have the potential to build a more optimal level of health. Ultimately, high complex carbohydrate diets do not suffice for good health, particularly if vegetables are neglected.

Today, in the 1990s, many people think that grains and complex carbohydrates should be the foundation for the human diet. Yet, history shows us that people who live on bread and rice were not particularly healthy, and this is true today. For a clear understanding how the Pro-Vita! plan is designed, keep in mind the nutrition pyramid illustration. The food-basis of human nutrition categorized by IMPORTANCE TO HEALTH consists of vegetables; followed by judicious and necessary use of proteins; followed by high quality oils; then compex carbohydrates, and finally, liberal use of fresh fruits in their natural season for enjoyment. This nutritional hierarchy, or nutrition pyramid, will be explained throughout this book.

The Pro-Vita! Nutrition Pyramid is a rational and creative approach to a food plan. It is based on biochemistry and keen insights into the human body through the microscope of bioenergy, the patterns of energy that support life. Our nutritional approach represents a balance of "right brain" and "left brain" approaches to simplify the complexities of diet.

We emphasize that the ideal diet for humans is based on VEGETABLES. Approximately 65 - 75% of the food program by volume should be vegetables as dictated by numerous facts and insights including the body's acid/alkaline (pH) balance, a major factor predisposing a person to health or disease. However, it remains crucial to focus on proper administration of PROTEIN as the difference between sickness and health.

THE PROTEIN MATRIX OF PHYSICAL LIFE

The fundamental principle of the vital body processes such as growth, repair and healing of tissue, is that the success or failure of the body is dependent on amino acids. Thus protein forms the matrix of physical life from the development of the embryo to the ability to survive immunologically. Proper dietary intake of protein is essential to a healthy life.

To reemphasize a point or two, The Pro-Vita! Plan is NOT A HIGH PROTEIN DIET. Instead, it is an optimal health nutrition plan based on both the body's energy and tissue needs. We focus here on protein because it is the most important, most costly to obtain and most needed nutrient for health. But just because we focus attention on HOW TO USE protein, this does not imply that a person should eat an excess of it. Remember the soybean story: MORE IS NOT BETTER!

Proper use of protein will allow a person to get more benefit out of less protein. This is good for health because it promotes efficient use of the body's digestive resources and provides more energy than was required to process the nutrients. And proper use of proteins reduces the toxicity associated with poor utilization of protein by the body.

Protein is the foundation of our body functions. Without a proper protein matrix, a person cannot have good health. Yet, most people today are deficient in protein at the cellular level—the nucleo-proteins—for the following reasons:

- Some people eat incorrect amounts of proteins. Some don't eat enough proteins in general due to deliberate protein-avoidance diets. Others eat too much animal protein, that is, red meat. Dearth and excess both cause less than optimal health.

- Some people eat proteins that are too complex and hard to digest, such as unfermented soybeans, raw nuts and peanuts. This eating habit causes stress for the liver, kidneys, lymphatics and immune systems.

- Some people incorrectly combine protein with carbohydrates or sugar which ruins digestion/ assimilation of nutrients and creates putrefactive toxins, stressing the organs.

- Some people worry while eating which inhibits proper digestion.

- Some people drink too much fluid with their proteins which dilutes the digestants consisting of acids and enzymes, resulting in inability to properly digest food.

- Some people often don't buffer proteins with vegetables, thus omitting needed enzymes, assimilation factors, chlorophyll and fiber.

- Some people eat too much volume for the stomach to digest properly.

- Some people don't exercise properly to move proteins from the lymphatic pool into the cells and to remove cellular wastes.

EATING EXCESSIVE PROTEINS IS DETRIMENTAL TO HEALTH. Many authoritative works on nutrition advise to use 100 grams of protein daily for every 100 pounds of body weight. But by following the guidelines of The Pro-Vita! Plan a person can use 22-30 grams of protein for every hundred pounds of body weight, get much more use out of it and avoid the toxic reactions associated with higher protein intakes.

The current minimum Recommended Dietary Allowance (RDA) for protein for males (155 lbs) is 56 grams/day; for females (120 lbs) 44 grams/day. These values are based on ideal weight. Excess weight due to body fat does not increase the protein requirement. Note that the above figures do not take into consideration the Pro-Vita! method of optimizing protein through low-stress food choices and protein synergism and could therefore be lower.

During PREGNANCY, the prospective mother should increase her protein intake to approximately 50 grams of Pro-Vita! protein per 100 lbs. of ideal body weight to support the developing baby and avoid toxemia. Few people understand that protein deficiencies during pregnancy cause toxemia in which cellular metabolic waste products are not eliminated. Symptoms of toxemia such as blurry vision, elevated blood pressure, protein in the urine, headaches and water retention are common and can progress into eclampsia (coma). Also, proper protein intake during pregnancy helps minimize morning sickness, provides steady energy, and in the latter stages (8th month) contributes greatly to the baby's mental development.

MORNING SICKNESS is primarily, but not exclusively, a liver/intestine problem. During the early stages of pregnancy, the woman's hormones increase dramatically. The liver has the responsibility for conjugating and processing the hormones. The first trimester is a time of great stress on the liver. If the liver cannot fully maintain the bile function via the gall bladder, the bile stays in the intestines causing the nausea of morning sickness. If bile gets into the stomach, vomiting of bile may occur.

For these reasons, nutritionists and naturopaths often recommend Wheelwright's Liver Triad program prior to conception. This information is discussed in the book, *Your Liver-Your Lifeline* (Tips, 1990). Wheelwright was very effective in helping women overcome morning sickness by having them supplement their diets with his BLDB herbal formula and adding a little vinegar in water to their diets. For morning sickness, the natural health-care provider may also recommend safe homeopathic remedies to help effect a rapid cure, such as Sepia, Tabacum, Nux Vomica, Anacardium, Cerium Ox., Natrum Phos., Kreosotum, Aletris Farinosa and Symphoricarpus, to name a few. Such remedies are chosen according to the person's specific symptom picture and are very effective.

Be wary of diet plans that downplay protein because they have only a partial perspective. The dry weight of the body is 70% protein. Bones are mostly protein, skin is protein, collagen is protein, the immune system and hormone system is based on protein. And these must be renewed constantly.

There is only approximately 6 to 12% carbohydrate in the body's entire make-up, and most of that is in transit for energy. Therefore, people who rely on too many carbohydrates (grains, potatoes, pasta) shortchange themselves. Their diet is too rich in a nutrient that makes up only a small portion of the body, and too lean in the nutrient that makes up the majority of the tissues. High carbohydrate diets avoid the potential toxicity problem of high protein diets, but they are not in accord with the human tissue matrix and the human bioenergy matrix. Proper use of proteins is essential.

Excessive carbohydrates turn into a sludge that provides a breeding ground for bacteria. As Stu Wheelwright said, "You are not a dough boy!" A steady stream of carbohydrates in the diet can contribute to weak tissue, since tissue is built from a protein matrix. The carbohydrates provide a superficial energy that can keep people with poor tissue integrity going from day to day, but carbohydrates cannot build or maintain strong tissue in the long run in the human being.

It is also important to recognize that many commercial grains are not what they used to be in nature, because they have been hybridized. For example, an anti-smut factor has been bred into wheat which now makes it more allergenic. Many grains have also been herbicided, pesticided, chemically fertilized and gassed until they hardly resemble a food at all. Organic grains, such as spelt, are far superior nutritionally and should be used whenever possible.

Food is also a matter of QUALITY. The proteins in sprouts, soaked seeds and other low-stress sources provide a nutritional quality that is sorely lacking in grains, baked potatoes and other starchy foods.

For all of these reasons, the high carbohydrate diets are ultimately unsuccessful. The body's tissues get weaker, while the shallow carbohydrate energy keeps the processes going. The superficial energy disguises the lower performance of the less-than-optimal quality tissues. Because of this, it often takes a while for people to notice the lack of vibrant health. Their less-than-optimal condition can be seen bioenergetically by nutritionists trained in such analysis. People who rely on beans and rice, pasta and cheese exclusively for their protein inevitably come up short. The Pro-Vita! Plan will show how to use such foods and build a vibrant state of nutritional health.

The only people who need higher than normal levels of carbohydrates are children and athletes. But the carbohydrates must be eaten

AFTER a proper protein matrix is provided for the body's integrity. Children are growing and working with a higher energy system. Athletes are working their bodies at a higher level and require more available energy. But most people's metabolisms burn at a rate that will not properly accommodate high levels of carbohydrates.

When I hear of professional athletes who heal slowly, I consider that this is often a sign that they do not have the protein matrix to heal quickly (either they are eating too much red meat or getting too little useable protein) and are using a lot of carbohydrates for energy-loading without a proper protein foundation. It has been my clinical observation that athletes who follow the tenets of The Pro-Vita! Plan have fewer injuries in non-contact sports and repair faster from contact injuries.

Proteins provide strength and stamina. Carbohydrates provide a ready source of energy for optimal performance when there is strong tissue-protein as a foundation. A proper food plan provides the body with high quality raw materials so that it can synthesize the proper fuel mix for its life-style.

Diet plans that advocate high carbohydrate diets, such as eating a lot of grains or potatoes, often erroneously base their insights on the nutrient breakdown of mother's milk, which has a relatively high carbohydrate content compared to many other protein-rich foods. Such diets take this fact as license to promote high carbohydrate consumption. But these diets fail to recognize the biochemical and metabolic differences between an infant and an adult, primarily that the infant can double its body weight in a few weeks, but the adult does not, or certainly should not.

When so-called health authorities criticize consumption of protein in general, they are doing so from a limited perspective, probably that of a limited perspective of biochemistry alone without the perspective of bioenergy. In other words, they do not understand the different qualities of protein, that some proteins are poor and some are valuable. What they say about protein is basically true, but their perspective is based on typical protein consumption—poor quality, prepared incorrectly and eaten improperly at the wrong time of day. Under such conditions, of course, protein causes problems. But we will learn how to use high-quality proteins in the proper fashion as we come to understand the Pro-Vita! Plan. Used incorrectly, protein causes many health distresses. Used correctly with a foundation of organically or bio-dynamically raised vegetables, protein creates abundant health. Thus, protein is a two-edged sword that can heal or kill, depending on how it is wielded.

Since the body is a protein system, proper qualities and quantities of protein must be addressed. This nutrition plan is basically a LOW PROTEIN plan considering that some health researchers and authorities have advocated up to 200 grams of protein a day. With the Pro-Vita! Plan an average person can prosper on 25-40 grams a day. One day of the week can and should be designated as a day of rest without protein. The amount of protein depends on body weight, age and activity level. Maybe even less protein is used when all systems are functioning well, including handling stress and maintaining an attitude of being at peace with the world and with life.

Protein is required to build strong cellular immunity and resistance to disease. A deficiency of available protein at the cellular level can be caused by a low protein, high carbohydrate diet; a high protein diet where proteins are not properly digested; and the wrong kind of proteins meaning those too complex to be assimilated. To restate, diets both too low and too high in proteins cause poor health. Obviously we want the right amount of protein, the right quality of protein, and the ability to use it in conjunction with other nutrients for optimal energy and optimal health.

Currently, protein is one of the most controversial areas in the field of nutrition. It is also an area fraught with contradictions, since each new finding can be interpreted as a case in point for opposing views. Let's take a quick look at the difficult areas. Then we'll see how the study of energy (bioforce) provides a rational plan for using protein usually overlooked.

The proponents of a high protein intake often claim that our tissues are mostly amino acids (the components of protein) and that amino acids are required for healthy glandular function and hormone production. The more they study protein, the more they see a critical need for it. They are alarmed that in a country where protein intake is very high, people still exhibit symptoms of protein deficiency, which, as we now know, is actually caused by poor use of protein foods.

In contrast, the proponents of a low protein intake state that protein is toxic, for example, raw egg white and rattlesnake venom are, chemically, virtually the same. Proteins that putrefy in the colon cause most of the diseases (such as cancer) and ailments (such as headaches) affecting people today. This is because the toxic burden of excessive dietary proteins creates the terrain for disease organisms, lowers the body's immunity and ability to overcome stress, and causes imbalances in the body's pH. Improperly digested proteins poison the lymphatic system, the bloodstream and vital organs. Low-protein advocates point out that the body can synthesize most amino acids, so it is better to go easy on protein and capitalize on vegetables, grains and fruits, our sources of energy and enzymes.

Every statement above is true! The solution does not come from either extreme—neither high nor low protein intake. Instead, it derives from proper use of the proper amount of protein, properly consumed. And these factors vary from person to person and even vary within a person's lifetime. We simply need to be aware of the damages of either excessive or insufficient protein intake and plan a diet in the middle.

EXCESSIVE PROTEIN consumption or improper protein use can result in:

- Osteoporosis (calcium loss from bones)
- Teeth and gum diseases (calcium loss)
- High cholesterol (from animal proteins)
- Acidosis
- Constipation
- Toxic lymphatic system
- Kidney infections and weakness
- Swollen, over-oxidized liver
- Water retention

- Chronic degenerative disease (arthritis, cancer, diabetes)
- Allergies
- Hypertension
- Poor immune response

PROTEIN DEFICIENCIES can result in:

- Glandular fatigue (adrenal burnout)
- Anemia (iron-poor blood)
- Inability to use amino acids for metabolic processes
- Weakened immune system
- Stringy muscles
- Degenerative diseases
- Inability to heal
- Slow metabolism (cold extremities, weight gain)
- Accelerated aging processes
- Hair loss
- Depression
- Memory loss
- Deep fatigue
- Infertility
- Alkalosis
- Hypoglycemia
- Catabolism (robbing amino acids from tissue)
- And many other conditions

People who consume large quantities of red meats are poisoning their systems, even though this protein source is complete in its amino acid structure. Besides, red meats are often loaded with steroids, antibiotics and preservatives, as Steinman (1990) has shown. People, such as vegetarians, who avoid meat, often eat foods that have an incomplete amino acid structure. Their body will attempt to complete the protein structure in the small intestine prior to absorption, which is additional work and causes an overall loss of amino acids. Often, their lymphatics are congested, usually with large molecular proteins from complex vegetable sources, such as unfermented soybeans, raw nuts, peanuts and cooked cheese. In these situations, the body will draw upon protein structures from the kidneys and other organ tissues, thus weakening vital body parts.

Not surprisingly, heavy meat eaters often have poor kidneys, because kidneys are abused by having to filter out the urea and protein acids. But vegetarians can also have poor kidneys, because their tissue is often robbed of protein to complete the incomplete foods they eat. And frequently, vegetarians already have a dietary tendency toward protein deficiency because of their high carbohydrate diet.

When people overeat proteins, massive quantities of unusable proteins are stored in the body. The causes of this toxic accumulation include eating unbalanced proteins, heavy proteins (meats, cooked cheese, nuts, peanuts, unfermented soy beans), improper protein digestion, poor food combinations, and a lack of exercise which is needed to spread the amino acids out of the lymphatics into the body cells and tissues. The cells desperately need nucleo-proteins, the small molecule amino acids at the cellular level. But this valuable cell food is largely wasted with resulting degrees of starvation and poisoning because of the improper use of protein.

As nutrition research continues, the importance of proteins, amino acids and protein subunits in diets will continue to grow. Neurobiological researchers have discovered that the cell's energy source (the mitochondria) jumps from area to area within the cell along an intricate network of sub-protein fibers. This network is formed and reformed according to the needs of the cell, showing that usable proteins at the cellular level represent a fundamental part of the life-energy processes. The Pro-Vita! Plan addresses this fundamental life-energy process more thoroughly than any nutritional plan available today.

Protein, more than any other food, with the exception of oil, requires attention for its proper and beneficial use. Therefore, it is high time for a rational and creative approach to food planning diet. The Pro-Vita! Plan considers the correct amount of protein, prepared properly, eaten properly, digested properly and the by-products eliminated properly. With this in mind, we now have a whole new perspective on diet, health and energy.

QUALITY OILS:
ESSENTIAL FOR OPTIMAL HEALTH

ESSENTIAL FATTY ACIDS ARE
A REQUIRED NUTRIENT

Oils, or fatty acids, are vitally important in a good nutritional plan. In fact, they are an important layer in the nutrition pyramid and are absolutely essential for our health. Before a protein can be used by the body, it must be made non-toxic by the liver, which adds a molecule of unsaturated fat (oil) to the protein molecule. Therefore, oil plays a crucial role in protein metabolism and ultimately in the whole body's metabolism.

Like the many different qualities of other nutrients discussed in this book, there are many differing qualities of oils. Some oils are beneficial and some are detrimental. So, for our discussion, we need to have a working definition of what oils are. Oils are a food substance found in seeds, vegetables, and other food sources of plant and animal origin. From a health perspective, we are primarily interested in oils from plant sources, though some people derive benefit from fish oils, such as salmon, shark, cod liver and other fish oils. When the term "oil" is used, it refers to the wholesome, fatty acid complexes found in vegetables in their natural, unprocessed, unheated state. This definition excludes oils such as in fried foods, mineral oil and hydrogenated oils. Industrial hydrogenation changes vegetable oils into hardened and saturated oils, like margarine, by adding hydrogen. References to such oils are as "detrimental" oils or "fats."

The body's nutrient requirement of oil is between one and two tablespoons a day. Few people realize that the body has a nutritional requirement for essential fatty acids, just like it does for Vitamin C. The current fear of oil instilled in the public by the medical profession under the guise of cardiovascular health is not rational because the real culprits are saturated fats, hydrogenated oils and fried foods.

Oil is used for energy metabolism, glandular integrity, skin, heart function and the immune system. Most of this oil should come from seeds and vegetables. The body requires both saturated and unsaturated fats for its life processes, but the proportions weigh very heavily toward the unsaturated fats. The most exciting recent bioenergetic research pertains to unsaturated oils or, as they are called commonly, essential fatty acids. We will discuss this research before looking at other aspects of oil consumption.

THE BUDWIG RESEARCH ON FATTY ACIDS

The unique effects on human health by the essential fatty acids contained in cold-pressed, fresh, organic flax seed oil, have been researched by Dr. Johanna Budwig (1988) in Germany. Her research concentrates on the importance of photo elements—the photons of solar energy and the pi-electron system for human health. Budwig considers the photons to be a principle of order in the life process of human beings. She bases her quantum biological research on Einstein's quantum energy theory.

Since pi-electrons and photons of solar energy are especially pronounced in seed oils, these oils are crucial for the maintenance of good health. According to Dr. Budwig, the electron-rich fatty acid of flax seed oil plays a decisive role in the functions of all body membranes, all sensory organs, the immune defense, the cardiac function, the lymphatic system, the cerebral and nervous functions and in growth processes. The fatty acids are active in the body's metabolism and are involved in the building of protein.

Budwig's theory is an example of the Sun Element—its light and heat—stored in a vegetable seed. When flax seed oil is used, one of the rarest five elements—fire—becomes available for human health. Along with it come other complimentary elements. This anti-entropic food slows down the aging process, prolongs health and contributes bioenergetically to vitality.

Budwig's research also indicates that fatty acids are crucial to overcome illness from cancer, because this disease has proven to be a problem of fat exchange. Ultimately, Budwig considers the sun-oriented electrons, as contained in fatty acids, to be the important anti-entropy factor, helping us to maintain the body's homeostasis.

Budwig's books discuss ground-breaking research about fats and their good and bad effects on human health. In her most recently translated book, *Flax Oil as a True Aid Against Arthritis, Heart Infarction, Cancer and Other Diseases* (1992), she explains how the metabolism of fat has an extensive effect on the vital functions of every organ of the body. Specifically, she notes that a lack of essential fatty acids is particularly noticeable in connection with nerve and brain functioning. The heart's function is also vitally affected by essential fatty acids. Equally dependent on the essential fatty acids are the cell membranes, that is, the external skin of the cell.

Dr. Budwig's book contains several discussions about the lack of essential fatty acids as the cause for the formation of cancers. She explains how optimal fats inhibit tumorous growths. She provides examples of her own clinical use of flax seed oil for successfully healing a number of diseases.

Dr. Budwig is a seven-time Nobel Prize nominee, a world-renowned nutritionist and biochemist, famous for her work about the relationship between cancer and fat metabolism. Unfortunately, much of her work remains untranslatable into English. We thank Charlotte Lodi, nutritionist (MD, Germany) for drawing our attention to the currently available English translations of Dr. Budwig's ground-breaking research.

OILS AND DIET

Dr. Budwig (1992) recommends that flax seed oil should be mixed into non-fat cottage cheese for optimal dietary use. The reason for this mixture is that the fatty acids easily associate with the protein of the cottage cheese and thus achieve water solubility in the fluids in the body. In other words, the cottage cheese easily dissolves the fatty acids which become easy to digest and easy to utilize for the liver. Non-fat yoghurt with acidophilus culture is a good substitute for the cottage cheese to make the recommended mixture.

A healthy person should consume two tablespoons of flax seed oil in this fashion; a person with chronic illness should take up to six tablespoons a day. It is best to work up to the maximal amount of flax seed oil slowly, because it has a slightly laxative effect for some people.

Our discussion of oils brings up a difference with the traditional food combining rule, "Do not eat oils and proteins at the same meal." So let's address this briefly. This is, in its traditional context, basically a good rule because some oils are poisons, like shortening, lard, gravy and fried foods. But this old rule is superseded in the Pro-Vita! Plan with its focus on high quality, healthful oils. The modified rule about oil now reads, "Use a small amount of high quality oil with protein and always accompany it with vegetables." It needs to be noted that fatty acids support the liver's process of humanizing proteins. The Pro-Vita! Plan which consists mostly of vegetables with some protein and a small amount of high quality oil, follows good rules of health and optimizes nutritional values.

Some of the biochemical values of oil are the following. Oils help the metabolic rate, also called the oxidation rate, to be optimal. In fact, oils render two or more times as much energy as proteins and carbohydrates. Oils are a rich source of acetate which prevents cellular exhaustion caused by the combustion of carbohydrates. For this reason, avocado (a food rich in oil) helps hypoglycemics to control and sustain the combustion of blood sugar and not have energy slumps. Since oils are absorbed slowly, they provide a steady energy supply.

Another important fact about oils is that phosphorus cannot be absorbed through the intestinal wall, or be eliminated by the kidneys, without the use of oils. The reason for this is that phosphorus moves into and out of circulation as phospholipids, or in an oil-based form. Finally, if used properly, oils are helpful with protein meals to humanize the amino acids by making them acceptable to the body.

A warning about detrimental oils is in order. Oils can be the most damaging food substance ingested if used improperly as in chips and fried food. In fact, if oils are rancid, they are quite poisonous. For this reason, the fast food industry is a leader in destroying human health. By patronizing fast-food french fry establishments – "over 10 billion sold!" – we all pay with high insurance rates for a generation marked with cardiovascular and bowel disease, and other chronic, degenerative illnesses.

The following section provides some insights into oils to better understand the issue of cholesterol and current trends in the nutritional use of oils.

A NUTRIENT CALLED VITAMIN F

Although oils are a very valuable nutrient, misused oils are the most potentially dangerous food substance we eat causing cancer, hardened arteries, high blood pressure and heart attacks. Therefore, we need to take a look at how to work with oils. In this way we learn about cholesterol, omega-3 oils, saturated and unsaturated oils to become familiar with the basic nutritional factors of fatty acids. Because cholesterol is a fatty substance, our discussion also relates to the hotly debated consumption of eggs which is another area where the public is being mislead by TV advertisers.

When too many detrimental oils (fats) are consumed, the likelihood of heart disease, cancer, hypoglycemia, allergies, obesity, food sensitivities, sluggish liver, gall stones and endocrine gland dysfunction is greatly increased. However, when a diet is low in beneficial oils, health problems ensue also.

Symptoms of too many fats in the diet include:

- Acne
- Bad breath
- Bloating
- Body odor, strong
- Cholesterol problems
- Constipation
- Dysmenorrhea
- Fatigue 2 hrs. after eating
- Gas
- Gall stones
- Menopausal symptoms
- Mood swings
- Oily skin
- Prostate problems
- Tension
- Yellow, white, or grey stool
- Water retention

Symptoms of a diet too low in oils include:

- Amenorrhea
- Hair loss
- Healing process slow
- Hormonal imbalance
- Immune system weakness
- Menopausal symptoms (hot flashes)
- Nerve weakness
- Platelet adhesions (sticky blood)
- Prostate, enlarged
- Reproductive organ dysfunction
- Skin problems, dry

Oils are fats, or lipids, which are composed of fatty acids also known as VITAMIN F, an essential nutrient as discussed at the beginning of the chapter. Vitamin F is vitally important for the thyroid and adrenal glands (our energy glands), the nerve sheath, the hair, skin and mucous membranes. It plays an important role in balanced cholesterol, blood clotting, proper blood pressure, glandular function and arterial flexibility. The symptoms of deficiencies in vitamin F include acne, allergies, arteriosclerosis, diarrhea, dry skin, eczema, hair loss, gall stones, nail weakness, nerve fray, inability to gain weight and varicose veins.

There are three major types of fatty acids—saturated, monosaturated and polyunsaturated—depending on how "saturated" or "unsaturated" they are. Saturation refers to the chemistry of fats, based on how many double-bonded carbon atoms are available to accept another atom, such as hydrogen or oxygen.

SATURATED OILS lack available slots for double bonds. These oils are short-chain molecules of 8 to 18 carbons, somewhat brittle and sticky. Examples are coconut oil and lard. They are usually solid at room temperature. Recently, medical experts have rightly warned people to avoid consuming products containing such fats, such as many processed foods, cookies and crackers. However, pure, properly-processed coconut oil is a wonderful oil for dietary use. It provides valuable medium-chain lipids that support intestinal and immune system health. Processed, partially-hydrogenated coconut oil is ruined by the processing and should be avoided.

A MONOSATURATED OIL has one double bond and can accept two new molecules. It is a somewhat flexible molecule, not as sticky as a saturated oil and is liquid at room temperature. Examples of monosaturated oils are olive, avocado, almond, apricot kernel, canola and peanut oils. These are valuable oils and their usage is recommended, if they are organic and processed properly. The wonderful effects of extra-virgin olive oil for the cardiovascular system and skin are well known.

A POLYUNSATURATED OIL has two or more double bonds and thus slots for additional molecules. They are very active molecules. Examples are safflower, sunflower and corn oils. Although polyunsaturated oils play a biochemical role and are of some nutritional benefit, they are not optimal for exclusive use because they become rancid so easily. The use of partially-hydrogenated corn oil, or margarine, is a destructive factor in many people's health.

Two important fatty acids have been designated as "essential fatty acids," although currently about twenty-two fatty acids have been identified that support the human body. The number of fatty acids will undoubtedly increase as fat research continues. Significantly, all but two of these fatty acids are synthesized by the liver. These two, the linoleic and linolenic acids, designated essential fatty acids, must be derived from diet. Linoleic acid is considered the most important one of the two essential fatty acids, because it is required to synthesize other oils. Consequently, these fatty acids all play important biochemical roles in human nutrition.

NATURAL SOURCES OF VITAMIN F include raw or soaked nuts, whole grains, beans, avocado and seeds, especially flax seed. Most people are deficient in good quality oil because their diets lack raw seeds. Many potential oil sources, such as grains, are cooked and as a consequence the oils are damaged. Nutritionists and biochemists recognize that high quality oils are a valuable nutrient. Most people need between one and two tablespoons of high quality, non-rancid, monounsaturated or polyunsaturated oil per day. For this reason, people who go on an oil-free diet run the risk of serious damage to their health.

There are diets that eliminate all oils, but these plans are only temporarily therapeutic and not for optimal health. People whose bodies are out of balance, may temporarily respond well to avoiding oil, since they cannot handle it in their ill state. But prolonged abstinence from oils results in the lean, sallow, scarecrow look that is now the trademark of such diets. Once again, balance is the key.

I once consulted with a man who had been on the Pritikin Diet for eight years, strictly avoiding oils. He was sallow, thin, shaky, cold, forgetful, weak and complained of symptoms too numerous to list. My sole recommendation was to add organic flax seed oil to his diet. He stared at me in disbelief since he was obviously convinced that oil was the consummate evil and he came to me for homeopathic counsel. He reluctantly consented to the idea mumbling some words to his wife about being killed. He missed his next appointment 30 days later, but came back into town two months later. I did not recognize him because he looked so well. He did not want any further treatment, and later embarked on a world cruise with his wife to "live it up." I was never given the opportunity to find a fundamental homeopathic remedy for him as the initial case-taking was too immersed in oil-deficiency symptoms.

Having established that oils are a necessary nutrient performing vital functions, let's address the issue that some people say that low-fat diets prevent cancer and tumor growths. As we have seen from Budwig's research this is not the case where fatty acids are concerned. It is also well known that diets high in olive oil and fish oil prevent cancer. Once again, we encounter the age-old issue of quality. High quality oils build health. Poor quality oils destroy health. One of the very real factors connecting oil to cancer is the RANCIDITY of the oil. Here is a discussion of dangerous rancid oils.

RANCID OILS, FREE RADICALS AND THE CARDIOVASCULAR SYSTEM

Rancid oils, as found in fried foods, cause "free radicals" which are electrically-charged atoms. This charge makes them extremely reactive and uncontrollable molecules which act like destructive maniacs randomly destroying cells. Consequently, they damage cells and encourage abnormal cell growth. Free radicals can be compared to people who go berserk, enter a restaurant and start shooting people at random. Until free radicals are controlled and neutralized by an enzymatic policeman, they wreak havoc in the body, particularly in the cardiovascular system.

Referring back to our lesson on the oil chemistry of fatty acids, the oils with the most double bonds (polyunsaturated) have the greatest likelihood of becoming rancid. This rancidity occurs when oxygen joins the molecules and, as a consequence the oil oxidizes. Since heating an oil causes oxidation, proper use of oils means minimizing the cooking temperature in stir-fry recipes (set the wok on 250° F), avoiding fried foods, and never reusing a heated oil. Also, it is best to use a 100% vegetable-source vitamin E supplement as an antioxidant if using heated oils.

As an aside about the quality of vitamin E, a terrible hoax has been played on the American consumer regarding "Natural" vitamin E. Wheelwright used to call attention to this situation frequently. A by-product of the Kodak photochemical process is used to make vitamin E. The same ingredients as moth balls, along with acetone and sulfuric acid can make a synthetic vitamin E (dl-alpha tocopheryl acetate). When the molecule is reversed in a magnetic field, d-alpha tocopheryl acetate results which the FDA allows to be called "natural." (Note that the "l" is missing from dl-alpha to designate the clockwise molecular rotation.) Wheelwright was adamant that people should use natural Vitamin E (d-alpha-tocopherol) from vegetable sources for human nutrition and thus manufactured such a supplement. (Please note that the "y" of tocopheryl is now an "o".) If you use vitamin E, be sure it is 100% from a plant source. The word "natural" does not guarantee the quality of the ingredients.

It is hard to avoid toxic, rancid oils particularly in such common foods as tortilla chips. Here in Texas, millions of pounds of fried tortilla chips are consumed as appetizers in restaurants to dip into salsa (hot sauce). They are also bought in bags for home use. It seems that many people are unwilling, or unable, to forego the crispy crunch and pungent taste of chips dipped in hot sauce, despite the cheap, rancid oils in which they are commonly fried.

There is a way, however, to make fine chips without frying and thus greatly reducing the amount of rancid oil in the diet. Whole wheat pita bread can be split in half into two disks of flat bread, toasted in the oven on low to medium heat (200 degrees F works fine) and broken into chips. Chapati whole wheat tortillas, corn tortillas, and organic blue corn tortillas can all be toasted into a crisp chip without frying.

There are also fat-free, baked, very tasty corn chips on the market. Two Austin-based companies marketing these non-fried corn chips are Guiltless Gourmet (the initiator) and El Galindo. A further improvement on the chip situation comes from Japan in the form of crackers (seaweed and rice) that are baked without oil. These substitutions for traditional fried chips are much more than make-do. They are delicious and crispy-crunchy, which is what people want and expect from a chip.

NUTRITION AND CARDIOVASCULAR DISEASE

When we understand how seriously free radicals damage the cardiovascular system, and how our bodies control and repair their damage, we recognize how important good oils are in addition to their basic nutritional values. The statistics on cardiovascular disease are appalling, particularly since this disease is predominantly a dietary issue. Medical science is spending millions of dollars to find a gene that predisposes a person to arterial plaque deposits. Yet, nutritionists already have the answer of how to avoid this life-threatening disease, since its process is clearly and simply one of basic nutritional biochemistry.

The medical research is missing the elementary point of the problem. Naturally, there is a gene responsible for arterial plaque build-up, because it is a healthy process of the body to prevent death by arterial lesion. However, the contemporary problem with plaqued-up arteries is one of nutrition as will soon be explained. But first, here are the national statistics on heart disease.

Although heart-and-cardiovascular disease is the number one killer of our population, this was not always so. Currently, cardiovascular disease kills two people a minute in this country. Last year, more than 1.6 million people in the United States suffered a heart attack, with more than 650,000 deaths. Those persons who did not die from the first heart attack, now have significant degrees of impairment. More than 200,000 people received by-pass surgeries. 155,000 people died of strokes, and thousands more now live lives of lower physical function.

However, insurance companies are delighted to pay thousands of dollars for by-pass surgery instead of paying a hundred dollars for a clinical nutritionist to help a person avoid such surgery!

Consequently, it is useful to know some facts about the cardio-vascular system. This information could very well save your life as well as the life of people around you. If there were a psychopath prowling your neighborhood streets, killing wantonly and randomly, you would willingly learn his habits and movements to protect yourself. According to the heart disease statistics, there is such a killer haunting your grocery stores' shelves and pharmacies, your fast food restaurants and most likely your pantry.

As we mentioned earlier, the plaque accumulation of arteries by cholesterol is actually a normal healthy process when it is needed. It is the mechanism the body uses so that an artery does not spring a leak and cause death. The real question here is NOT if there is a gene that allows plaque; it is NOT how do we reduce cholesterol in our diets; it is NOT how to reduce all oils in our diets. The real question is WHAT CAUSES DAMAGE TO THE ARTERIES SO THE BODY HAS TO KEEP APPLYING PLAQUE TO PATCH THEM UP?

This crucial question leads us to discuss the cardiovascular system and nutrition. Let's start with a model of a healthy artery which must be strong as it functions in the body's high pressure system. Just like the radiator hose in your car, your arteries must be strong, flexible and elastic to deal with the pressure and flow of blood from the heart. Like car hoses and tires, arteries are made up of layers.

The body must protect and care for the arteries because death results if the arteries spring a leak. The body cares for the arteries with several systems:

- nutrition to the arterial tissue

- enzymes that clean the blood

- enzymes that halt the terrible damage caused by free radicals

- the plaque-applying system to cover over any damage so that lesions do not rupture, causing the person to die.

69

Looking at each system above, we should be interested in what foods nourish the arteries. Dr. Wheelwright found the herb, or food, pimiento to be very supportive of arterial tissue. Thus, he often recommended that people eat pimiento as found stuffed in olives, or use his Hcv (Heart/Cardiovascular) herbal formula which contains Italian pimiento and other herbal nutrients as food for the arteries.

The next two protective body systems listed above are based on enzymes. They are another reason why vegetables must be the foundation of human nutrition. Only raw vegetables, and fresh fruit, contain living enzymes. Eating living enzymes in raw vegetables with every meal reduces the amount of enzymes the body must provide to the digestive processes. This situation is a simple matter of economy.

If your enzymes have to leave the arteries to take care of digestion, or if they have to work with the white blood cells as a back-up digestive system in the blood, then the arteries are more susceptible to damage. If you provide enzymes with every meal, then your arteries are better protected. A meal without some raw vegetables causes Leukocytosis, or the activation of white blood cells, and arterial enzymes to take over the digestive function. The research on this situation is more thoroughly presented in Appendix C. Dr. Edward Howell found that food enzymes can replenish the enzyme banks in the body as well as conserve existing enzymes, thus prolonging life and protecting health. Howell's book, *Enzyme Nutrition* (1985), is a nutritional classic.

To date, over 100 enzymes have been identified with their specific duties of maintaining the quality and integrity of the arteries. These enzymes primarily need an amino acid (protein) to do their job. A few rely on a fat or carbohydrate molecule to be activated.

The fourth body system to care for the arteries, the plaque system, is the last defense against cardiovascular disease. When damage is done to an artery by ingested substances, such as sugar, free radicals from food preservatives, chemical additives to foods, prescription medications, cigarette smoke and rancid oils, a lesion occurs. The damage and pressure cause the inner lining of the artery to rupture leading to an open sore, or lesion, inside the artery. Consequently, the artery is weak in that particular area because it now has fewer layers of protection.

The body's vitality quickly responds to the problem by sending platelets to plug up the area. Platelets, blood cells responsible for clotting, are sticky cells so they quickly adhere to the damaged area. Also, by being sticky and electrically charged, they attract other material such as elemental calcium, low density lipids and cholesterol to adhere and help plug, or cover over, the wounded area. This patch on the artery is called "plaque." Hardening of the arteries occurs when calcium gets embedded in the artery tissue like a patch on a tire.

In a healthy body, the slight obstruction to the arterial system during repair would present no problem. The artery heals, the build-up dissipates like a scab, and soon everything is back to normal. Just another minor episode, a day in the life of the body's arterial maintenance. But it does not happen this way now-a-days because people ingest many damaging substances including rancid oils, cigarette smoke, pasteurized milk, prescription medications, sugar and alcohol, to name only a few. Chemicals in the air can cause damage to the arteries. What we are dealing with here is an overload of stresses on the arterial system.

Many people experience irreparable damage to their arteries. Free radicals can damage the DNA identity of cells causing mutations, abnormalities and cancer. Inferior rebuilding materials in the blood are used by the body to repair damage, because high quality materials are not contained in many people's diets. Sugar can reticulate the blood vessels, making them more susceptible to clogging.

Free radical damage to blood vessels weakens their electrical charge. Normally, the vessels carry a negative magnetic charge and the red blood cells carry a slightly negative charge. Thus, the vessels and the cells repel each other slightly, which makes the blood move through the capillaries with ease. When free radicals damage the vessels, they impart a neutral or positive charge. In this way they encourage the attraction between the vessel wall and the blood cells resulting in clogged vessels and greater strain on the heart to pump the blood. This situation is a cause of heart attacks.

All of the following questions lead to the scary statistics presented earlier. What happens when there is no nutrition for the arteries to maintain their integrity? What happens when there is a dearth of enzymes in the food, and the arterial enzymes must occupy themselves with digestive processes instead of protecting the arteries? What happens when the diet is loaded with free radicals and other damaging chemicals, preservatives and rancid or hydrogenated oils as are found in margarine, meats, crackers, cakes, chips, cookies? What happens when the blood is full of sludge and inorganic elements that get involved with the patching up process? What happens when the entire arterial system is overworked, stressed and failing? What happens when prescription medications damage the arteries and contribute to abnormal healing of arterial lesions?

Well, what happens are the appalling national statistics and the heartbreak of deaths. Of course, you could take an aspirin a day as advertised on TV, bleed your stomach and do other damage to prevent heart attacks. Then you could keep right on eating the way America eats!

Hopefully, you do not want to wait for medical research to discover the gene we already know exists. Instead, you can protect and build your health with the Pro-Vita! Plan right now. Obviously, we want to eat right and not even be concerned with cardiovascular problems. After all, our bodies were made to take care of our cardiovascular systems on their own.

Here is a quick check list of common symptoms of people experiencing cardiovascular stress:

- Cold hands and feet
- Couperose, spider veins
- Leg cramps when walking
- Burning sensations in hands and feet
- Discoloration of fingers and toes
- Slurred speech
- Temporary loss of balance
- Poor concentration
- Tingling in hands and feet

- Migraine-type headaches
- Ringing in ears
- Pins and needles sensations
- Slow healing of superficial wounds

This is a summary of how to protect your cardiovascular health:

- Feed your arteries with whole foods
- Eat vegetables with every meal
- Use good quality oil
- Avoid poor quality oils
- Exercise

COLD PRESSED OIL

While discussing the poisonous effects of heating our dietary oil, let's look at one of the biggest jokes that the health food industry has played on consumers. We all know the commercial food industry has tricked us for years but, even the HEALTH FOOD industry has "pulled the wool" over our eyes a few times. This joke concerns the term "cold pressed" on the label of oils.

To many people, "cold pressed" oil brings up images of the old mill house and stream, the stone wheel pressing nature's bounty on a lovely fall day. But this image is far removed from the actual high-tech, fast-paced world, where cooking oils are treated with solvents, heated in blast furnaces, bleached and deodorized in a process that makes crankcase oil more desirable than "cold pressed" oil. By the way, a little crankcase oil is used by the food industry to impart that wonderful "smoky" flavor to some processed foods!

Actually, the initial use of the term "cold pressed" was not in a positive context. In his book, *Food Products* (1933), Columbia University professor Henry Sherman stated, "The so-called 'cold' pressed or expeller oil differs mainly from the 'hot' pressed (hydraulic presses) oil in that the former required longer agitation with caustic soda solution before heating in subsequent refining operations."

In 1953, a product promoter decided that "cold pressed" was a good marketing term to sell poor quality oil to the newly growing health food movement at a higher price. The embarrassing fact is that 25 years later people are still falling for this hype.

Cold pressed oil is often heated to 470 degrees F. This is done after the solvent (hexane) extracts the oil instead of an expeller press doing the extraction, a process that generates heat at the time of pressing. No reputable company puts "cold pressed" on the label of their food oils. However, some oil companies make a reputable product. They focus on "cold-processing" in which they strive to avoid heating the oil, since heat is damaging to the quality of oil.

Yet, there is actually such a product as genuine cold pressed oil. And it does indeed involve the good old days. The first pressing of olives in small Mediterranean mills yields a tiny bit of oil that does not exceed 80 degrees F in the pressing. This wonderful oil, called "extra virgin" and selling for a premium price, is a highly desirable source of Vitamin F.

Another cold processed oil (at 80 degree F) is organic flax seed oil. Organic flax seed oils carry the endorsement of Dr. Budwig only if the manufacturers use a special extraction process and do not expose the oil to the heat of the conventional "cold pressed" methods which exceed room temperature and result in damaging the oil and altering its healing qualities. Additionally, Wheelwright's son has introduced an organic cold processed flax seed oil in capsule form to the American market.

FATS: THE CHOLESTEROL ISSUE

THE CHOLESTEROL MYTH

In the latter part of the 1980s, cholesterol became a household word. Whether it really deserved it or not, cholesterol was made the nemesis of health—the boogey-man—whose fault it was when someone had a heart attack.

Once there was a culprit to blame, few people took time to understand the facts about cholesterol and look at diet in a more comprehensive light. Compounding the confusion were manufacturers with a product to sell who seized the opportunity to allay people's fears with their low-cholesterol products. Many of these low-cholesterol products, such as margarine and other hydrogenated vegetable oil products, as well as products containing tropical oils, do much more damage to the cardiovascular than the cholesterol-containing foods.

Before examining the so-called dangers of eggs and the alleged benefits of milk, here are some general facts about cholesterol.

- There are beneficial cholesterols that the body must have to be healthy.

- There are detrimental cholesterols that lead to cardiovascular disease.

- The liver makes cholesterol out of lipids for the body's needs.

- Non-cholesterol fats, such as saturated fatty acids and tropical oils, can cause more cardiovascular disease than moderate use of cholesterol-containing foods.

- In normal digestion, the body does not absorb cholesterol from foods. Any cholesterol in foods is digested into lipids before being absorbed.

Now, we look at several topics involving cholesterol to learn how to better manage it for our health. Let's look at some myths about cholesterol in eggs and milk as well as gain an understanding of the ratios of the different kinds of cholesterol in the body.

EGGS: THE CHOLESTEROL FALLACY

Cholesterol is a subject of much misunderstanding. Caught up in this situation are eggs because they contain cholesterol. Such statements as, "Don't eat eggs, they'll put cholesterol in your blood," border on the ridiculous. But millions of people believe these messages, largely due to TV advertising. People also have forgotten basic biochemistry which teaches that the cholesterol in eggs (wholesome yard eggs) is broken down to the nutrient lipids before it can be absorbed. The liver decides what to do with lipids, whether to make cholesterol or not.

Yard eggs do not put cholesterol in the blood as the research of Simopoulois & Salem (1989) has shown. In fact, yard eggs contain lipoproteins to help emulsify the cholesterol. In the digestive process, yard egg cholesterol is broken down to lipids, and egg lecithin becomes choline and inositol. It is up to the liver to decide if the lipids are reassembled into cholesterol or used for some other function, such as the myelin nerve sheath.

However, the commercial cage eggs are suspect from a nutritional perspective. Food chemists have discovered that the eggs produced by chickens cooped up in cages, exposed to artificial day/night rhythms, and fed on feed that is laced with steroids and antibiotics, are indeed different from the old-fashioned yard egg. The commercial cage egg may well be an aggravating factor in cholesterol problems. So, when you buy eggs, get yard eggs from the farmer or health food store.

Avoid commercial eggs as inferior and inhumane. The inhumane production methods of the commercial poultry and egg industry have been discussed eloquently by John Robbins in his famous book, *Diet for a New America* (1987).

MILK: THE NUTRITIONAL MYTH

Like commercial eggs, pasteurized and homogenized milk is also a suspect food. Actually, milk is more than suspect because it is directly linked to cardiovascular disease, as Sampsidis has shown in his book *Homogenized!* (1983).

Whether or not a person should drink milk is a subject of much discussion. Many nutritionists strongly oppose the use of milk for numerous reasons including cholesterol concerns. Yet, we hear on the television that milk is a "health kick." Let's examine some facts and understand the concerns because, generally speaking, commercial milk is not fit to drink and not a good food for most people. Although there may be some people who do well with milk, when we examine what the grocery stores sell as milk, it's hard to think of it as a good food.

First, let's figure out what real milk is. From a natural health perspective, milk would have to be in its natural form. Thus, it would originate from a human breast from a woman free of drugs and on a healthy diet. Since breast milk is not used as a food for people other than infants, we then must look to the animals—cows, goats, sheep, yaks—that produce an abundance of milk.

From the natural health perspective for public consumption of milk, we could say that milk derives from a cow or goat in its natural state. Should we find such an animal that is fed a healthy diet and kept free of pesticides, growth hormones and antibiotics, we would have a sample of whole, raw milk. This milk would be a superior food, particularly for the offspring of that animal, but could also be a food for human beings.

An assay of the raw milk from a certified dairy's organically raised animal would show that it contains an abundance of vitamins, minerals, fatty acids and other nutrients. It would contain fewer bacteria than the pasteurized milk people buy at the grocery store. This is MILK! Sampsidis (1983) suggests that certified raw milk has many nutritional advantages. It is most likely a good food for many people, if they wish to continue using milk after weaning. We've defined milk to be a product as it is found naturally. But this natural product is certainly not what people are buying, as "milk" in the stores.

So what's different about commercial milk? Well, it's pasteurized, homogenized and contains added synthetic ingredients. Let's examine pasteurization from a nutritional perspective. Pasteurization is a process of heating the milk to around 150 degrees Fahrenheit for 30 minutes. A newer method of pasteurization heats the milk to around 170 degrees for about half a minute, killing some of the bacteria in the milk and reducing the chance for infectious diseases.

However, it takes a temperature of around 190 degrees Fahrenheit to kill b-coli and the bacteria causing typhoid and tuberculosis. So from a sterilization perspective, pasteurization is only partially effective. Although pasteurization does kill some of the streptococcus bacteria, it also kills the beneficial lactobacillus acidophilus which is a beneficial bacteria provided by nature to keep the harmful bacteria in check. In this way the milk loses its inherent germicidal control and soon contains many more bacteria than if it were left in its raw state.

If raw milk is left to stand, it clabbers or turns into curds. As long as the acidophilus is present, it inhibits the harmful, putrefactive bacteria, and the milk curdles. But if pasteurized milk is left to stand, it rots since pasteurization leaves the milk unprotected and the putrefactive bacteria reign. If you drink pasteurized milk and your body does not have the ability to digest it properly, you end up with bacteria-laden, rotten milk in the bowel.

Dr. Royal Lee found many cases of undulant fever in consumers of pasteurized milk. There are also many cases of salmonella poisoning from pasteurized milk. We need to know that pasteurization does not really protect us completely, and that it harms the nutritional value of milk.

Why is milk pasteurized? Like so many detrimental things that have happened to our food, pasteurization is primarily done as a convenience for the dairy industry and the grocer. If the milk is cleaned up by the heat of pasteurization, then lower sanitation standards are required in the earlier stages of handling the milk. For this reason, the certified, raw milk dairies are so meticulously clean—much cleaner than the commercial dairies—and raw milk has a lower bacteria count than commercial milk. Since raw milk is not pasteurized, its bacteria counts must be kept low at all times or the milk will not be fit to drink. Also, if raw milk starts to spoil or curdle, it smells bad and warns the consumer. However, pasteurized milk takes longer to give off a bad smell since it does not have an active curdling potential, thus it has a longer shelf life.

Much nutrition is lost to pasteurization because heat kills enzymes. In the case of milk, the enzymes killed by pasteurization are the very enzymes needed to assimilate the calcium and properly digest the milk. We hear a lot of advertising hype about milk supplying calcium. How can it supply calcium when pasteurization kills the enzymes needed to assimilate it? It is noteworthy that the U.S. ranks as one of the top ten countries in the world in drinking pasteurized milk, and also ranks in the top ten for calcium deficiency diseases!

There is much vitamin loss due to pasteurization. Over two thirds of milk's inherent vitamin E and vitamin A are lost as well as large amounts of the vitamins C and B complex. Then synthetic vitamin D is put back into the milk to fortify it. Along with the vitamin loss, there is significant mineral loss. The heat also causes the minerals to form ionic bonds, meaning the body cannot break the bond to use the element or mineral.

The calcium in pasteurized milk is much harder for the body to use, if it can use it at all.

Since fats are sensitive to heat and should not be heated, pasteurization alters the milk's fat molecules. Pasteurization also damages the proteins, and milk is a protein food.

Pasteurized milk is a commercially damaged product. What that damage really means can be seen when calves are fed only pasteurized milk. What do you think happens to calves fed only pasteurized milk for two months? Well, they die. This research was first conducted by Dr. Frances M. Pottenger, the famed nutritional researcher, and has been duplicated by other researchers. Dr. Pottenger's research about the ill effects of pasteurized milk on children's teeth, cats and calves was presented in 1945 at the Second Annual Seminar for the Study and Practice of Dental Medicine. The research established that raw foods sustain health and prevent disease, but pasteurized and processed foods ruin health and cause disease. It raises the question why we use pasteurized milk to feed our babies.

People keep giving commercial milk to their children after weaning them because they are concerned about a calcium source for their bone development. But commercial milk is not a good source of calcium for several reasons:

- Milk alkalizes, yet calcium is absorbed only in an acid medium.

- The enzymes needed to assimilate calcium are destroyed by pasteurization.

- The heat of pasteurization hardens the calcium molecularly, making it very difficult, if not impossible, for the body to break it down to elemental calcium.

- The natural vitamin D is replaced with synthetic vitamin D which is less effective in transporting calcium into the body.

The best source of calcium for human infants is breast milk. If the mother can't nurse, a wet nurse should be provided. If that's not possible, raw goat milk, diluted a little, should be used. If raw goat milk is not available, here is a recipe which is certainly superior to the infant formulas in the grocery stores since they contain sugar, synthetic vitamins and inorganic minerals and are cheaply made.

Substitute baby milk-formula. Get the powdered goat milk (usually in a can) and other products at the health food store. Mix the ingredients in a blender. Mix six tablespoons powdered goat milk in a quart of pure water. This is a little less than the eight tablespoons recommended on the can. (The can gives measurements for baking.) We do not want to mix the goat milk as thick as suggested because goat milk is inherently thicker than breast milk. And, since goat milk is nutritionally different than breast milk, we want to compensate several ingredients. Add a spoonful of colostrum-based bifivia culture such as Eugalan-forte or Systemic's Bifivia. Add a drop of liquid minerals or a few drops of sea water. You may add one drop of children's liquid vitamins for a tiny amount of natural vitamins D, A and E. Then add three drops of Aerobic 07 stabilized oxygen to keep the milk fresh. Pour this milk into bottles, and you are set for the day. You won't even have to refrigerate the milk, because the Aerobic 07 acts as a preservative.

The best source of calcium for humans after weaning is in green leafy vegetables, carrots, cabbage, bok choy and Chinese cabbage. If you are really worried about calcium, or need to improve your intake, make your own calcium citrate. Simply put a whole egg in a narrow jar. Squeeze lemon juice over it so the egg stays covered in lemon juice. Put this in the refrigerator for eight hours. The lemon juice absorbs the calcium from the egg shell. After doing this, you may use the egg for cooking. Then, use the lemon juice as a readily bio-available source of calcium. Just add it to water or put it in orange juice.

The most famous and extensive research on the ill effects of pasteurized milk on children's teeth, cats and calves was conducted by Dr. Frances M. Pottenger and formally presented in 1945 It the Second Annual Seminar for the Study and Practice of Dental Medicine. The research established that raw foods sustain and prevent disease, but pasteurized and processed foods ruin health and cause disease.

Pasteurization is only part of the damage done to the white liquid people buy as milk. Homogenization, another processing of the milk, is done so the consumer will not have to contend with the cream separating to the top of the milk. Homogenization breaks down the fat globules so the milk and the fats (including cholesterol) are mixed together and won't separate into layers.

Unfortunately, homogenization produces a root cause of coronary heart disease. Milk fat naturally contains a substance called xanthine oxidase (XO) which is digested together with the fat into smaller molecules which are useful for human nutrition, IF the milk is not homogenized. However, Sampsidis (1983) reports research which discovered that the homogenization process is responsible for allowing some of the xanthine oxidase to pass intact through the wall of the intestine and from there into the blood circulation. If this foreign XO—coming from homogenized cow's milk—enters the bloodstream, it creates havoc by attacking tissue within the artery walls. The result of such attacks are lesions in artery walls. XO can also directly attack parts of the heart muscle.

Furthermore, the heat-altered fats (lipids) of the homogenized milk may well cause auto-immune reactions. According to Dr. Emanuel Revici (1961), a doctor with thousands of cancer cures to his credit, abnormal lipids are part of the process of cancer. His research shows that when fats degenerate into unrecognizable forms, abnormal reactions occur that can lead to tumors and cancerous cellular replications.

It is all right to drink raw milk from a healthy, organically-raised nanny goat or cow. Such milk is probably a very good food, provided the individual is able to properly digest it. There have been clinics around the world that have treated many diseases with raw milk. Years ago, sanitariums treated tuberculosis and gastro-intestinal disorders effectively with whole milk. But the pasteurized, homogenized, commercial milk from the American Dairy Association dairies is laden with antibiotics, growth hormones, pesticides and plaque-causing xanthine oxidase. Therefore, many knowledgeable nutritionists do not recommend commercial milk for consumption.

RATIO OF LIPOPROTEINS

Some cholesterols are beneficial, some are detrimental. People's overreaction to cholesterol has resulted in discarding the good foods with the bad ones. As with so many topics in nutrition, the balance of elements provides health, which is also true of cholesterols.

Actually, it is the ratio of the different kinds of cholesterol that speeds health or disease. There are three kinds of cholesterols depending on the protein content of the lipoproteins that are carrying it. Cholesterol is never floating around in the bloodstream alone. It is escorted by lipoproteins, which are specialized fatty-protein structures.

The high density lipoproteins (HDL) are known as good lipoproteins. They can collect the cholesterol from the arterial walls, bringing it back to the liver and gall bladder for processing by bile. Thus HDL can clean up a body full of junk food, provided that the liver function is strong.

The low density lipoproteins (LDL) are known simplistically as bad cholesterol, carrying the dietary fats and cholesterol from the liver to the bloodstream. The very low density lipoproteins (VLDL) are known as the very bad cholesterols. They have very few proteins and are very effective in transporting cholesterol into the bloodstream.

If a person has a high cholesterol level in the blood, it is an indication to increase the body's liver and thyroid function and provide HDLs to the diet. A moderately high LDL cholesterol rating is really too high for good health, because the accepted cholesterol standards have grown more lenient during the last twenty years. Actually, the standards established by medicine represent the average of all the sick people in this country.

Few people are aware that there is a difference between "dietary cholesterol" and "blood cholesterol." Dietary cholesterol is the actual cholesterol molecule in foods of animal origin. Blood cholesterol is, of course, cholesterol in the blood. Let's clarify the relationship of these two types of cholesterol.

Eating a food with a "dietary cholesterol," such as an egg, does not necessarily put cholesterol in the blood as many people have been lead to believe.

However, eating a "no cholesterol" food, such as partially-hydrogenated coconut oil or palm oil high in saturated fats, although containing no cholesterol, can elevate blood cholesterol. However, a tropical oil such as pure, unaltered coconut oil, does not raise cholesterol and can serve to lower elevated cholesterol. This fact is fertile ground for misleading the public. Often, the products that do the most damage, are labeled "no cholesterol" to trick he public. Pretty soon consumers will be able to buy "no cholesterol" batteries for flashlights, no cholesterol apples and no cholesterol paper towels!

It is easy to be misled about cholesterol. Therefore, the Pro-Vita! Plan arranges nutrition to automatically balance cholesterol over a period of time. This nutritional program is rich in the right kinds of oils without going to extremes.

ESSENTIAL FATTY ACIDS AND MONO-UNSATURATED OILS

Essential fatty acids, known as omega-3 oils, emerged in 1987 as an anti-cholesterol measure. These oils, most commonly fish oils, are known as EPA and DHA. They came to the forefront as healthful oils, when scientists learned that the Eskimos have an extremely high fat diet and an extremely low rate of heart disease. Initially, scientists ignored the excessively high rate of osteoporosis for a diet with excessively high protein. The omega-3 fatty acids, found in cold water fish, were discovered as the balancing factor in the Eskimos' high fat diet containing whale blubber and polar bear grease. Unfortunately, many EPA/DHA supplements are poorly processed and do not impart the health that fresh fish does.

But fish is not the only source of EPA and DHA. Flax seeds are the finest source, rich in alpha-linolenic acid that the body can process into EPA and DHA. Pumpkin seeds also have some of this nutrient. It is best to use the actual seeds rather than the traditional pumpkin oil due to the problem with rancidity from heat in processing.

Several companies now provide organic flax seed oil to retailers around the country. Be careful, though, which product you buy. Numerous companies have begun to produce and market flax oil because the consumer demand for it has gone up. Make sure that the oil is pressed at very low temperatures, not to exceed room temperature, and without oxygenation. If in doubt, buy the best product available.

One of the readily available oils is Barlean's flax seed oil which is produced by a bioelectron process at pressing temperatures not to exceed 80 degrees F. The result is a truly "honest," cold-processed flax seed oil with a smooth, subtle, nutty taste. Barlean's oil is one of the flax seed oils recommended by Dr. Budwig. Do not hesitate to use it liberally mixed into non-fat cottage cheese or yoghurt and on salads, because virtually everyone is deficient in omega-3 oils.

Udo Erasmus, author of the book, *Fats and Oils* (1986) and the condensed version, *Healing Fats...Killing Fats* (1990), studied with Dr. Budwig in Germany. He describes in his books many of Budwig's cures of cancer using flax seed oil. He also notes additional research and cures from the USA. Moreover, Erasmus writes that research has shown the beneficial action of omega-3s in the following situations: heart disease, cancers, diabetes, arthritis, asthma, PMS, allergies, skin conditions, water retention, inflammatory tissue conditions (e.g. bursitis, meningitis, tendonitis, tonsillitis, gastritis, colitis, otitis), stress and lack of vitality.

Monosaturated oils also have good qualities. They can be used to get around the rancidity problem with vegetable source omega-3 and obtain the benefits of HDLs. The best fatty acid is oleic acid, most commonly found in good quality olive oil. Oleic acid is an omega-9 oil by its chemical structure, the double bond is formed at the 9th carbon atom on the molecule, whereas in omega-3 it is formed at the 3rd carbon, if you happen to be interested in this sort of thing.

The current position of nutritionists is that the monounsaturated oils (oleic acid) are superior to polyunsaturated oils in preventing heart disease. Research has shown that polyunsaturated oils reduce cholesterol, both HDL and LDLs. But monounsaturated oils have the ability to remove more of the LDLs (bad lipoproteins) while leaving more of the HDL (good lipoproteins) alone.

To summarize the importance of essential fatty acids (EFAs) in nutrition, here are a few key points about their role in human health.

- EFAs regulate cholesterols and triglycerides.

- EFAs support cell membrane structures, without which the cells become subject to infections, die quicker, fail metabolically and become allergy prone.

- EFAs are essential to brain function and brain development, adrenal function, vision and the nervous system.

- EFAs increase the body's ability to absorb oxygen for energy, reduce the time for fatigued muscles to recover, increase metabolic activities and decrease degenerative conditions.

- EFAs are the parents of prostaglandins which regulate blood stickiness, sodium and water retention and the inflammatory process. For every "-itis" there is a fatty acid involved in the immune response.

The best advice is to use flax seed oil on a daily basis and to use a variety of the best oils sparingly, and most importantly to AVOID RANCID OILS.

To work healthfully with oils, throw out lard, shortenings, margarine and old bottles of commercial oil. Resupply your refrigerator with small can or bottles of grape seed oil, sesame oil, peanut oil for cooking, extra virgin olive oil, flax seed oil, and alternate a few others, such as safflower and some of the new high-oleic sunflower oil.

Udo Erasmus passed on the following two tips for Pro-Vita! advocates when I interviewed him for the "Health Tips" TV show in 1989.

HOW TO PAN-FRY AT LOW TEMPERATURE. First put water in your skillet. Then add a little oil, then add your fish or stir-fried vegetable mix. This is similar to the way Stu Wheelwright woked vegetables when he put 2 tablespoons of water in the wok, applied the oil to his hands and worked it all around the vegetables to protect the enzymes, dropped them in the wok and put the lid on. When the lid pops up from steam, Stu turned off the heat. Three minutes later he served crispy, delicious, nutritious vegetables.

BALANCED BUTTER. Let a pound of butter made from organically-raised raw milk get soft at room temperature. Add 1/2 cup flax seed oil. Mix and put back in the refrigerator to harden. This mixture balances the cholesterol and adds omega-3s to your diet. The big problem is how to get organic butter. Steinman, in his book, *Diet for a Poisoned Planet* (1990), lists butter as a highly toxic food. The reasons for its toxicity are that the dairy industry uses steroids, vaccines, pesticides and antibiotics which end up in the milk. Since butter is an end product of milk, it has a high concentration of toxins. Public demand should create a good market for organic butter soon. Ask for it! The Alta Dena Dairy in California produces raw milk, organic butter.

As an alternative to balanced butter, you can mix flax seed oil with French goat milk feta cheese or non-fat cottage cheese, even use it in this form as a spread. A mixture of non-fat yoghurt with flax seed oil makes a good dressing with added herbs or a touch of organic jam. Or this yoghurt mixture is simply a healthful snack.

Oils are a valuable nutrient, but few people use good quality oils. Most people abuse oils by frying or overheating foods. The hydrogenation and processing of oils turn this nutrient into a poison.

Therefore, the general state of society's health today is that oils contribute to heart disease. But we should not blame the oils, instead we should blame the abuse of them. This abuse is largely done by food manufacturers who chemically extract oil, heat it, hydrogenate it and sell us rancid oil.

These poisonous products are sold as "oil" in our grocery stores, and so we blame oil for poor arterial health. To make it even worse, we heat the oil and fry with it. Fried foods lead to heart attacks! Not the delicate stir-fry method of fine oriental cooking, but the deep-frying of American fast food places is the problem.

Here is a brief introduction to grape seed oil, since it is yet to be properly introduced to the U.S. consumers. More widely used in France, grape seed oil, or raisin oil, is proving to help reduce high blood pressure and not promote cancer since it resists rancidity. Grape seed oil is one of the richest source of the essential fatty acid, linoleic acid, thus it can nourish many aspects of a person's metabolism and tissue function. It also makes a fine cosmetic oil or massage oil. In our initial testing, the grape seed oil in cans tested well (hopefully there is not a lead seam), but the kind in glass bottles with a branch of herbs in it tested poorly. This oil probably had some rancidity due to the clear glass bottle and the branches of added herbs. Look for, or request, grape seed oil in natural or whole food markets. More information on the proper use of oil in your kitchen is provided in the chapter on "Protein Humanization."

To summarize the various factors in comparing dietary oils, the following chart is provided. Here you can see that flax seed oil is the richest source of alpha-linolenic acid, grape seed oil is a rich source of linoleic acid, and olive oil (preferable extra-virgin) is a rich source of oleic acid. People who use these oils receive much-needed fatty acids and their benefits. For variety, you can see where other valuable oils such as sunflower, sesame and pumpkin seed fit in. You can also see that you need to avoid partially-hydrogenated coconut oil, lard and partially-hydrogenated palm oil.

A COMPARISON OF DIETARY OILS			
Type	Alpha-Linolenic Acid (Omega 3) Polyrunsaturated	Linoleic Acid (Omega 6) Polyunsaturated	Oleic Acid (Omega 9) Monounsaturated	Saturated Fat
Butter	2%	2%	3%	66%
Canola	10%	24%	60%	6%
Coconut		2%	6%	92%
Corn		60%	27%	13%
Cotton Seed		54%	19%	27%
Flax Seed	57%	18%	16%	9%
Grape Seed		71%	17%	12%
Lard	1%	11%	47%	41%
Olive	1%	8%	80%	11%
Palm		10%	39%	51%
Peanut	15%	30%	51%	19%
Pumpkin Seed		42%	34%	9%
High Oleic Saffower		16%	76%	8%
Regular Saffower		79%	13%	8%
Sesame	8%	41%	46%	13%
Soy		50%	28%	14%
High Oleic Sunflower		11%	81%	8%
Regular Sunflower		69%	19%	12%

Chart from T. Kuss, *A Guidebook To Clinical Nutrition For The Health Professional* (1992).

USE OILS WITH CARE

The following are some suggestions for proper, healthful use of oils.

- Flax seed oil is optimal for cold use. Grapeseed oil and sesame oil (unrefined) are also good for salads because of their anti-rancid factors. Extra virgin olive oil, rich in oleic acid, offers protection to the heart by reducing the low density lipoprotein (LDL cholesterol is often called "bad cholesterol"), while leaving the high density lipoproteins (HDL is often called "good cholesterol").

- Use sesame oil with other oils. It prevents rancidity inside the body.

- Use cooking oils very sparingly.

- Use grapeseed or peanut oil for cooking. They have high flash points and thus do not turn toxic as quickly as other oils. Never save heated oil and never reuse heated oil.

- Occasionally use extra virgin olive oil to obtain monounsaturated acids. Green olive oil is known to help prevent gall stones if used once a week. It also has anticandida properties and anti-LDL-cholesterol factors.

- The very best sources of oil are those locked inside the cells of a plant. Next best are cold-processed flax seed oil, grapeseed oil and extra virgin olive oil.

- Expeller-pressed oils are preferred. "Cold pressed" is a meaningless term since the oil is pressed cold, but heated when it is not being pressed. The term is simply a marketing hoax. "Cold-processed" is a more meaningful term because the oil's temperature is kept low. However, the processing may involve skelly oil (hexane) as a solvent. Expeller-pressed oils are consistently high quality. To insure high quality, buy oils from the health food store. But even then check the oil's quality since many "health food" oils are "cold pressed" to temperatures of 140-180 degrees F.

- Store oil in the refrigerator in dark colored bottles or cans. More companies provide this consideration these days. Do not expose oil to heat or light. Do not shake the bottle because this contributes to oxidation.

- Wipe the rim of the bottle and cap off after each use. Avoid rancidity.

- Never choose fried foods. Avoid them. They're not fit to eat.

- Avoid wheat germ oil pearls, seed meals, dry lecithin or commercial wheat germ. They are usually rancid. Use brown rice sparingly because it contains rancid oils Basmati and Texmati rice do not have the rancidity of brown rice. Cottonseed oil usually contains pesticides.

- Use natural vitamin E from 100% vegetable sources as a protective dietary supplement when using oils.

- Avoid margarine and any oil that stays solid at room temperature (shortening). These hydrogenated oils are unnatural and are linked with cancer. Instead, use organic butter balanced with flaxseed oil sparingly. Tahini can be a good butter substitute. Olive oil is a good butter substitute and is featured in top Italian restaurants for dipping bread.

- When stir-frying, heat the skillet or wok to a low temperature first, (250 degrees F) then add two Tbsp. water rather than oil. Many fine cooks simply toss the vegetables in a little oil and add them to the wok with a little water. This minimizes the oxidation of both the oil and the vegetables.

We now turn our attention to complex carbohydrates.

COMPLEX CARBOHYDRATES:
THE BASIC FUEL FOR ENERGY

THE ROLE OF COMPLEX, SIMPLE
AND REFINED CARBOHYDRATES

Since carbohydrates are the most abundant component of many people's diets, obtaining them for energy is not a critical concern. It is highly unlikely to find a person with a nutritional deficiency of carbohydrates, whereas we do find people deficient in other nutrients such as protein, essential fatty acids (oils), vitamins and minerals. However, as with all areas of nutrition, there is a big difference between quality and quantity of carbohydrates. It is common to find that people lack the quality carbohydrates and have too much quantity of poor quality carbohydrates.

First, let's be sure we know what carbohydrates are. Carbohydrate is a word to describe a molecule which our bodies can readily use for cellular energy or to store it for future energy requirements. The CARBO part of the word refers to the element carbon, which is the differentiating element between organic and inorganic chemistry. Most people think carbohydrates mean starchy food. Actually, carbohydrates include all starches and sugars: alcohol is a carbohydrate; squash is a carbohydrate; bubblegum is a carbohydrate; spaghetti is a carbohydrate; and apple pie is a carbohydrate.

When we mention carbohydrates we are referring to a class of foods that the body digests and metabolizes in a certain way. Foods such as potatoes, breads, pasta, grains (grits, rice, breakfast cereals), candies, jellies, boiled beans and strawberry pie are all carbohydrates.

Carbohydrates are the basis of our cellular fuel system. Glucose, which is blood sugar, is another term used to describe this basic fuel. Carbohydrates make up a little more than half of our fuel burned by the cells for life functions. Since the remaining percentage is divided between protein and fat, carbohydrates are our most abundant fuel. A gram of carbohydrates yields four calories of cellular fuel.

In addition to providing sugar for energy, carbohydrate foods can furnish other valuable nutrients such as cellulose (vegetable fiber), vitamins, amino acids and minerals. To further understand the quality vs. quantity issue with carbohydrates, we need to examine two classes, the COMPLEX carbohydrates and natural simple sugar vs. the REFINED carbohydrates. The difference between carbohydrates is generally the dividing line between health and disease from a nutritional perspective.

Complex carbohydrates are starches in their most natural state, as found in potatoes, whole grain foods, tubers, starchy vegetables and legumes. This molecule is more complex and larger with more elements than a simple carbohydrate such as the sugars in raw fruit. Complex carbohydrates require several steps in digestion before they are ready to be used as glucose for cellular fuel. These several steps are necessary for the body to properly handle the fuel and thus make complex carbohydrates a controllable fuel source.

If a carbohydrate food is a simple carbohydrate such as sugars in raw fruit, then the body has less processing to do to get the fuel ready for the cells. Although natural, simple carbohydrates still undergo processing in the body, they do not inflict the damage that refined sugars do. A fruit is only 15% simple carbohydrates (sugars), whereas a refined grain pasta can be 75% simple carbohydrates.

If the carbohydrate is refined, as sugar in candies, the fuel can be too explosive, or too ready as a fuel source, thus causing metabolic stress. The impact of refined sugar on many people's metabolisms could qualify it as a drug because it dramatically alters body chemistry and can be addictive. It causes changes in behavior and dramatic changes in the body's metabolism; and it has damaging side effects. Yet, a stroll down the aisle in a supermarket reveals large quantities of this substance on children's breakfast cereals. Of course, the manufacturers tell us, "That's O.K. We've fortified the food with eight essential, very common vitamins in synthetic form, and we now admit this substance resembling food is only part of what anyone would call a complete meal."

However, we know that Mom and Pop both work, or that Mom or Pop is a single parent, and that Mom and Pop are too tired, stressed and overworked to prepare a real meal. After a couple of boxes of dry cereal, the kids are hooked on sugar for breakfast. It is time now to reevaluate our value system. In this book we learn how to prepare a wholesome, nutritious breakfast. When your children help, breakfast becomes quality time in more ways than one.

To emphasize, carbohydrates come in varying degrees of complexity. The most complex carbohydrates require a system of disassembly, based on enzymes, which is easily controlled by the body; the more simple carbohydrates are ready sources of energy; but refined sugars are injections of fuel with low nutritional value demanding cellular response.

The complex and simple sugars can be wholesome, natural foods such as a potato or an apple. Refined sugars are unnatural foods and cause metabolic stress, resulting in tissue damage particularly to the liver and blood vessels over time. More information on the addictive qualities, metabolic stress and tissue damage to the pancreas, liver and adrenal glands caused by refined sugar, is presented in the book, *The Next Step To Greater Energy* (Tips, 1990).

CARBOHYDRATE METABOLISM

Since complex carbohydrates provide glucose gradually to the body, it has a controllable supply of energy. Deriving from whole foods, they also provide valuable nutrients such as minerals, enzymes (if eaten raw), fiber, B and C vitamins. Controllable energy is important to health. If our bodies cannot control or regulate the cellular fires, then we do not have good health. Complex carbohydrates provide fuel at the proper rate for human metabolism. However, refined carbohydrates put jet fuel into a diesel engine, so to speak, resulting in the cellular fires burning too hot. In this condition the body is stressed to adjust its metabolic processes, often resulting in hypoglycemic distress.

An improperly burning cellular fire ultimately means a lack of energy. When we burn too hot, we have let-downs and greater systemic stress. After years of these conditions, a person can become burned out and absolutely dependent on quick energy fixes.

Unfortunately, refined carbohydrates dominate the diets of most people in industrialized nations. Sodas, candies, jellies, cakes, ice cream, alcohol, pies, cookies, donuts, pastries, processed breakfast cereals and syrups are luxury foods which many people use daily. These luxury foods tax our bodies, and the coin rendered is our health. Many other products have hidden sugars in them, including some brands of canned beans! Read the labels and know the products.

The degeneration of our health as well as the rise of cancer and diabetes, can be directly related to the industrial revolution and our consumption of refined foods. The industrial revolution brought us the ability to mass-produce foods, mill out all the fiber and nutrients, and "enrich" them with a couple of common, synthetic vitamins. This does not mean that refined foods are the sole cause of chronic degenerative diseases. Similar correlations can also be seen between the expanded use of vaccinations, antibiotics and chemical pollutants in our external environment, and a rise in chronic, degenerative disease. All factors add up to a toxic burden of substances for our bodies.

It is not necessary to become fanatical and eliminate all refined sugars all the time. A strong body should be able to enjoy a fun food or dessert on occasion. But we need to put refined carbohydrates in their place which is occasional rather than daily use. Furthermore, there are ways to enjoy a tasty sweet food and minimize its damage as we discuss in this book. The simple inclusion of a raw vegetable or two can minimize the impact of the refined sugar on the body and safeguard health when the occasional treat is enjoyed. The basis for this insurance policy method of enjoying a treat is presented in Appendix C.

Carbohydrates play a major role in the body for proper energy metabolism. Carbohydrates do not build healthy tissues, or the immune system or antibodies. They do not build enzyme systems, nor do they make hormones. Around 15 grams of carbohydrates are in the bloodstream all the time, in transit for the body's energy requirement. A supply of concentrated carbohydrate fuel, called glycogen, backs up this necessary, life-supporting supply of glucose. Excess carbohydrates are stored for future use as fat.

However, excess carbohydrates can cause a sludge in the blood, forming a breeding ground for bacteria that Wheelwright called "paste." Here again we find a basic principle of nutrition. Too little is a problem. Too much is a problem. Poor quality is a problem. But the right amount of good quality complex carbohydrates maintains the body's energy requirements without excess stress, and thus is fundamental to good health.

Now that we understand the role of complex carbohydrates in the body, the question has to arise, why do some nutritionists claim that our diets should be built on carbohydrates? It appears such a statement would be like saying, "Let's build a car around the gasoline rather than the quality of the steel and durability of the moving parts."

Since carbohydrates are such a common food and their role in the body fairly superficial as fuel, it is certainly correct to challenge the idea of building a diet on grains or other complex carbohydrates. For this reason the Pro-Vita! Plan is built on VEGETABLES as a foundation. Vegetables contain plenty of carbohydrates, but they have the added bonus of being able to be eaten raw, thus giving the body enzymes and vitamins unaltered by heat. Further, the vegetables are often much richer in minerals than grains.

Complex carbohydrates as a focus of nutrition certainly have advantages over many people's diets, particularly when such diets are too high in animal proteins and too low in fiber. Introducing more grains to a diet focused on meat will bring many improvements, such as help to prevent colon cancer and osteoporosis. Grains can also help with constipation. Actually, grains will help in a thousand ways, but it still is not an optimal food. For this reason our health pyramid is not founded on grains.

Many people with a macrobiotic background have begun the Pro-Vita! program with great success, rediscovering the energy and spark that exemplifies good health. Often, questions arise in trying to reconcile apparent differences in diet philosophy between the macrobiotic and the Pro-Vita! Plan. My reply to such queries is that macrobiotics is an excellent diet system for some people, and since the Pro-Vita! Plan does not have to be radically different, there are many elements that are quite compatible.

With any formalized nutrition plan, some people are simply not cut out for it. There are too many individuals with unique biochemical and bioenergetic characteristics to factor them into a formalized dietary equation. For example, in clinical study, I have seen where a hygienic or "fit for life" type diet of fruit for breakfast is successful for only one out of eight people trying it. And this diet worked only for a transition period, until the toxic backlog was corrected and a more suitable Pro-Vita! approach implemented. To accommodate different folks, the Pro-Vita! Plan teaches principles of nutrition, so that the individual can tailor them as needed.

The person who is metabolically a fast oxidizer (meaning the cellular combustion of glucose is too fast), will struggle health-wise with a grain-based diet. The reason for this problem is that cooked grains cause an acidic reaction, since they are high in phosphorus which binds calcium and increases lactic acid. According to my observations, this acidic reaction is the reason why many people suffer while adapting their lives and bodies to a macrobiotic lifestyle. The phytates in many grains interfere with calcium, magnesium and zinc absorption, the very minerals needed to keep people from burning out their adrenal glands. By my personal observation, a macrobiotic diet is only suitable for one out of five of the people who try to eat that way.

On the other hand, a slow oxidizer (meaning the cellular combustion of glucose is too slow), will prosper on some grains in the diet, because these will allow increased sodium and potassium intake. Therefore, the metabolism does not drag so much.

From an oriental yin/yang perspective, the Pro-Vita! Plan is not excessively yang or acid-forming, although its focus is on yang proteins, such as fish, scrambled eggs, or seeds. The small amount of yang proteins in the early part of the day is buffered by the vegetables, creating a synergistic, balanced and dynamic energy. Later in the day, the grains can be added if they are the appropriate food for the individual.

Let's take a moment and learn about a superior complex carbohydrate, Spelt.

AN ANCIENT GRAIN: SPELT

Spelt, *Triticum spelta*, is a recent introduction to the American diet and is probably the most superior grain food available today. This little-known staple food is a grain like wheat, but it is many times more nutritious than wheat, much less allergenic, and often can support health improvements due to its numerous, inherent healing properties. If you are not yet familiar with spelt, try to find it and products from it at your health food store. It is currently available as flour, delicious pasta and a wonderful pancake mix.

Spelt is an ancient grain, dating back ten thousand years to Southeast Asia and nine thousand years to Europe. It is mentioned several times in the Old Testament as well as in medieval European manuscripts. As an ancient grain unaltered by civilization, spelt has not been degenerated by hybridization or generation-after-generation of exposure to pesticides and chemical fertilizers as have wheat, rice and oats. Thus, it retains more of its pristine and original genetic blueprint as a naturally-evolved, bio-available food for human nutrition.

Spelt's benefits as a nutritious food for superior health can be discussed in three categories: high-quality, bio-available nutrients; its specific nutrients for the immune system; and its excellent fiber.

As a superior nutritional food, spelt provides more important vitamins, minerals, fatty acids and amino acids than other grains. Even more importantly, the inherent nutrients are water-soluble (unlike soybeans in unfermented form), thus easily digested and absorbed by the body. Spelt is exceptionally high in protein for a grain food, providing eight amino acids.

While still a carbohydrate food, spelt offers more protein to vegetarians trying to subsist on grain-based amino acids. It is more than 14% protein and seems to have the capability to impart needed amino acids to the body because it can be digested easily. In my opinion, spelt is a necessary food for vegetarians (as are soaked seeds and beans prepared the Pro-Vita! way) to provide the important amino acid matrix for vital cellular processes. Without these few key foods, I have seen very few people prosper in good health on a strict vegetarian diet. Vegetarians must consider using spelt to improve their health.

Spelt's second major benefit concerns the immune system. It contains special nutrients, such as mucopolysaccharides, which help with proper blood clotting and stimulate the immune response. In this way, spelt helps to increase the body's resistance to infection by supporting the immune system. Dr. Wighard Strehlow writes in his book *The Wonderfood Spelt* (1989) that, "the immune-stimulating properties of spelt are in its cyanogenic glucosides or nitrilosides, called the 'anti-neoplastic' Vitamin B17. They support the body's cancer fighting system."

Spelt's third nutritional benefit is its content of fiber which is one of the best available. Not only does spelt provide lubricants via its essential fatty acids, it also furnishes the fiber for proper bowel function. The importance of fiber is stressed throughout this book and in a section of its own. The fiber in spelt, like other fibers, functions to buffer and remove toxins and cancer-causing chemicals from the body; maintain proper blood sugar; alleviate constipation; lower cholesterol and triglycerides if they are too high; promote good digestion; neutralize excessive bile; and help prevent obesity.

It is important to point out that spelt provides nutrients for brain chemistry and thus can help prevent depression and promote emotional stability. It is particularly high in the amino acid phenylalaine which is a precursor to dopamine, a neurotransmitter, as well as epinephrine and noradrenalin which are both hormones. Dopamine deficiencies can result in Parkinson's disease, while the hormones dependent on phenylalaine are essential for a positive mood.

Spelt also provides the essential amino acid, L-tryptophan, which is a building block for the neurotransmitters and absolutely essential for sleep. L-tryptophan was the subject of international news as the FDA successfully sought to take this nutrient away from the American public. Instead, in the hands of a drug company for use by prescription only, tryptophan now costs three times as much. The fact that spelt provides tryptophan is important to know because it is a vegetarian source of this rare amino acid. Therefore, spelt is critical to vegetarians who choose to avoid meat-based sources of this vital nutrient such as turkey. A further discussion about the FDA's action on L-tryptophan can be found in Appendix B.

We are aware of at least two ancient literary sources about spelt. The first source is in the Old Testament, Exodus 9:31, 32 and Ezekiel 4:9. An interesting dietary experiment took place involving Daniel— of the lion's den fame—some 2600 years ago and what most-assuredly included spelt.

Daniel refused to eat King Nebacadnezer's royal diet of meat and wine, because he did not wish to defile himself since his Jewish religion and common sense prohibited these foods. Instead, Daniel and three companions lived on pure water and a sprouted grain and vegetable diet. The king was so impressed with Daniel's radiant health, intelligence and wisdom at the end of three years, that he appointed Daniel to an important advisory position.

Usually, this story is considered valuable because it demonstrates Daniel's obedience to God. And from a nutritional perspective, it teaches the value of whole foods.

Another old source about spelt is the work on medicine by the famous medieval Saint Hildegard von Bingen (Strehlow and Herztka, 1988). Primarily known for her mystical and theological books, she also wrote about the natural medicines she used to heal people. However, this work was only discovered in the current century. Diet is an important part of Hildegard's healing system, and spelt is a major factor of her nutritional prescriptions to correct faulty digestion and to heal a sick intestinal track.

For more information on spelt and availability of certified organic spelt products, such as spelt-spaghetti, flour, pancake/cupcake mix, you may contact Purity Foods, 2871 W. Jolly Rd., Okemos, MI 48864.

A major key to health is flexibility, not rigidity. The Pro-Vita! Plan is flexible enough not to cause feelings of deprivation. You can go ahead and add a little cheese to your bean enchiladas. If the cheese is not heated, and if it is properly buffered with fresh vegetables, it probably will not upset the balance of the meal. Restriction will cause failure. Find substitutions and work with moderation, when you have to stretch the rules while dining out.

The Pro-Vita! Plan builds your strength and health at the cellular level. Once a person is strong at the cellular level, health becomes the norm. Then the body is much less reactive to dietary indiscretions. It is a simple fact that a young, healthy, robust person can get away with dietary indiscretions for a while. However, a sensitive, allergy-prone, immune-compromised person cannot. As a person builds health via the Pro-Vita! Plan, the ability to enjoy occasional nutritional indiscretions increases. Pro-Vita! leads to better health and the ability to enjoy life more fully. It builds the foundation for abundant health every day it is practiced. Your personal experience is the proof of the Pro-Vita! nutrition plan. Let us know how you fare with it!

CARBOHYDRATE FOODS

In the Pro-Vita! Plan we categorize starches and fruit together, although fruits are a major classification of their own. First, we provide a list of carbohydrates, then we look at fruit.

COMPLEX CARBOHYDRATE FOODS

Vegetables (High in Carbohydrates)

beans, boiled	Jerusalem artichoke	potatoes
cactus	jicama	pumpkin
carrots	lentils	rutabaga

Cereals and Grains

amaranth	grits	quinoa
barley	hominy	rice
bear mush	lentils	rye meal
breads, whole	grain millet	spelt
buckwheat	oatmeal	triticale
corn	popcorn	wheat
granola		

Simple Carbohydrates

bread, white, refined	cookies	honey
cakes	crackers	pie
candy	fruit juices, bottled	sugar
chewing gum	fruit juices, canned	sugared drinks
syrup		

OPTIMAL USE OF FRUIT

A well-known fruit diet prescribes fruit for breakfast for all people. Is this a good idea? In fact, for a few months to a couple of years, toxic people will feel better on a "fruit for breakfast" hygieni-cally-based diet, because they are getting poisons out of their system, if they avoid consumption of protein late in the day. Some persons will lose weight, but they will not build strong immune systems, strong organs and glands, or experience a strong, vibrant life for an extended time.

I saw this pattern first hand when I studied with Dr. Herbert Shelton, the early advocate of the hygienist philosophy at his clinic outside of San Antonio. I continue to see this pattern in clinical practice today. Many of the followers of this hygienist philosophy test out to be low in vital force which consists biochemically of amino acids and minerals held in electrostatic suspension in the tissues and extracellular matrix. It is correct that such people do not have the toxins that many other people have. They also do not have the mucus-related concerns which other people complain about. In effect, for the first couple of years they feel much better on their diet. But they do not have the vitality and energy that mineral-rich, amino-acid-rich people display. Dr. Shelton died of chronic, degen-erative nerve disease.

Many people following a diet which consists of fruit for breakfast, have stated, for example, "For a while, I loved it. It felt great to eat fruit when I got up. And it was a quick meal. I could eat two apples while driving to work and be done with breakfast. I'd get a slump around 10:30 am, but then I'd eat more fruit, or get a muffin. But as time went on, I started to develop a desire for sweets in the afternoon. Furthermore, now I get very cold in the winter and don't have the energy I used to have."

This statement is exemplary of the initial benefits of cleansing and the long-time detriment of not following the body's natural cycles. The man who reported the above experience, was diagnosed hypoglycemic prior to consulting with me. Six weeks of the Pro-Vita! Plan corrected his condition and brought back a mental clarity which he had missed for two years. The Pro-Vita! Plan takes the best of the hygienic philosophy and applies it within the matrix of bioenergy to provide the best of both practices.

It is not a matter of choosing sides and thinking that one diet plan is right and another is wrong. The fact is, foods are our tools. In certain instances, fruit for breakfast can be a valuable tool. Suppose that you eat out at night and have a heavy meal. Then it might be a good idea to have fruit for breakfast the next morning, continue the cleansing period and give the digestive system a rest. But then get back on the body's natural schedule the next day.

As a rule, fruit for breakfast as a way of life is detrimental in the long run. The reason is as follows: During the latter part of a person's sleep cycle the body is in an alkaline state. During this alkaline pH state the best sleep, best dreaming and best body repairs take place. Then the body heads for its acid pH swing, which brings the activity and productivity of morning. The acid side is required for enthusiasm and energy, just as the day follows the night.

But if fruit is eaten first thing in the morning, it pushes the body back toward an alkaline pH when the natural body cycle is heading for a more acid swing. This inhibits the digestion activity of future meals. It tranquilizes the brain leading to low productivity and the use of stimulants (coffee, tea, tobacco, refined carbohydrates) to bring energy to the body. And by inhibiting the acid pH cycle, fruit pushes the alkaline cycle further into alkalosis, thus contributing to greater stress on the blood sugar.

People who say that they need fruit for breakfast, because "it's the only thing my stomach is ready for," are usually low in cellular protein. Or, they have consistently eaten heavy suppers, and it is quite correct that their stomachs are not ready for more work. Such people are either exhibiting the symptoms of weak adrenals and crave the quick, but shallow, energy fix; or they have worn-out digestive processes with congested lymphatics. Their digestive systems lack the power (acids) to digest the nutrients which they so desperately need.

Because of its high sugar content, fruit generally appears in the carbohydrate family, but it actually falls into a class of its own dietarily. A general dietary rule regarding fruit is to eat it by itself, although there are many exceptions. The food combining plans divide fruit into subcategories of sweet, acid, sub-acid and melon, a tedious division for general use. But for those people who want to work with the subcategories, we list them here. Separating fruits, however, is not a major factor in health. The following are suggestions how to use fruit:

- Eat fruits alone or as a meal, not with a meal of other foods (proteins, carbohydrates, oils).

- If eating several fruits, it is best to mix fruits within their own subcategory, but this is not a major concern. The main concern is that most people do better eating melon by itself.

- Use fresh fruits when your urinary pH registers excessively acid (5.5 or below) since most fruits are alkalizing (some excessively so) and can help balance the acid pH. Even though fruit may taste acid due to the citric acids, to the body's metabolism they are mostly alkalizers. Cranberry is an exception and is an acidifier. This is why people often drink cranberry juice to overcome bladder infections. The acids discourage bacteria proliferation which occurs best in an alkaline urine.

- Fresh fruit meals are great for supper, particularly in summer, or in the fruit's natural season.

- Using fruit "in the season thereof" works with the natural, seasonal cycle of nutrition.

FRUIT CLASSIFICATION ACCORDING TO THE FOOD- COMBINING SCHEMA

Acid

blueberry, cherimoya, grapefruit, lemon, lime, loquat, orange, pineapple, pomegranate, sour plum, sour cherries, strawberry, tangerine, tangelo

Sub-Acid

apple, apricot, blackberry, cherry, grape, kumquat, mango, nectarine, papaya, peach, pear, plum, prune, kiwi

Sweet

banana, dates, dried fruit, raisins, persimmon

Melon

banana melon, cantaloup, casaba, crenshaw, honeydew, musk, Persian, watermelon

Fruit is an enjoyable, refreshing food that can often be used for between meal snacks. Fruit, more than any other food, brings to the body the "essence of the seasons" or the particular minerals and enzymes for the body to adapt to the change of seasons. This is why "eating fruit in the season thereof" plays an important role in the body's overall health.

Fruit is considered by many health experts to be the ideal food because of its ease of digestion, high water content, rich supply of living enzymes and organic minerals, and general cleansing effect. Fruit can add a vital dimension to a person's diet.

PRO-VITA! FOOD COMBINING GUIDE

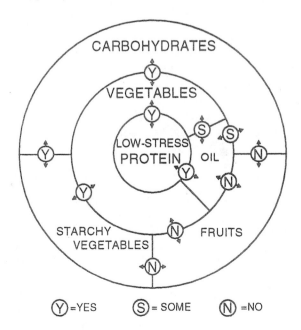

Ⓨ =YES   Ⓢ = SOME   Ⓝ =NO

NATURAL BODY CYCLES
AND NUTRITION

BODY CYCLES AND HEALTH

Understanding the natural body cycles provides a fundamental perspective on important factors governing a person's health and longevity. Whenever we learn to work with nature rather than figure out how to get away with unnatural lifestyles, we find it easy to accomplish our goals in health and in life. If we eat, exercise and sleep in cooperation with our innate, natural rhythms, we experience greater effectiveness in our endeavors. Usually, we also earn the right to continued survival in this world to the full span of our years.

The ancient Chinese had a profound knowledge of the order of nature, as did many other cultures. One of the more poetic portrayals of this sense of order and natural cycles is found in the King James translation of Solomon's Ecclesiastes:

"To every thing there is a season, and a time to every purpose under the heaven;

A time to be born, and a time to die; a time to plant and a time to pluck up that which is planted;

A time to kill, and a time to heal; a time to break down, and a time to build up;

A time to weep, and a time to laugh; a time to mourn, and a time to dance;

A time to cast away stones, and a time to gather stones together; a time to embrace, and a time to refrain from embracing;

A time to get and a time to lose; a time to keep, and a time to cast away;

A time to rend, and a time to sew; a time to keep
silence, and a time to speak;

A time to love, and a time to hate; a time of war, and a
time of peace."

We need to understand that there is order in the stars, in the earth's
rotation around the sun, in the earth's daily spin on its axis, in the body's
gestation, birth and maturation. Then we can understand better why
there is so much chaos in our lives because such orders are generally
ignored. In effect, chaos is philosophically a result of being out of step
with the natural cycles and order of life. We find that we are not eating
what and when we should. We are not working in healthy environments
and our desires are beyond what we need. We are not sleeping a restful
sleep cycle. Then we wonder why we have stomach ulcers, prostate
cancer and premenstrual depression.

People most often seek quick palliation of their symptoms via a
drug that is incapable of healing the body. For example, women with
PMS do not have a deficiency of Ibuprofen in their bodies. Nor do
people with ulcers have a deficiency of Tagamet. Thus, with such
palliations people continue to be out of sync with the natural order
of life. They wonder why a cancer develops and cry out: "Why me,
Lord?" The allopathic doctor then wants to cut out the offending part
and treat the ailing body with cancer-causing chemicals (chemotherapy) and lethal radiations. The body's impaired vitality responds
to this major onslaught by surging to stay alive with the help of the
artificial stimulation of numerous drugs.

There is an old saying, "For want of a nail, the kingdom was lost."
As the story goes, the king needed a sword in a battle. But the horse
could not run to get one, because it had lost a horseshoe. The shoe
was lost, because it lacked one nail. Thus, the king was killed, the
battle was lost, and the country conquered by the enemy.

The point is that it is important to take care of the "loose nails"
in our health. The condition of PMS, for example, means that the
individual needs to find and correct the cause of it. The best way to
heal it naturally is with diet, herbs, homeopathic remedies and
cooperation with the natural laws of life, rather than to suppress the
symptoms of PMS with drugs and call it a cure. The condition of an

ulcer suggests that a person should heal the cause of it, not suppress hydrochloric acid with a drug instead. If the cause of an ulcer is improper diet, then the body is crying out for the correct nutritional solution. If, however, the cause of the ulcer is a stressful lifestyle, then the body is crying out for peace and harmony with the natural cycles, resulting in happiness and satisfaction.

The natural body cycles are a vital aspect of effective nutrition. Every body process is cyclical and nothing in health is truly linear. For example, there are inherent cycles that operate the digestive system, turning on hydrochloric acid production and making digestive enzymes such as pepsin, lipase, cathepsin, amylase, protease, turilic acid, trypsin, chymotrypsin and ribonuclease.

This means the body cycles function like the wheels-within-wheels clockwork of a city carrying on daily functions such as manufacturing, warehousing, distribution, law enforcement, power and light, heating and cooling, water works, sanitation, construction and postal service.

Much of what the body does occurs within 24-hour cycles, with larger cycles of 7 days and 28 days. For example, a 24-hour cycle is the metabolism of food; a 7-day cycle is biorhythmic; a 28-day cycle is the menstrual cycle.

In turn, the 24 hour food processing cycle contains three 8-hour cycles that fall approximately as follows:

> 7 a.m.   -   3 p.m: Process nutrients (eat, digest)
>
> 3 p.m.   -   11 p.m: Use nutrients (build, exercise)
>
> 11 p.m. -   7 a.m: Cleanse cellular wastes (rest)

In a constant rhythm, one cycle flows into the next while all cycles happen to some extent at the same time. Of course, the body is not rigid in its cyclic functioning, but each cycle's keynote marks the activity best conducted during that time period.

TIMING: WHEN TO EAT

The following key philosophies provide the larger matrix for any food plan to promote health. Understanding these concepts will help you find the plan that's right for you without needless wear and tear on your body or on your lifestyle.

No single diet is right for everyone. Different people have different nutritional requirements. Not only are people biochemically individual, but at different times in life and in different climates and in different lifestyles, people's nutritional requirements vary greatly. For example, infants, teenagers, men, women, Pigmies, pregnant women, athletes, computer programmers or Eskimos all have different specific, nutritional requirements.

However, THE PRO-VITA! DIET IS THE HUB AROUND WHICH YOU CAN DESIGN YOUR OWN HEALTHY NUTRITIONAL PROGRAM, regardless of age (after weaning), environment, race, occupation or lifestyle.

For good health, diet must conform to the body's natural laws. These laws include such factors as the body's pH (acid/ }alkaline balance), cleanse/build cycles of the cell, body type, bioenergetic pattern, enzyme supply, oxidation rate and the body's assimilation/elimination process. It is difficult to reconcile these different concepts from a limited viewpoint. However, applying the bio-energy perspective of the natural laws of health, these various wheels-within-wheels facets fall into line and function like clockwork.

As a general rule, Wheelwright taught WHEN you eat a certain food is often of greater importance than WHAT the food is. Poor quality foods eaten at the "right" time do less damage than good foods eaten at the "wrong" time. Basically, there is a time to eat, a time to live, and a time to sleep. All eating causes the body to work and adapt. This activity occurs best at certain times of the circadian rhythms.

Of course, we can make absurd exceptions to this rule such as whether it is really better to eat commercial ice cream at the "right" time, than to eat alfalfa sprouts at the "wrong" time. However, timing of food makes a big difference for good health as discussed here and in a subsequent chapter. Therefore we have to exercise prudence and judgement regarding this rule. A little common sense is needed to derive full benefit from our understanding of this point about the timing of when we eat and what we eat.

This general rule stresses the importance of eating when it is time to eat and not eating when the time is not right. If we make our example between two foods in the same category such as protein, then we could say that eating a piece of turkey for breakfast causes less stress than eating a tofu patty before bed. Yet, the goal of the Pro-Vita! Plan is far more than eating detrimental foods at the best time. It is eating the best foods at the best time for the best health.

Constant preoccupation with diet and what is wrong with foods precludes health. Such attitudes keep health beyond arm's length, always out of reach. We need to learn to eat properly, do the best we can and relax. Wheelwright taught, "Keep the liver healthy and it will keep you healthy. For more information about the liver see *Your Liver-Your Lifeline*, (Tips, 1990).

GLANDULAR TYPING

Some people are advised that they are a certain glandular body type, based on which endocrine gland is dominant in their system. They are told that their body type is such that they are not ready to eat until lunch time; that they should eat fruit in the morning, because their systems are not ready for anything heavier until later in the day.

Wheelwright was very familiar with body-typing based on glandular dominance, but was reluctant to accept its premises as completely accurate. In our first discussion on this topic, he simply said that too often such categories and diets to accommodate them, "played into the body's weaknesses," rather than building genuine health.

In another discourse, Wheelwright admitted that some people were glandularly sluggish in the morning and could have their Pro-Vita! breakfast as late as 11 am. But he also said that as such people became more healthy and vital, they would naturally shift to an earlier breakfast time.

In yet a third discussion on this topic of glandular body types, six months before his death, Wheelwright affirmed that people could endeavor to correct glandular dominance by supporting both the dominant gland and the opposing glands with his precise herbal-glandular nutritional formulas. This would bring better balance and overall health.

Subsequently, in 1990, I worked clinically with people who exemplified a glandular dominant pattern. Specifically, I worked with one pituitary, one thyroid and one adrenal type. All three persons reported improvement in their many diverse symptoms applying Wheelwright's ideas and herbal formulas. Most important for these people was the knowledge that they were not locked into a system of having to cater to their glandular dominant pattern.

Later, in my own homeopathic studies, I found that many characteristics of glandular dominance are, in fact, listed as symptoms in Kent's *Repertory*. These symptoms are then matched to homeopathic remedies which correct them. This means that glandular imbalances and dominance, or compensatory patterns, are really a disturbance of the person's vital force. Therefore, balance must come from within the individual to eliminate the need for a tailored diet to overcome glandular imbalance. Consequently, special dietary patterns to accommodate such glandular dominance can help, but are not at all required. Perhaps this is what Wheelwright meant when he explained that a diet designed to accommodate a glandular pattern was "playing into a weakness." It makes the situation better, but does not correct the fundamental issues of the limitation to health.

In clinical practice we see that the people who neglect the Pro-Vita! Plan principles and continue with fruit or sugary cereals for breakfast, are those who fail to build strong energy glands (thyroid, adrenals). They remain slightly tired, with dark circles under their eyes, and continue to battle allergies despite supplementation therapies. If their cellular protein levels were higher, they would not swing into lower blood sugar levels and crave the sugars to get going. It is simply a nutritional fact that fruit for breakfast will not build adrenal tissue.

Another fact is that eating fruit or refined carbohydrates (donuts, croissants, pancakes) for breakfast disrupts the body's natural pH cycles and interferes with proper protein use. This kind of a breakfast sets an altered metabolic pattern which is far less than optimal for people who wish to be active, enthusiastic, joyous and productive.

Save fruit for afternoon snacks, supper and evening enjoyment. At such times it will give the digestion a well-earned rest and promote better sleep. Used correctly, "fresh fruits in the season thereof" are wonderful, enjoyable, rejuvenating foods.

We now look at two of the major cycles at work in our bodies: the meridian clock and the pH (acid/alkaline balance). The meridian/organ clock provides us with bioenergetic insights for our body; the pH cycles are the basis of our biochemical life processes. If we work in accord with these natural cycles. Nature rewards us with better health and longevity. If, in contrast, we fight or live in conflict with our natural cycles, then dispassionate nature allows only the survival of the fittest.

THE MERIDIAN/ORGAN CLOCK

The Chinese Acupuncture "Meridian Clock" is an example of a 24-hour cycle which portrays the body's complete functions as well as its relationship with diet. There are 12 meridians, each taking the lead for two hours during the 24-hour period. Each of the 12 meridians has a dual flow, a coming and a going, or a yin and yang rhythm, marking 24 cycles per day. The clock delineates which meridian system is activated and dominant at a specific time.

The Chinese have known of these cycles for several thousand years. In the last twenty years, Western science has proven the validity of these cycles using piezo-electrical equipment commonly called "electro-acupuncture."

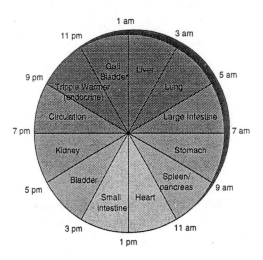

COMMENTARY ON MERIDIAN CLOCK

TIME	MERIDIAN	COMMENTARY
5-7 a.m.	Large Intestine	Drinking water triggers bowel evacuation making room for the new day's nutritional intake. Removes toxins from night's cleansing.
7-9 a.m.	Stomach	Stomach energies are the hieghest so eat the most important meal of the day here to optimize digestion/assimilation.
9-11 a.m.	Pancreas	The stomach passes its contents on. Enzymes from the pancreas continue the digestive process. Carbohydrate energy made available.
11 a.m. - 1 p.m.	Heart	Food materials enter the blood stream. The heart pumps nutrients throughout the system and takes its lipid requirements
1-3 p.m.	Small Intestion	Foods requireing longer digestion times (proteins) complete their digestion/assimilation.
3-5 p.m.	Bladder	Metabolic wastes from morning's nutrition intakeclear, making room for the kidney's filtration to come.
5-7 p.m.	Kidney	Filters blood (decides what to keep, what to throw away), maintains proper chemical balance of blood based on nutritional intake of day. Blood to deliver useable nutrients to all tissues.
7-9 p.m.	Circulation	Nutrients are carried to groups of cells (capilaries) and to each individual cell (lymphatics).
9-11 p.m.	Tripple Warmer	The endocrine system adjustthe homostasis of the body based on electrolyte and enzyme replenishment.
11 p.m. - 1 a.m.	Gall Bladder	Initial cleansing of all tissues, processes cholesterol, enhances brain function.
1-3 a.m.	Liver	Cleansing of blood.Processing of wastes.
3-5 a.m.	Lung	Respiration. Oxygenation. Expulsion of waste gasses.

The ancient meridian clock teaches that the bioenergetic cycles of the body have rhythm and order. Since these cycles happen automatically, we do not have to be preoccupied with them. However, if we know of these cycles, then we can make better decisions when it is generally best to eat, exercise and sleep. We will examine the meridian clock again, when we investigate the optimal times to eat, exercise and rest.

THE pH CYCLE: YOUR ACID/ALKALINE BALANCE

The following material on pH is the most technical discussion in this book. I have endeavored to make the information easy to understand, yet detailed enough to be useful. Your perseverance in reading this material can pay a big dividend to your health.

The acid/alkaline swing (the pH cycle) is a natural body cycle that occurs two times a day. This cycle is another major force of nature, or body dynamics, that we can cooperate with, ignore or oppose. Of course, when we cooperate with this natural cycle, we experience conservation of energy and an enhanced degree of health.

The pH cycle is a major process of the body and one of the large wheels within which the multitudes of other wheels turn. The term pH (potential of a solution to accept Hydrogen) refers to the parts, or percentages, of hydrogen ion concentration in a solution (blood, urine, saliva). The pH is a logarithmic scale that runs from 1 to 14, with 7 in the middle denoting a neutral state. Any reading below 7 means an acid condition; any reading above 7 is indicative of an alkaline condition.

For those not familiar with the term "logarithmic," it means that the pH scale is based on a multiplicity of 10. A pH of 8 is ten times more alkaline than a pH of seven. A pH of 9 is a hundred times more alkaline than a pH of seven. One more example, a pH of 5.5 is a thousand times more acidic than a pH of 8.5.

Dr. Arthur Guyton, the world-renowned author of the *Textbook of Medical Physiology* states that

> Only slight changes in hydrogen ion concentration from the normal value cause marked alterations in the rates of chemical reactions in the cells, some being depressed and others accelerated.

For a long time, the pH cycle has been an area of knowledge tinged with mystery and complexity. Because of its complex electrical and chemical ramifications, many nutritionists have completely avoided dealing with the pH factor. This is unfortunate because the pH cycle is a major governing factor in a person's health. Ignoring the pH is like ignoring the oceans in a planetary study of weather. A person's energy level, immunity and emotional outlook are all based on pH.

THE IMPORTANCE OF pH IN HEALTH

To understand the importance of pH in health and disease, we begin with the general statement that when pH is right, then everything works well; but when pH is wrong, then nothing works well. This simply means that the process of pH is vitally important for our health, perhaps the most important biological process in our lives.

The acidity or alkalinity of our cells and fluids govern what metabolic activities can take place and how effectively they function. If pH is too acid, then our body's chemical reactions and electrical responses are too fast. Consequently, we can wear out or "burn up." The cliche phrases "adrenal burnout" and "stress burnout" are frequently used. On the other hand, if pH is too alkaline, then our chemical and electrical processes are too slow and we have autointoxication or self-poisoning. Thus, we have the expressions "sluggish liver," "sluggish bowel," and "congested lymphatics."

pH governs the rate and effectiveness of two essential life processes: our enzyme reactions and our rate of burning fuel for life's energy needs. The latter is also known as "oxidation rate." Consequently, pH is the medium in which our most fundamental life processes occur.

Enzymes which digest our foods can only function within a certain range of pH. For example, the enzyme pepsin in our stomach is not active in a pH environment higher than 5. Consequently, pepsin only works in a strong acid medium. If our stomachs or foods are too alkaline, then pepsin cannot work. Therefore, we miss the food values we would have received if pepsin were able to function properly. For example, meat requires pepsin to digest properly. After initiating partial digestion, pepsin will later activate the pancreas' protease enzymes to complete the meat's digestion. If milk which has an alkaline pH of 7.2 is ingested, it neutralizes the pepsin and ruins the entire digestion of the meat. Hence, there is the age-old rule to avoid milk if meat is eaten.

Furthermore, without pepsin's ability to digest proteins, the food passes undigested into the intestinal tract where it putrefies and releases toxic chemicals into the bloodstream before it is discharged. The basic understanding of how pH works with digestion establishes rules of proper eating which limit the consumption of milk with a meat meal. Yet, people often eat gravy with meat, or drink a glass of milk with a hamburger.

The body's ability to assimilate nutrients cannot occur when the pH is out of the proper range. Vitamins and minerals can only be assimilated within certain pH values which collectively range from 5.3 to 7.4. This means that people with pH deviations can eat food and not take in nutrition.

pH is critical to proper enzyme function. Every one of our thousands of enzyme systems has an optimal pH range which governs its function. When pH is not in the range for the enzyme to function, pH keeps the enzyme dormant, and the processes of that enzyme cannot occur.

Through the cycles of pH, the body orchestrates the complex biochemical activities of life according to natural and optimal rhythms. Every enzyme required for an activity is held in check until the appropriate time at which the pH adjusts for the enzyme's activation and maximum effectiveness. If the proper pH is inhibited, as can happen by improper diet, stress and lack of exercise, then the body enters an existence that is less than optimal. If normal pH swings are inhibited for an extended period of time, disease results as consequence.

Another reason why pH is so important to health is that it governs the rate at which our cells burn glucose for energy. In days past, the wood-burning fireplace was the central focus of the home. The fireplace makes a good analogy for us to understand the combustion, or burning of fuel, for our bodies' life processes.

Every cell in our bodies has a miniature fireplace, called the mitochondrion where glucose and oxygen mix and burn to keep us warm, active and alive. If the fuel mix is correct, it contains a mixture of mostly glucose, some amino acids and fat, and the right amount of oxygen for proper combustion. When this mixture is present, then the cellular life fires burn properly, providing stable health and energy. Thus, in our analogy of the fireplace, we have a merry little blaze with the right type of wood (not too hard, not too soft), with minimal ashes, the right updraft through the chimney and oxygen to keep the fire burning brightly. Everything is fine as long as these elements can be maintained.

Problems occur in our fireplace if someone throws gasoline on the fire. Then the fire burns too hotly and dangerously, finally catching the house on fire and burning it down. Or a problem can occur if the ashes build up and smother the fire with the result that the house gets cold. Consequently, in our bodies with their billions of tiny cellular fires, pH is a governing factor, controlling how well the fire burns or conducts its physiological oxidation.

pH governs all aspects of cellular combustion. It governs the fuel supply which is derived from glucose from our dietary carbohydrates, proteins and fats. pH also governs the oxygen supply used to control the rate at which the fire burns.

Glucose production is controlled by a complex system of checks and balances which include the pancreas, adrenal glands and liver. The primary regulator is the hormone insulin, produced by the pancreas. Insulin controls how much glucose enters the cells and thus regulates the fuel supply. Like other hormones and enzymes, insulin functions best within a certain range of ph which is 7.79 to 8.02. Consequently, the extracellular fluid (lymph) which bathes every cell, should be in a pH range of 7.8 to 8.0 to have optimal effectiveness of the hormone insulin.

The blood delivers insulin, glucose and oxygen to clusters of cells. Each individual cell is in contact with extracellular fluid which is the medium in which the cell lives. The blood is best oxygenated at a pH of 7.40 - 7.46 because at this pH blood is able to transport the most oxygen and to carry off most of the metabolic wastes.

Different people have individual tendencies toward pH irregularities which affect their health and lives. Thus, people can be categorized according to how their pH cycles work. Some persons drift high and become too alkaline; others waver up and down the pH scale with too much slack; and some sink low and become too acid, before the buffer system holds the pH in check. Such determinations can be found after an analysis of the venous blood pH which must address pH swings of 1/100 of a percent, or more practically via measurements of the urinary and salivary pH.

Nutrition can help to stabilize an inherent irregularity and bring an element of stability. This is one of the reasons why vitamin, mineral and herbal supplements can improve how well people feel. The right ingredients can help to stabilize the pH factor. On the other hand, a diet or supplement that plays into a pH weakness can make health worse. Consequently, if a dietary or supplemental regimen is implemented without regard for pH, then the results will just be "hit or miss," and most often will miss.

From a homeopathic perspective, an imbalance in pH causes symptoms which affect many aspects of health. For example, pH imbalances affect sleep patterns, energy level, appetite, food desires, perspiration and mental state. Overt symptoms such as tingling in the extremities, headaches, cold hands and feet, odor of the urine, aches and pains, all give testimony to errors in pH and the body's attempts to correct or compensate.

Many of the homeopathic remedies impact the individual's vitality to correct inherent pH deviations. The remedies affect the person's metabolism at the deepest, most vital level and can restore health where other methods ultimately fail. Many of the remedies convey elemental energy to the body and are derived from elements such as Sulphur, Phosphorus, Cadmium, Platina, Magnesium, Iodum, Silica, Zincum. Additional remedies derive from combined elements such as Calcarea carbonica (calcium + carbon), Calcarea fluorata (calcium + fluoride), Natrum muriaticum (sodium + chlorine), Calcarea phosphoricum (calcium + phosphorus), Kali iodatum (potassium + iodine), Magnesia carbonica (magnesium + carbon). The remedies' effectiveness to initiate cure lies in their ability to help the body adjust its pH and metabolism to a more optimal rate.

As a clinical example, a well-mannered, shy, twelve year old boy suffered chronic allergies, stuffy nose with clear discharge, irritated eyes and dyslexia. His pH reading was 5.5 when it was taken. He began the remedy Natrum muriaticum (LM-1), one dose per day. On day 20, a bad bout of sneezing and nasal discharge began, but the following day these symptoms unexpectedly subsided. The boy's pH broke out of its 5.5 range, and swung to 8.5 for a few hours and then stabilized between 6.5 and 7.1. Since this change, the boy has been free of allergies and has added previously aggravating foods back into his diet. He has no nasal discharge, irritated eyes, or stuffiness. The remedy has been continued at higher potencies because other constitutional and maintenance considerations exist.

With the Pro-Vita! plan we design, as much as possible, a safe and supportive "all things for all people" type of foundation for nutrition. Then, with further understanding of your personal pH tendencies, you can add or delete foods to bring a greater enhancement to your metabolic processes as you tailor the principles for yourself.

For example, people who drift toward the acid, or catabolic range (meaning the metabolism is in a tearing down mode), can benefit by adding lemon juice to their water to pick up the anionic element which their system requires. People whose pH floats too alkaline, or anabolic (meaning the metabolism is in a building up mode), can introduce, or focus on more acidic foods such as nuts and seeds. The people who waver in their pH can focus on stabilizing, non-extreme foods as are commonplace in the Pro-Vita! Plan. In this way the individuals tailor the Pro-Vita! Plan to their unique pH system. Often, this tailoring can be an instinctive decision as people notice that they feel better when eating certain foods and worse when eating others. Or some foods may work better at a certain time of day as they compensate or offset extreme pH swings.

Proper pH of the blood is critical for life. The body has many buffer systems to ensure that the pH of the blood is maintained in a range of 7.36 - 7.46. The blood pH is so important that the body will sacrifice the calcium in its bones to maintain the necessary blood pH. This situation gives us the metabolic cause of the disease osteoporosis which is too much acid in the diet, such as from red meat, sodas, sugar and the extensive use of many drugs like antibiotics and steroids (cortisone). More information on this topic is contained in *Osteoporosis: The Preventable Disease* by Jack Tips (1990).

To summarize our analogy of the fireplace, we find that pH controls how much fuel and oxygen are made available to the cell to operate its life fire. If a cell burns too hot, it burns up too quickly. However, if the cell burns too slowly, then the incomplete combustion results in excessive ash which burdens the lymphatic system with metabolic waste products.

For proper cellular activity we require correct fuel, the correct oxidation rate and the clean removal of the ashes. To get the correct fuel, our diet must provide the quality foods (complex carbohydrate, protein and fat) in proper amounts, as the Pro-Vita! Plan teaches. To have the correct oxidation rate, we need both insulin and oxygen provided by the blood and proper extracellular pH to optimize introduction of the fuel to the cells. In turn, to have proper disposal of the metabolic ashes, which are acids, the alkaline extracellular fluid must be circulated by exercise to carry off wastes. Altogether, pH is a crucial factor in this entire process.

The importance of the pH cycle is stressed by Dr. M. Ted Morter (1988) in his nutritional research. In effect, Morter claims that no other single indicator than the body's pH is encountered as often in assessing health and disease. As well, he comments that most researchers have consistently missed the true relationship between pH and good health. The major point of confusion about the function of the pH is the paradox of some acidifying foods producing an apparent alkaline condition. For example, acid citrus fruits actually produce alkalinity in the body because citric acid is a weak acid and readily metabolizes to alkaline when an enzyme splits the molecule. Another example is that apple cider vinegar contains enough citric acid to cause an alkalizing effect whereas other vinegars are acid throughout the metabolic processes.

A brief summary of Morter's research suggests that monitoring the pH is important to obtain an accurate picture of biochemical health. When the pH varies radically, the person is not in the optimum state of health. According to Morter, excessive amounts of protein in any form—animal or vegetable protein—are debilitating to the body, affect the pH and ultimately lead to chronic diseases like arthritis, diabetes, cancer and osteoporosis. However, Morter emphasizes that protein is essential to health, but not an excess of it. He recommends adding a good amount of vegetables and fruits to an effective food plan.

We also point out that predecessors to Dr. Morter, for example, Dr. Royal Lee, Carey Reams and Dr. George Goodheart, were very much preoccupied with understanding health and disease through the pH of the body. Dr. Wheelwright claimed that Carey Reams learned the fundamentals of diet and pH in his class, then went on with the research to develop the Reams Biological Theory of Ionization. This theory is a specialized series of pH tests of the urine and saliva and other tests to analyze a person's state of health. When Reams' research and program bore fruit with people claiming cure from cancer, the medical and governmental authorities started a program of persecution that included incarceration of Reams leading to this great man's demise as had happened with Dr. Royal Lee previously.

From the court proceedings against Reams we learned that the medical establishment has a copyright on the word "cure." Further, that anyone proclaiming to "cure" is practicing medicine. As much as we would like to say that "the body cures itself," or that "God can cure an ailing heart," we are not allowed to say this unless we are licensed to practice a system known for its iatrogenic, that is, doctor-induced, diseases. Fortunately we can use the word "heal." We have this word left to us because the Biblical account of the life of Jesus states that he "healed" the sick and lame. Thus, the word "heal" is available to us through historical usage or what is known as public domain.

A *caveat emptor* for any claim of "cure" should be the knowledge that the word is copyrighted by the medical cartel. An example is the claim made on TV that the drug Gyne-Lotrimin "cures" vaginal yeast. By now we should know that no drug can cure. A true cure can only take place when the body becomes immunologically strong enough to control and prevent yeast infection by itself. An antifungal, poisonous drug does nothing to correct the reason why the vagina became susceptible to infection by opportunistic yeast. In effect, to achieve a cure, the imbalance of the vaginal environment, which is influenced by hormones, pH and an inherited or acquired tendency of the vaginal environment to be weak in its tissue, must be corrected from within for the body to heal and be healthy.

When we hear the claim that a certain drug can "cure," we can understand that the manufacturer has a license to make that statement in the context that the drug effectively suppresses the symptom. Instead of learning how to "cure" our symptoms at the expense of our health, we need to learn how to HEAL. We find that those who can help us best, live accordingly to the natural laws of health.

ANALYZING pH: YOUR WINDOW TO YOUR METABOLIC PROCESSES

Here are the most important facts about pH for an introductory understanding of how it functions. The body has a preference for the pH of the blood, which is generally established at 7.4 on the pH scale, that is, slightly alkaline. A venous blood pH of 7.46 is considered optimal. If the pH deviates even a little bit, this creates great metabolic problems. Deviations too far from the body's normal range result in convulsions and death. However, the body has several fail-safe mechanisms to regulate the blood pH and keep it suitable for life, primarily through buffer salts. Many other tissues that deal with the external environment (colon, living skin, vagina, stomach, lymph node fluid), rely on an acid pH for their proper function.

The pH is a dynamic state of ebb and flow like the ocean tide. One difficulty people have in understanding pH is that they try to make it a static, or linear, rather than a cyclical condition. The pH scale most often appears linear like this:

1-2-3-4-5-6-7-8-9-10-11-12-13-14

But in effect, in body health pH is actually circular. If pH becomes too alkaline (too high) such as 9, the body automatically switches into an acid-fast condition at 5 for self-preservation. Since we know this, the pH scale looks more realistically like this:

5-6-7-8-9-5

And, for self-preservation in an over acid condition such as a consistent pH of 5 which depletes the body's alkaline reserves, the body will access bicarbonate and ammonia to buffer the acid and the pH shifts to the alkaline. Thus, the pH scale looks like this:

9-5-6-7-8-9-5

So extreme pH values often have underlying opposite deviations. A very acid pH can be the body's effort to control alkalosis. A very alkaline pH can be the body's effort to control acidosis.

Simply put, the pH wraps around itself rather than staying in a straight line. Therefore, such concepts as "alkaline pH is better than acid" or vice-versa, limit an understanding of the dynamic principles of pH. Dr. Morter's memorable quote on pH is, "We are alkaline entities by design, but acid-generating beings by function." This helps explain the interplay between these two polarities inherent within each of us.

Since it is natural for the pH to shift like the tides, if it dips too acid during the acid cycle, then the compensation is to rise too high during the alkaline cycle. Often, a deviation to one extreme simply causes a deviation to the other extreme like the pendulum on a clock.

pH can be measured easily via the urine and the saliva, each fluid providing specific insights to what is occurring in the body. The most accurate fluid to measure is venous blood, but this process involves phlebotomy and a centrifuge.

Urinary pH. The pH of the urine indicates how the body is working to maintain the proper pH of the blood. Concurrently, it shows what is occurring in the building (anabolic) and tearing down (catabolic) cycles. The pH of urine indicates the efforts of the body via the kidneys, adrenals, lungs and gonads to regulate pH through the buffer salts and hormones.

Urine provides a fairly accurate picture of body chemistry, because the kidneys filter out the buffer salts of pH regulation and provide values based on what the body is eliminating. Urine pH can vary from around 4.5 to 9.0 for its extremes, but the ideal range is 5.8 to 6.8 with slight variances for climate. The warmer the climate, the lower the pH median. For example, in the warm southern United States a urine pH of 6.4 promotes activity and offsets lethargy. In colder climates, optimal pH will climb to 6.45 or 6.5.

Salivary pH. While more acidic than blood, salivary pH mirrors what is occurring in the blood and is also a fairly good indicator of health, because it tells us what the body retains. It also is a fair indicator of the health of the extracellular fluids which is indicative of the alkaline mineral reserves.

Optimal pH for saliva is 6.4 to 6.8. This reading is taken upon arising before anything is put into the mouth. A reading lower than 6.4 is indicative of insufficient alkaline reserves. After eating, the saliva pH should rise to 7.8 or higher. Unless this occurs, the body has alkaline mineral deficiencies and will not assimilate food very well.

To deviate from ideal salivary pH for an extended time invites illness. Acidosis, an extended time in the acid pH state, can result in rheumatoid arthritis, diabetes, lupus, tuberculosis, osteoporosis and most cancers. If salivary pH is not in optimal ranges, the diet should focus on fruit and vegetables as well as remove strong acidifiers such as sodas and red meat.

Alkalosis, an extended time in the alkaline state, results in most other diseases, such as the symptoms of constipation, flu, heart trouble, indigestion, and bacterial and viral infections.

CHARTING YOUR pH FOR ANALYSIS

Here is a pH chart for visual comprehension of its function.

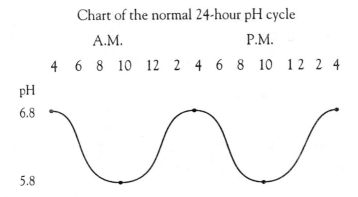

Chart of the normal 24-hour pH cycle

The body goes to great lengths to regulate the homeostasis, or equilibrium, of its preferred blood pH. Yet, as seen by the general health of most people, the body's environment needs some assistance. An imbalance in the blood chemistry means that many of the natural functions will be inhibited at the atomic level by the presence of too many acid hydrogen (H) or alkaline hydroxyl (OH) ions.

Most people are not particularly interested in understanding, or monitoring, their pH. But for the persons who understand how the pH functions, it can be a turning point in their health. People who are environmentally sensitive, or are affected by chronic fatigue, may find that metabolic balancing of the pH provides a degree of energy and stability that is critical to their daily function. If you are interested in this vital knowledge about your health, here are the instructions how to monitor your pH. Using "pHydrion lo-buff" pH paper available from your natural health professional, follow these guidelines:

- Measure the pH of the second (or any subsequent) urination of the day. The first urination is a composite of the acid/alkaline swings during sleep and is analyzed separately. Log the first urination and designate it as such. Measure the saliva at the same time. Urine and saliva pH do not always coincide—one may be acid and the other alkaline.

- Allow the urine to run on a small piece of the pH tape. It is best to measure salivary pH by spitting saliva on the tape rather than putting the tape in your mouth. Immediately compare the color of the pH tape with the color chart provided with the tape and log it on your pH chart.

- If your urinary pH is not within a 6.4 to 6.8 range, take a gentle step to assist it. IF TAPE IS TOO YELLOW, indicating an ACID pH, select one of the following which, according to Wheelwright, will help to alkalize your pH.

    ◆ Cool bath or shower.

    ◆ 6 oz. pineapple juice or most other fruit juices, but not cranberry.

    ◆ Fresh vegetable juice.

- Herb teas: chamomile, peppermint, fenugreek, red clover, hibiscus.

- Deep breathing, rapid exercise.

- Salt and baking soda bath, or Epsom salt and baking soda bath. (2 lbs salt, 2 lbs baking soda in full tub. Soak for an hour.)

- 1/2 tsp. citro-carbonate (available in drug stores) in water, but only use this when that other means listed here are not available, or the pH is unresponsive to the other means.

- Lemon juice in water.

- 1/2 tsp. baking soda plus 1/4 tsp. cream of tartar plus juice of 1/2 lemon in 4 oz. water.

Foods considered by nutritional researchers to be alkaline-forming and thus helpful to people with consistently acid pH include: Almonds, aloe vera, apples, apricots, bee pollen, buckwheat, cabbage, cantaloup, celery, carrots, cucumbers, dairy products except hard cheese, dates, dulse, poached eggs, figs, grapefruit, honey, lettuce, millet, parsley, raisins, peaches, fresh red potatoes, pineapple, soy products, sprouted seeds, raw spinach, turnip tops.

People who remain too acid often display symptoms such as:

Anxiety
Diarrhea
Dilated pupils
Extroverted behavior
Fatigue in early evening
Headaches, occipital to frontal
High blood pressure
Hyperactivity
Hypersexuality
Insomnia
Nervousness
Rapid heartbeat
Restless legs
Shortness of breath

Strong appetite
Warm, dry hands and feet

If pH remains in the yellow range consistently, contact your health professional for assistance.

- **If TAPE IS TOO GREEN OR BLUE**, indicating an ALKALINE pH, select one of the following, according to Wheelwright, to acidify the pH:

  - Hot bath or shower.

  - Mustard bath (1 oz. dry mustard in warm bath for 14 minutes—no longer!).

  - Drink unsweetened cranberry juice (dilute in water).

  - Vinegar bath (2 cups vinegar to full tub. Soak 30 minutes).

  - Herb teas: desert herb, spearmint, shave grass (horsetail), raspberry leaf, buchu.

  - Eat low-stress proteins: soaked seeds, sprouts, sesame tahini, 5+5 protein meal.

  - Eat sauerkraut, sour pickles, olives.

  - Take brisk walks with long strides.

Foods considered by nutritional researchers to be acid-forming and thus helpful to people with consistently alkaline pH include: Brown rice, hard cheese, chicken, cranberries, fried or scrambled eggs, fish, whole grains, (wheat, oats, corn, brown rice, rye), lentils, meat, nuts (except almonds, Brazil), mayonaise, pomegranates, tomatoes, seeds and vinegars.

People whose pH is too alkaline often display some of these symptoms:

Cellulite

Constipation

Cold, clammy hands and feet

Fatigue in mornings, hard to arise from bed

Headaches, sides of head, temples

Indigestion, fermentation

Introverted behavior

Leg cramps

Low blood pressure

Paleness

Slow pulse

Sluggishness

If your pH consistently remains in the blue area, contact your health professional for assistance.

Since it is often difficult to control and correct an acid pH through diet, a homeopathic remedy can be used. M. L. Tyler (1989) writes that Natrum phosphoricum (Phosphate of Soda) is a useful remedy for "that modern bogey 'acidosis' supposed to need very careful dieting." Nat. phos. is one of Schüssler's cell salts and useful for conditions arising from excess of lactic acid.

Clark (1986) reports Schüssler's explanation how Nat. phos. helps with acidosis. Through the presence of Nat. phos. lactic acid is decomposed into carbonic acid and water. Nat. phos. is able to bind to itself carbonic acid which it conveys to the lungs. Here, the oxygen flowing into the lungs liberates the carbonic acid which is exhaled and exchanged for oxygen. Clark also notes that Nat. phos. is necessary for dissolving uric acid in the blood. If uric acid is not dissolved and deposited from its solution in the joints, then arthritic rheumatism occurs. Clearly, if acidosis can be checked by the remedy Nat. phos., serious illness can be prevented.

For alkalinity, homeopathic remedies based on the potassium salts can be effective. Such Kali remedies impact the fundamental state of the vital force and therefore also the pH factor.

Balancing the pH is a major step toward well-being and greater health. Therefore, the Pro-Vita! Plan builds proper pH, both the alkaline reserve and the acid activity. This food plan builds a depth of resources and stability rather than causing radical swings in the pH cycle.

The following chart will help you to map out your pH so that you can understand your cycles and tendencies. From this chart you can then plot a graph.

URINARY AND SALIVARY pH JOURNAL					
Date	Time	Urine pH	Saliva pH	Food/Drink	Feelings, Reactions

Wheelwright conducted extensive research on the ionization potentials of foods, that is, whether a food was predominantly positive or negative energetically. This is important in health because our energy level is directly related to the resistance between the positive (anionic) and negative (cationic) molecules and atoms. In our automobiles, resistance consumes energy and generates heat. In our bodies, resistance creates our energy and body heat. For this reason Wheelwright taught that diet must provide more energy than it takes to digest and process it. Because we live on the ENERGY created by our food and not on the food itself, the ionization of food is an important factor in health.

Wheelwright used this principle to design his remarkable herbal formulas. He catalogued thousands of herbs according to their ionization potential and established patterns of compatibility. He formulated cleansing formulas by combining compatible cationic herbs. In turn, he formulated builder formulas by combining anionic herbs. He also identified polyionic herbs which he felt were best used by themselves and not in combination with other herbs.

An anionic (negatively charged) molecule rotates clockwise and carries a measurable amount of energy of 1-499 Millhouse units, like a battery. On the other hand, a cationic (positively charged) molecule rotates counterclockwise and carries 500-999 Millhouse units of energy. The rotation identifies in which direction the outer shell electrons spin around the nucleus of the atom or molecule. When an anionic and a cationic molecule meet, there is resistance due to the opposite spins, and thus our physical life energy is generated.

pH is a way to measure the resistance, or energy, we have at our disposal. If our foods are too acid or too alkaline, then our anions and cations exist in less than optimal ratios. Consequently, our cellular energy and ability to function is impaired.

Impairment of cellular function over an extended period of time means disease. In human health this state of dis-ease means a shortage of anions needed for good health in the predominantly cationic diet that most people eat. Foods, with the exception of fresh lemon, are mostly cationic, though all foods have elements of both polarities. pH readings outside the optimal 6.4-6.8 range for an extended period of time show an impairment of energy and cellular function.

Dr. Emanuel Revici (1961) is a great researcher who built a model of healing on the two opposite, yet complementary, processes of anabolism and catabolism. He founded the Revici System of Medicine which is based on three fundamental principles of healing and healthcare. These principles serve as a fitting conclusion to this chapter.

- The dynamics, manifestations and mechanisms of the physical body are based on its blueprint or energy pattern, and not solely on its chemical and physiological reactions.

- The body has a dualistic (anabolic/catabolic) nature that is always attempting to move towards a state of balance, or equilibrium, like all other forms of life. The more we can facilitate the natural rhythm, the better the body can draw on its own innate wisdom and resources to experience a higher quality of life.

- The development of any pathology is due to disequilibrium of the host or environment, and is not directly caused by a pathological organism.

In concluding this chapter about life energy at the biochemical level, we emphasize that the Pro-Vita! Plan will help you to correct your pH and to derive energy and health from your foods. If you study your pH, you will be able to adapt the Pro-Vita! Plan more specifically to your individual needs. Otherwise, it will work on its own to bring or maintain pH in an optimal, balanced state.

UNDERSTANDING
THE ENERGY METABOLISM

PRINCIPLES OF ENERGY METABOLISM

The energy metabolism is the complex system the body uses to convert the primal five elements of earth, water, fire, air and ether into essential life processes and products. The interrelationship of these elements was established by the ancient Chinese and remains valid today. For our nutrition plan, we are concerned primarily with the element of earth which is food. By bearing fruit and vegetables, the earth element is sustenance for our bodies.

The other four elements of the metabolism also have an effect on our bodies. Water is important for our vitality. Fire is provided as heat for us by the sun. Air is essential for our breathing, providing vital energy. Ether is the most refined of the elements. It is the substance of our connection to the animating life force and the resulting electrical flow and magnetic field. Ether constitutes our etheric bodies, the bioenergetic matrix in which we exist.

The focus in our nutritional plan is on proper food for proper energy. To achieve this goal we need to consider an important natural law, the Law of Entropy. According to the principle of entropy, nature moves and changes along a path of least resistance. To follow this vital principle, we want our earth-based energy system strong, sustaining and causing as little stress, or waste products, as possible. Our energy system should function in a state of balance or homeostasis. Consequently, we need the right mixture of earth fuels to provide the proper energy system for a dynamic life.

An important law of physics states that energy cannot be created or destroyed. Energy is merely transformed. How we transform our foods into energy determines the quality of our energy. The transformation also determines whether a certain food is an optimal fuel for our bodies.

Many of the biochemistry books oversimplify the energy process when they teach it as a carbohydrate system of the glucose-galactose-galactogen-peruvic acid cycle. These texts do not show that proteins (Kreb's cycle) and oils are also involved in the process. Nutrition books are particularly guilty of this omission or oversimplification.

In fact, the pure carbohydrate-burning cycle exhausts the adrenal glands, because these tiny glands become the chief regulator of this fuel during the metabolic cycle involving the blood sugar. This process creates the need for more quick energy fixes as the body loses its ability to work with more complex and more optimal energy systems. The adrenals have other functions besides stabilizing the carbohydrate metabolism. They function as energy glands, pH regulators and play a vital role in our immune system. Therefore, weak adrenals mean inability to have sustained energy, handle infections and control allergic reactions.

To provide a more correct understanding of the energy metabolism, here is a brief overview. There is no perfect energy system for the physical body at this time; if there were, we would have a perpetual motion machine for our body and eternal physical life. The process of having energy is the combustion of molecules for energy, causing waste residues which the body has to recycle or eliminate.

The three basic food energy suppliers are carbohydrates (sugars), proteins and oils. Each group has its nutritional shortcomings. Pure carbohydrates burn out the adrenal glands; pure protein systems are quite toxic; and oils are rich, but laborious to access, thus making them costly in terms of energy. The waste products from oil combustion tax the kidneys. But the proper availability of all three energy sources provides the optimal energy system, consisting of a good amount of energy efficiency, low stress and clean burning.

For our explanation of the energy metabolism we find a good analogy in the combustion engine. The diesel engine is strong, durable and delivers a lot of power. It is a lot like what most people want their bodies to be—strong, durable and around for a long time in good working order. In contrast, high combustion gasoline engines wear out quicker, cost more to maintain and need more repairs.

If we compare the food groups to engine fuel, we find that proteins could be likened to diesel fuel. They have many carbon molecules with the potential for long, strong and deep energy reserves. In turn, complex carbohydrates (cereals, potatoes, whole grain bread) could be likened to gasoline or butane. They have fewer carbon molecules, shorter burning time, higher energy, but at a cost of lower reserve power. Refined carbohydrates (candy, sugar, pastries) and alcohol could be likened to jet fuel or hydrogen. They feature even fewer carbon molecules, much shorter burning time, high energy, hot burning and no reserves. Finally, oils could be likened to crude oil. They have great energy potential and storage, but are difficult to use and must be processed laboriously.

With this analogy of the combustion engine, it becomes clear that people who rely solely on complex carbohydrates (grains, breads, pasta) for their primary fuel are putting gasoline in their diesel engine which will work somewhat, but not without stressing the system. In contrast, refined carbohydrates (sugars) keep the body revved up on its adrenal supercharger.

According to Wheelwright and many other researchers, the ideal human energy system is founded on a complex carbohydrate-based fuel mix with the primary dietary focus on vegetables and low-stress protein. This does not at all mean that we should eat a lot of protein. Instead, the focus on protein means that we must recognize it as a key to health. Consequently, we must learn how to properly use protein. The focus on protein is explained by the fact that the body consists of protein with a bit of carbohydrate to provide the spark of energy. Although no energy system is perfect, proteins in addition to the combustion process build tissue and healthy immune systems, while carbohydrates do not build, and refined sugars destroy.

To obtain an efficient energy system, the first choice has to be for the fuel that controls the combustion rate. This energy fuel further must provide the nutritive capability to build tissue, make hormones and antibodies. It must also impart quality and integrity to the body tissues instead of shallow energy without substance. Proteins represent this nutritive factor.

Just as combustion engine fuels are mixtures, the optimal energy system for the human body is based on having a mixture available. Of course, the big question is, "What to base this mixture on?"

The fuel system of the Pro-Vita! Plan is based on the structure, biochemistry and energy systems of the body. As a result, the program advocates high quality, low-stress protein with a small amount of carbohydrate in transit for energy and a lot of vegetables for fiber, vitamins, minerals and enzymes. The plan's PRIMARY FOCUS IS ON VEGETABLES WITH PROTEINS. We need to remember that our foods provide more than metabolic energy. They also provide building blocks, buffers and biochemical catalysts for the function, maintenance and repair of our body systems. Thus, physical energy is only one, but an important, piece of the dietary picture.

PROTEIN FOODS

Before we discuss protein foods in more detail, we want to reemphasize that the Pro-Vita! Plan promotes light use of low-stress protein sources. A recent study, as reported by Kirk Johnson (1991), provides excellent insights into the connection between effective protein consumption and a well-functioning immune system. Conducted by James Hebert, a nutritional epidemiologist with the University of Massachusett's Medical School, this study demonstrates that proper nutrition plays a major role in the body's resistance against infectious agents, like the AIDS virus. Diets which lack protein have a direct impact on the immune function. The lack of dietary protein is specifically responsible for protein malnutrition, according to Hebert. Such protein malnutrition has a destructive effect on the structure and function of the important, but overlooked, thymus gland which plays a major role in immune functions even in the later years of a person's life.

Moreover, Hebert is not the only researcher expressing concern about people with protein malnutrition. Although these recent studies have evolved from research on the AIDS virus, (or more correctly, viruses), they clearly have implications for a general nutritional plan. Nutrition for an effective immune system needs to contain proteins which can be digested and assimilated as short chain amino acid structures, as discussed earlier in the soybean story.

The following discussion pertains to identifying low-stress proteins as required by the Pro-Vita! Plan. Protein foods such as nuts, seeds, eggs, meats, fish, unprocessed cheese, beans, raw milk and others are predominantly composed of amino acid structures. We will differentiate these protein sources according to their stress potential for the digestive system. However, no natural food is 100% protein. Instead, natural foods are combinations of amino acids, carbohydrates (starches, sugars), oils and other factors (fiber, cellulose, enzymes, vitamins, water and minerals).

Foods that are predominantly rich in amino acids are classified as protein foods. But as we learned from the soybean story, not all forms of protein foods are beneficial to health. Also, we need to keep in mind that when some foods are cooked, their category changes. For example, dry beans are protein, but boiled beans are carbohydrates as we explained.

The protein foods include the following foods, although not all are optimal protein sources:

avocado (Not a true protein, mostly an oil.)
beans, dry, sprouted, or Pro-Vita! cooked
beet leaf
cheese
chlorella (algae)
coconut milk, from young, green coconuts only
    (Mature coconuts are mostly fat.)
conch
cottage cheese
dulse
egg
fish
gelatin
meats (beef, chicken, duck, lamb, pork, etc.)
milk
miso
nuts, nut butters
peanuts
peas, dry
pine nuts
seafood (fish, shrimp, algae, scallops, squid)
seeds (sunflower, squash, pumpkin, radish, sesame, flax,
    chia)
seitan

shrimp
soybeans
sprouted seeds (alfalfa, mung, sunflower, pumpkin flax,
    chia, radish)
ahini
tempeh
tofu
wild rice (a seed and not the same as brown rice)

Some of these listed proteins are high-stress and some are low-stress proteins. The value of a protein source depends upon the ease with which its minerals and amino acids are made available to support the body's energy and life processes. To furnish this vital support, the protein's minerals and amino acids have to undergo digestion and the enzymatic processes of reducing the original proteins to small nucleo-proteins.

If a protein is bound by heavy oils, it stresses the body and takes more energy to be processed than it gives. Pork is an example of a protein bound by oil that takes more energy than it gives, unless a person's digestive system is exceedingly strong. Recently, several German practitioners in Biological Medicine agree that pork should be eliminated from a healthy diet, because pork is bioenergetically unsuitable for human consumption.

Crab and lobster proteins also stress the body. Due to the oil content of avocado, some people have difficulty processing this food. The fact that avocado contains oil does not mean that it is a poor food choice, because it has other redeeming features. But for people with a slow metabolism, called slow oxidizers, this means only occasional use of avocado.

Slow oxidizers are persons who break down nutrients for cellular combustion slowly due to very alkaline pH and weak, or underactive, thyroid and adrenal glands. The oxidation rates of other people can fall into a "fast" category. Fast oxidizers burn fuel too quickly, because their body does not apply the breaks to the combustion process. In turn, mixed oxidizers alternate between fast and slow rates of metabolism. Finally, normal oxidizers have a metabolism rate with optimal supply, combustion, effective utilization and successful removal, or recycling, of waste products. Personal oxidation rates can be determined by a hair tissue analysis. Check with your health professional to see if such a test is beneficial and insightful for you.

If a protein is too complex, or cooked to a point where the amino acid structures are irreparably altered or destroyed by heat, it is of little use to the body and results in toxic stress. We are referring here to the fact that heat or cooking alter the molecule structure of foods. Cooking foods can be both beneficial and detrimental to nutrition, depending on the foods, and how heat affects them.

Cooking is considered beneficial when heat is used to break down complex or destructive/toxic substances in food into more assimilable substances. Examples of this include cooking inedible foods, such as plantains, dry beans, peas, Lima beans, rice and other grains. Although the beans could be sprouted and thus become available as a raw alternative, some foods must be cooked to be used as nutrients. One example is the Akee fruit of Jamaica which is poisonous when raw, but as a cooked food is a staple, resembling scrambled eggs in texture. Soup is another example of a highly assimilable source of minerals derived by cooking food.

More often, though, cooking destroys food values with a critical loss of the enzymes inherent in the food which would have been helpful with its digestion. Cooking also alters the protein molecules into unusable forms. To understand the damage of cooking to the protein molecules, we will use the egg as an example, since its chemistry adjustments to heat are visible. In its raw state the egg is composed of protein, lipids, minerals and other factors. The egg in its raw liquid form can thus mix with water and other liquids.

Once exposed to heat, the egg changes dramatically because it solidifies. When this occurs, the egg cannot be changed back into its former liquid state. Unlike liquid water which can be heated in steam and condensed back to a liquid or cooled further into its solid form of ice and then heated back into liquid again, the egg's response to heat is to form unchangeable bonds.

From this example of the egg we can see that heat alters the egg's molecules, causing a chemical reaction which forms strong molecular bonds in eggs. For this reason, a hard-boiled egg is difficult for the body to digest. Later we will discuss why raw egg-white is not optimal for human nutrition either, and how to lightly cook an egg to produce maximum nutritional value from it.

Relying on grains or protein sources such as rice, millet, barley, rye, wheat, triticale, quinoa and amaranth for nutrition also presents challenges. They all are well cooked before they can be eaten. The proteins contained in these foods are compromised by the cooking process. Concurrently, these foods become stronger in their carbohydrate values when cooked. Thus, the focus of a cooked grain is carbohydrate rather than protein.

While on the subject of grains and protein values, we want to acknowledge the ground-breaking research by Frances Lappe as presented in her book, *Diet for a Small Planet* (1971). Lappe's information teaches people how to combine beans and rice to get complete protein values for better protein nutrition from non-animal sources. Her research has helped thousands of vegetarians to maintain better health by obtaining better protein values from their grain-based diets. Lappe recommends combinations of beans and grains. However, currently a debate is in progress in the vegetarian communities whether the seeds and grains must be eaten together at one meal, or can be eaten separately within a 24-hour period.

Although Lappe's nutritional approach is a major improvement over plans which do not combine grains and seeds, it still has some flaws. We find it important to address these points. The first point is that the protein values of COOKED beans and rice are not the same as those of raw beans and rice, because cooking alters the molecules, making some of the original proteins unusable in human nutrition.

The second point concerns the immutably bonded proteins in cooked foods which reduce the effectiveness of the foods as proteins and render a stronger carbohydrate volume to the body. When the body recognizes cooked grains and beans as carbohydrates, it will digest them as such and thus further reduce the effectiveness of the protein assimilation. The key to assessing protein values is to know which protein is assimilable, not which protein is contained in the raw and uncooked food according to assays.

For all of these reasons, we often see clinically that vegetarians on a grain-based existence are still deficient in nucleo-proteins. This deficiency is usually evidenced by poor "sphere" of a drop of blood and by other related health disorders, such as cravings for carbohydrates and spices, fatigue, overweight and lowered resistance to infections. It is also common knowledge that cooked beans, for example, can be associated with obvious digestive problems in processing carbohydrates as evidenced by flatulence. If you are a vegetarian, the Pro-Vita! Plan will teach you how to cook beans to retain the value of their wonderful protein instead of continuing to overcook the beans.

Another serious concern is that proteins are increasingly bound by toxic substances. When proteins are bound with toxic chemicals, fertilizers, growth hormones, antibiotics or steroids, they become less available and more toxic. Therefore, a serious concern for vegetarians is the high level of pesticides, fungicides and herbicides that come from eating large quantities of commercial fruits, vegetables, legumes and dairy products. Crucial research on the subject of toxicity in food is contained in David Steinman's book, *Diet for a Poisoned Planet: How to Choose Safe Foods for You and Your Family* (1990).

Unless people are eating from their own organic garden exclusively, they should clean their produce as explained later in this book. Also, they should consider taking a homeopathic or herbal therapy once a year to release any accumulated toxic residues. Dr. Wheelwright established a 13-day program, called the "ACX/CTV/CLNZ Pesticide Detox Program." (See your natural health professional to determine if such a program would benefit you.)

Proteins can be classified according to their bioenergy, mineral content, ease of assimilation—how loosely the amino acids are bonded—and amino acid content. We are providing below a list of the finest protein sources in the world. The difference between this list and the previous list of proteins is that we have removed the detrimental or high-stress foods from this new one. The proteins in the following list are called low-stress proteins which promote health. They have a 15 to 90-minute digestion time, burn cleanly if properly prepared and eaten, conserve energy and return more energy and nutrients than they take.

Digestion time is one measure of a food's stress potential. For example, breast milk requires a 30-minute digestion time; goat's milk about 1 1/2 hours; and cow's milk about 3 to 4 hours. For this reason and many other reasons, numerous nutritionists are against using cow's milk in our diets. The large fat molecule of cow milk puts stress on the infant's digestion and can establish that pattern for life. So here we are looking for proteins that can digest well and be properly broken down to nucleo-proteins.

LOW-STRESS PROTEINS

Low-stress proteins are superior foods for health, when used as outlined in this book, and include the following:

- Beans, sprouted, cooked without boiling. (Boiled beans arecarbohydrates.)

- Beet leaf (A little goes a long way.)

- Chicken, organically grown, range, without the skin; a borderline medium-stress protein

- Chlorella and some other sea algae, if free of mercury

- Coconut, green, young, the clear milk (almost a gel), not the mature coconut which is a fat

- Conch

- Cottage cheese, raw milk, low or nonfat; borderline medium-stress to some people, but not to others

- Dulse, a sea vegetable

- Eggs, yard egg; yolk cooked between 180 and 200 degrees F

- Feta cheese; a low/medium-stress food made from sheep or goat milk

- Gelatin (It is not a complete protein and should be used with other proteins, but has similar energy-matrix as kidneys.)

- Miso, fermented soybean paste (low to medium stress)

- Nuts, a medium to high-stress protein whose value is improved when used as nutmilk (nuts soaked in water and blended for liquid form); makes an excellent base for salad dressing

- Ocean fish, Steinman's (1990) list of "green light" seafood includes Cod from Denmark, Canada, Iceland, New Zealand; Dover Sole from California, Washington, France; English Sole; Flounder (not from Boston Harbor!); Grouper; Haddock; Halibut from Alaska or Iceland; Mahi Mahi; Marlin; Red Snapper; Pacific Salmon

- Potato juice, raw; use all potatoes except Russet bakers which are a fine carbohydrate when cooked. (Remove eyes and green spots.)

- Octopus

- Scallops

- Sesame tahini

- Shrimp, cooked in garlic or beer to remove puricines (Buy U. S. shrimp.)

- Soy ferments, tofu, miso (medium stress)

- Sprouts, especially sunflower

- Squid

- Tempeh (medium stress)

- Tofu, a medium stress food

- Wild rice, cooked without boiling

We recently noted with satisfaction that David Steinman (1990) lists the LOW-STRESS SEAFOOD PROTEINS octopus, shrimp (U.S. shrimp!) and squid as VIRTUALLY POLLUTION FREE! These proteins are free from pollution for the same reason that they are so easy to digest.

In his lectures, Wheelwright taught that shrimp—as well as oysters, squid and scallops—were healing proteins when properly prepared and used. Inevitably his theory would be challenged on three points. Shrimp are the scavengers of the sea; shrimp contain cholesterol and puricines which are detrimental for health; shrimp have no scales and are thus not to be eaten according to the Old Testament Bible.

But Wheelwright would reply that shrimp are, in fact, primitive creatures and loosely bonded protein structures. This loose bonding means that toxins pass through the shrimp. The toxins do not stick in the shrimp's tissue but are instead eliminated. The shrimp should be deveined. Regarding the cholesterol in the shrimp, this is not a concern in the low-stress protein plan. If the cholesterol is digested, it enters the body as lipids. Puricines are neutralized by cooking shrimp in ginger and garlic (the Chinese way!) or by boiling shrimp in beer (as Texans do!). To counter the third point, the structure of the shrimp shell is similar to a scale on a fish. Wheelwright was also quick to point out that the New Testament rescinds the Old Testament law.

Wheelwright never presented any other research or rationale for his theory of the loosely bonded proteins. But he told me personally that in 1984 he was able to heal his body of a colon cancer brought on by an incident when someone poisoned him. He effected the healing through fasting, herbs and a two-week rest in Hawaii where he lived on green coconut milk, squid, octopus and shrimp combined with innumerable vegetables. He attributed the renewal of his tissue integrity, meaning the regaining of healthy, strong tissue, to the primitive proteins.

Now, a year after Wheelwright's death, we find the confirmation of his theories by the evidence that toxins are not harbored in the loosely bonded tissue of the primitive sealife contained on his low stress protein list. We are most appreciate of David Steinman's fine research!

We should mention here that early in his nutrition career, Wheelwright spoke against eating shrimp, because it burned too quickly, giving too much energy at the cellular level. He taught this principle to others who went forth to establish careers in Natural Health and who thus perpetuated this concept. However, in 1980, Wheelwright rescinded this concept in favor of the healing attributes of properly prepared shrimp eaten with a good amount of vegetables. He taught that the key to reaping the benefits of the loosely bonded shrimp protein was contained in the buffering agents in green vegetables.

Wheelwright explained to me personally that, "Shrimp is a very important nutritional resource, even though conch and scallops are superior, because shrimp is a primitive protein and is readily available. When you talk about feeding the world, two shrimp correctly prepared and eaten with both raw and lightly cooked vegetables can do more for the body than all the rice in China."

Many proteins are MEDIUM-STRESS and may be used sparingly. These include avocado, turkey, game birds, such as cornish game hens, pheasant, quail, doves, soaked nuts (i.e., nutmilk) and French feta cheese, or organic Greek feta cheese.

HIGH-STRESS PROTEINS should be reduced and preferably avoided because they take more energy than they provide. Such proteins include pork, lamb, veal, beef muscle, peanuts, most raw nuts if eaten in large quantities, non-fermented soybean products like soymilk, soy flour, protein powder, sardines, brewer's yeast (except in small amounts), cow's milk. Note that miso, tofu, soy sauce, seitan and tempeh are fermented soybean or grain products and therefore are excellent vegetarian protein sources.

After discussing the high quality protein sources, we look at the rules governing the proper digestion of protein, its use in the body and the elimination of the acid by-products of protein metabolism.

GUIDE TO OPTIMAL PROTEIN USE

The following are Wheelwright's guiding rules of optimal protein use. Each rule will be explained in more detail in subsequent chapters.

Please note that the use of the word "rule" does not imply dogma! These rules are simply the way to maximize protein use. Some people need to follow the rules closely because they are weak or overcoming an illness. Others can have some slack because optimal nutrition is not essential for their high vitality.

By following the most important rules of protein use most of the time, people will greatly enhance their nutrition and energy. However, optimizing protein use perfectly is not essential and may not be practical. Besides, our bodies are designed in such a way that optimal nutrition is not absolutely essential. For thousands of years nutrition has been a "catch as catch can" matter. But today we are in a position to experience the freedom and vitality of optimal nutrition.

143

Once proper protein use is integrated as a way of life, this guide is amazingly simple. According to Wheelwright, here are the key considerations to maximize nutrition into a low-stress, Pro-Vita! 5+5 meal.

Eat protein foods:

- without carbohydrates/sugars,
- with a variety of vegetables,
- in complete protein groups,
- early in the day,
- with a small amount of good quality oil,
- as the focus of a meal (do not snack on proteins), in small portions.
- without liquid beverages.

The following chapters will discuss these guidelines in more detail.

PART II

HOW THE
PRO-VITA! PLAN WORKS

This part of the Pro-Vita! Plan focuses on Wheelwright's laws of protein nutrition. The next seven chapters are the rules Wheelwright thought essential for proper protein digestion, absorption and utilization. The explanations of these guidelines were the main body of his lectures.

EFFECTIVE PROTEIN DIGESTION

Wheelwright believed that once protein nutrition was properly handled, good health would follow. Around his view of protein as the hub of diet revolved the other foods, the critical focus on vegetables, the inclusion of oils, the separation of carbohydrates from proteins, the enjoyment of fruit. Around the hub of protein Wheelwright planned the timing of eating, activity and rest.

If you learn the principles in this section and have one Pro-Vita! 5 + 5 meal a day, your health will improve. This was Dr. Wheelwright's promise which has been verified time and again.

For some people it is easy to have a Pro-Vita! meal for lunch. This meal alone results in improved nutrition that should bring a number of possible benefits such as increased energy, sharper mental clarity and better elimination, depending on the individual and lifestyle. It is even better to have a 5 + 5 meal for breakfast.

With this chapter we will focus on the first rule for mastery of the protein meal, to make it work optimally for health.

BASIC REASONS FOR NOT
MIXING PROTEIN WITH STARCHES

The first rule of good digestion and assimilation of protein is: DO NOT MIX MAJOR PORTIONS OF PROTEIN AND STARCH AT THE SAME MEAL. This first rule is the most important one, and it is most often broken. If protein is eaten with too many carbohydrates (bread, crackers, potato, rice, pasta) or with fruit (sugar), digestion is severely compromised. Consequently, the body becomes a breeding ground for bacteria in the gastro-intestinal tract. Moreover, such a combination contributes to higher levels of cholesterol. Wheelwright taught that EATING PROTEINS

WITH CARBOHYDRATES IS A MAJOR CAUSE OF CHOLESTEROL PROBLEMS.

In a recent article in the German journal *Biologische Medizin* (Biological Medicine) dated February 1991, Dr. Med. W. Frase specifically blames overnutrition in carbohydrates as a coronary risk factor, that is, for the occurrence of arteriosclerosis. In effect, Frase actually discusses not the consumption of carbohydrates but the combination of protein and carbohydrates, because he cites the "McDonald-Kids" referring to the fast-food generation, as well as the high consumption of ice cream. In Frase's opinion, these foods cause serious metabolic disturbances, already apparent in young people. They lead increasingly to liver and kidney ailments as well as accumulation of plaque in the arteries. Incidentally, Dr. Frase also makes a strong argument against the use of pork, white flour products as well as sugar.

Perhaps one reason why cow's milk causes so many allergies is that it is a protein and carbohydrate (sugar) combination. Separating these two types of food is one of the first steps to being free of allergies.

Separating proteins and carbohydrates is basic food combining as taught by many leading nutritionists, too numerous to mention. They find that the digestion of protein and the digestion of carbohydrates are physiologically separate and conflicting functions.

The proteins are digested in an acid medium which means that the enzymes function in an acid environment. Combining protein and carbohydrates impairs the proper digestion of one or the other food. Historical and current observations show that the body opts for the digestion of the carbohydrates if both foods are present, perhaps after the principle of a "path of least resistance." Or the body opts for the digestion of the carbohydrates in mixed meals to meet immediate energy and survival needs. In this way, the body will function effectively and will be able to obtain proteins at another time.

When carbohydrates (starches) are eaten, the digestive system sends forth alkaline or neutral gastric juices, such as amylase which is most efficient at an alkaline pH of 7.1-7.2. However, when proteins are eaten, the digestive system sends out acid gastric juices at a pH of 3, for example. If these food groups are eaten simultaneously, the gastric juices (if both are provided) cancel each other out and poor digestion results.

But the body is concerned with conservation of energy and does not send for conflicting digestive enzymes.

Protein digestive enzymes are much more costly to the body to manufacture. If both protein and carbohydrate are eaten simultaneously, the body may only respond to the easier carbohydrate digestive process and let the protein pass through. This results in poor absorption of amino acids and poisoning of the body due to putrefying/decaying protein (i.e. rotten meat in the intestine).

Dr. Royal Lee, one of this century's most outstanding biochemists, investigated the digestion process in detail. He found that when a food is chewed, the ptylin and amylase enzymes in the saliva begin processing the carbohydrates. If carbohydrates are prevalent, a signal is sent via the hypothalamus to the pancreas to produce more alkaline amylase enzymes to further process carbohydrate food. If protein is prevalent, the signal is sent to the pancreas to produce more protease enzymes to further process the protein.

The pancreas mass produces one or the other enzyme at a time. If both proteins and carbohydrates are eaten simultaneously, Dr. Lee found that the pancreas opted for pancreatic amylase (the easier enzyme to produce) for the digestion of carbohydrates and neglected the protein digestion.

The purpose of this book is not to win you over to a rigid or strict food combining plan. I have never seen strict food combiners enjoy good health, since they are always worrying about what not to eat. However, the basic tenets of food separation are quite valid and essential for good health, the primary rule being DO NOT eat proteins together with carbohydrates (starches, sugars). Anything that inhibits digestion is an enemy of health.

Of course, some carbohydrates will be eaten in any protein meal, because the vegetables so strongly advocated as absolutely essential in a protein meal contain carbohydrates. Thus, the meal will not be devoid of carbohydrate. We can also add a tortilla or a few croutons to the meal and not exceed the body's ability to digest the protein. Wheelwright taught that if the carbohydrates were less than 18% by volume, the body could still recognize the focus of the meal as protein and digest it accordingly.

As mentioned previously, some protein foods and some vegetables become starches when cooked for an extended period of time or at high temperatures, particularly above 200 degrees F. These foods include beans, corn and peas. Although dry or sprouted beans and peas are proteins, they become starches when cooked.

For beans to retain their excellent protein values, soak them, allow them to begin to sprout, then slowly cook them below 200 degrees F. A crock pot works well for this process. By cooking beans this way, a small portion of beans may be included in a protein meal and not interfere with digestion. Otherwise, use beans away from the protein meal. See the detailed instructions for cooking beans in the section "How to Work with Protein."

Many people soak the beans overnight, then put them on a terry cloth towel to keep them moist. They save the initial soak water in the refrigerator to cook the beans in. Sprout the beans until a tiny white nub shows on 10% of the beans. Then they are ready to cook without boiling. If the soak water is used, boil it first to rid any bacteria, then reduce heat. Beans prepared in this manner provide wonderful proteins, cell-scrubbing minerals and no gas!

IMPROVING VEGETABLE PROTEIN DIGESTION AND ASSIMILATION

Wild rice also qualifies as a food fairly high in protein if cooked without boiling. It is a seed that has higher protein values than brown and white rice.

Although brown rice contains more nutrients and fiber than the refined, nutrient-depleted, milled, white rice, the brown husk contains rancid oils and gives brown rice its characteristic nutty smell. The Chinese understand this problem with the rancid oils and therefore use the white rice. If you eat brown rice, a carbohydrate, be sure to use additional natural vitamin E. Basmati or Texmati rice, which is white in color, is superior in nutrition, low in rancid oils, and thus a good complex carbohydrate food. But it should not be used in large amounts with proteins.

Some people attempt to combine beans and rice to obtain a full protein value. I have not seen such people have good protein values at the cellular level. This determination of their cellular protein is based on both a bioenergetic analysis as well as the specialized lab test known as amino acid profiling. A drop of blood from their finger exhibits a poor sphere revealing the poor amino acid qualities of their body. One reason for these people's low protein values is that they boil the rice and beans, thus making them into starch. Then the body digests rice and beans as carbohydrates, and the proteins do not become as available as they would if the beans were prepared to protect the protein values.

Also, the amino acids in rice and beans are complex and not easy for the body to break down into nucleo-proteins. Proper use of legume and grain products is dependent upon cooking with low heat and a strong digestive system. Poor digestion of plant proteins often results in congested lymphatics and its associated health concerns.

The combining of beans and rice helps somewhat with nutrition because it is a better plan than not combining at all. But this mixture does not provide optimal nutrition. Other reasons why a beans and rice diet does not work well are found in the energy matrix. It takes a strong liver for this plan to work well. Perhaps adding soaked seeds to properly prepared beans and some wild rice to the brown rice would help. This mixture would quadruple the protein values which would still not be optimal but much better than before. For people following such a diet philosophy, I highly recommend soaked seeds plus sprouted beans (cooked without boiling) along with a little miso to make a meal rich in protein. If an array of fresh vegetables is added and bread avoided at this particular meal, then this meal can deliver an excellent supply of amino acids.

THE NUTRITIONAL ENERGY
LINE OF FOOD GROUPS

Let's now look at the nutritional energy lines of carbohydrates, proteins and oils. This is a portrayal of how the body renders metabolic energy from a food group.

•**Simple and Refined Carbohydrates.** The chart on the next page reflects the energy lines of refined carbohydrates, such as sugar, fructose, alcohol, candies, sodas, sucrose, ice cream and typical junk foods, e. g. sugary cereals. These foods give quick energy, excite the system and drop off quickly, leaving an energy deficit. This topic is discussed further in the book *The Next Step to Greater Energy* (Tips, 1990).

THE SIMPLE AND REFINED CARBOHYDRATE ENERGY LINE

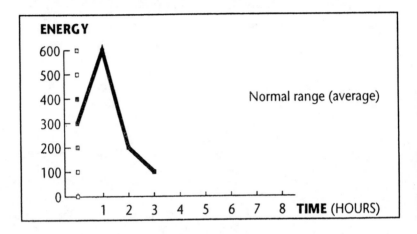

• **Complex carbohydrates** take longer to metabolize and do not leave as great an energy deficit. They are the foundation of proper metabolic energy as the body is best adapted to convert complex carbohydrates to glucose for the cellular files. Examples of complex carbohydrates are grains and potatoes.

THE COMPLEX CARBOHYDRATE ENERGY LINE

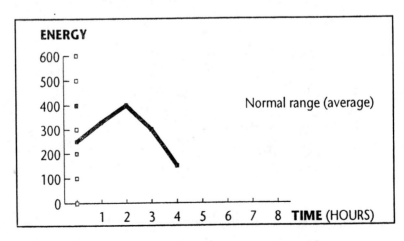

• **Proteins** take longer to metabolize, but they provide a sustained energy matrix within which the carbohydrates, in transit in the body fluids, can operate without spiking and causing deficits.

PROTEIN ENERGY LINE

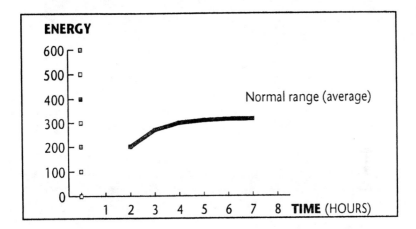

• **Oils** (fats) are storage houses for energy. When glycogen levels are low in the liver, the body will convert carbohydrates to fat to provide an energy reserve for later. Fats are rich in energy, metabolize slowly and give up energy grudgingly.

OILS ENERGY LINE

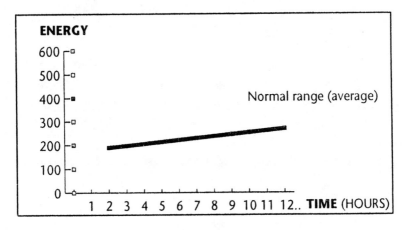

In an optimal food, the best feature of each graph would be present. If we could combine the best elements of each graph in proper proportion into a single food, we would have the perfect food. However, there is not one food that is perfect. This fact makes sense since each person is biochemically an individual. Thus, nutrition is a group effort and the result of a full and varied diet tailored to the individual. Since no one food is perfect, it is up to us to create the perfect diet from combinations of foods. The Pro-Vita! is the only nutrition plan today that does exactly that!

From the graph of simple and refined carbohydrates, we pick their higher value of energy that is readily available. We do not want the quick spike effect which leaves a nutritional deficit. We want our food to be easily combustible, but not injected into the metabolic fires explosively.

From the graph of the complex carbohydrates we choose their smooth, controllable availability of glucose and the ease of digestion. We leave behind the slight deficit at the end of the curve where it plays out without reserve.

From the protein graph we choose protein's sustaining and nourishing features as well as the minimal drop in energy. We leave behind the slower availability and extra digestive processes required. From the graph of oils (fats) we take their endurance and concentrated energy, leaving behind the difficulty in accessing their reserve.

In making these choices we will have the best of the fuels, carbohydrates, protein and oil. The next step is to put the fuels in the optimal proportions to have the most effective nutrition plan. This plan can easily be tailored to the individual's metabolism, lifestyle and time of life.

It is obvious from the fuel perspective that generally we want a good amount of complex carbohydrates, some protein and a touch of high quality oil to pick up as many energy attributes as possible. This plan will optimize our fuel intake. Ultimately, for the complete health of the body and its needs for enzymes, minerals and vitamins, we place our optimal fuel on a large foundation of vegetables.

ENHANCING PROTEIN ASSIMILATION WITH VEGETABLES AND HIGH QUALITY OIL

HOW VEGETABLES ASSIST PROTEIN DIGESTION

Many people have been fortunate enough to hear Wheelwright's lectures on nutrition. What they remember foremost is his admonishment against eating large amounts of carbohydrate foods at the same meal in which protein foods were eaten also. But an equally important rule of good digestion is this: ALWAYS HAVE VEGETABLES WITH A PROTEIN MEAL. In fact, if you wish to live long and vitally, you will have organic vegetables with every meal.

The discussion in this chapter will add to our information from the chapter about "Glorious Vegetables." In this section we learn why vegetables are critically important for proper digestion and assimilation of proteins, as well as elimination of the metabolic byproducts of proteins.

To be truly healthy, we must have good quality proteins available for our cells. Getting carbohydrates for a ready supply of glucose for cellular fuel is no problem. Vegetables and starchy foods, such as grains and potatoes, easily supply the body's energy needs, even if eaten in small amounts. But getting good quality protein is a nutritional challenge. Moreover, obtaining good nucleo-proteins without sacrificing more energy than they provide, is an undertaking which needs nutritional planning. However, the rewards for learning the principles of the Pro-Vita! Plan are more energy, less toxic stress, a stronger immune system, automatic weight control, and better overall health and quality of life. With this in mind, we learn how to have a meal which focuses on protein so that we can build our health.

Proteins pose a unique challenge for the body, because they are probably the most potentially toxic natural food required by the body. To process proteins from the start to the finish, vegetables are

155

absolutely essential. Few people understand that all foods are basically toxic because they are foreign to our bodies until they become "humanized" by the liver. "Humanization" is a word for the body's process of disassembling a food through digestion; matching it with other nutrients so that it can be absorbed (assimilation); and making it "self" or a molecule which becomes the body and used by the body.

All natural foods grow in a hostile environment and have built-in resistance to insects and fungus. We could say that they have their own internal insecticides and fungicides. Consequently, all natural foods have properties which our livers must decode and make acceptable for our bodies.

The human immune system reads protein as the important property in any food, be it fruit, vegetable or meat, to determine whether the protein is "self" or a threatening "non-self." This check occurs because viruses, bacteria, parasites, paramecium as well as airborne pollens are essentially protein. For our survival, the immune system is quickly alerted to foreign proteins.

Little protein is contained in fruit, because fruit consists mostly of water. Therefore, as a rule, fruits are less challenging immunologically than other foods though we occasionally hear of hives from strawberries or peach fuzz. Most vegetables are also low in protein and thus present less stress. Overall, foods high in protein have more immunologically recognizable molecules which the body must process. Thus, these foods are more toxic until the liver humanizes them.

Simply put, a pound of meat or nuts places a greater toxic stress on the body than a pound of apples, provided they are organic and free of pesticides and fungicides.

As a consequence, it only makes common sense that proteins should form a smaller part of our nutritional intake than fruits and vegetables. Yet, even though proteins are logically a smaller part of an optimal diet and hence occupy second place to carbohydrates for our fuel supply, proteins are still a critical link in our dietary health. For nutritional need other than fuel, proteins occupy a primary position when accompanied by vegetables.

Vegetables are essential because they assist the body with all phases of protein digestion and assimilation; and elimination of protein metabolic wastes. The first role of vegetables is to serve as buffers of the pH. As we have already discussed, the human GI tract is mostly suited to a vegetable diet with a small percentage of other foods. But foods containing a concentration of protein generate digestive acids to begin their digestive cycle. Since protein foods are concentrated foods, the vegetables add enzyme-rich bulk to dispense and buffer the protein.

Vegetables spread out the concentrated proteins and assist in their digestion. Vegetables also protect the colon from the protein's non-assimilated fibers, thus preventing putrefaction. Altogether, vegetables help to prevent future health problems, such as colon cancer, prostate problems and reabsorption of bowel gasses.

In addition to their high nutritive value, raw and lightly cooked vegetables serve to buffer dietary proteins and provide protection from the acids of the proteins. Vegetables play a vital nutritious role because they help to digest and assimilate protein by providing enzymes and minerals. In addition, they protect the body from metabolic side effects of protein digestion through their mineral buffer salts. For these reasons, proteins should always be eaten with a variety of vegetables. Following this one essential rule of the Pro-Vita! Plan will improve nutrition and health. As a good measure, of the entire amount of vegetables consumed, 65% should be raw and 35% lightly cooked.

RAW VEGETABLES FOR ENZYMES

Raw vegetables provide enzymes that help digest proteins. They also supply roughage to disperse proteins, as well as help lower cholesterol and provide good form to the stool. In addition, they function as an escort service for improved assimilation and also provide valuable vitamins and minerals. Vegetables like bok choy, cauliflower, kale and cabbage supply much more calcium, for example, than milk, plus anti-cancer factors, according to the National Academy of Sciences.

Raw vegetables provide a source of enzymes to the body which are critically important nutrients. If any part of a balanced eco-system can be determined to be the most important, enzymes would surely be it for numerous reasons. Enzymes rule over all other nutrients, because they are responsible for nearly every facet of life and health, far outweighing the importance of other nutrients.

Because enzymes are needed to help control all mental and physical functions, each body cell has in excess of 100,000 enzyme particles, necessary for metabolic processes. Enzymes cannot function properly without the presence of other substances, known as coenzymes which are minerals, vitamins and PROTEINS. Once enzymes have completed their appointed task, they are destroyed. Thus, for life to continue, a person must have a constant enzyme supply which requires CONTINUAL REPLACEMENT OR RECONSTRUCTION OF ENZYMES.

Enzymes are found in all living cells, including raw foods, or those cooked at a temperature lower than 116 degrees Fahrenheit (temperature of the food item itself, not the heat source). Enzymes begin to perish when the temperature of the food substance exceeds 116 degrees. Different enzymes perish at different temperatures. Therefore, some enzymes can only last a short while at skillet temperatures of around 250 degrees F. The degree of enzyme destruction is a function of time and temperature.

Primarily, enzymes are proteins; yet enzymes need amino acids for normal function. Hormones are primarily proteins which require interaction with enzymes to regulate body processes. Enzymes aid in transforming proteins into amino acids. Protein does not perform its function unless broken down into amino acids. Amino acids can be considered as enzyme carriers whose function is to transport enzymes to various functions in the body.

Enzymes help to extract minerals from food. They transform chelated (amino acid bound) minerals into an alkaline detoxifying agent which combines with acid cellular wastes and toxic settlements within the body, thus neutralizing them and preparing them for elimination. Enzymes use minerals to create an even balance of dissolved solids both inside and outside of the cells, thus equalizing both internal and external pressures which is called "osmotic equilibrium."

Vitamins are required as coenzymes to work with enzymes in every chemical reaction in every cell of the body. Without minerals extracted from food by enzymes, vitamins would be unable to perform their function. Consequently, we have a hierarchy of nutrient importance with enzymes at the top, followed by proteins, minerals and vitamins. Such a hierarchy can make a person wonder why health-conscious people take vitamin supplements when, in effect, vitamins are the least important nutrients.

Finally, enzymes play an important role in cardiovascular health. There are specific enzymes to protect the arteries from the damaging effects of free radicals which are the cause for the build-up of arterial plaque. Therefore, cardiovascular disease is directly associated with the quantity of enzymes versus the quantity of free radicals. Free radicals occur especially when people eat fried foods, or foods with chemical additives. If people subsist on diets depleted of enzymes, such as cooked and processed foods, and if they have a steady intake of free radicals, they are subject to cardiovascular disease and early death.

So, how will you get enzymes for your body today? All you have to do is eat some raw fruit and vegetables! Because enzymes are so important for good health, it is a fine, health-promoting practice to have 6 ounces of diluted, raw vegetable or fruit juice a day from a variety of organically grown fruit or vegetables, provided that adequate fiber is included in the diet. Juices do not substitute for eating vegetables with every meal.

It is important to note that people who change their diets to ONLY RAW FRUITS AND VEGETABLES often experience temporarily improved health as they detoxify and purify the blood and lymph. But after a period of time, they waste away from inside the cells. It takes several years to notice this trend, but the electrostatic charge in the inner cell diminishes in the absence of renewed chromatin factors (RNA, DNA), amino acids, and colloidal and elemental mineral factors. The ability of the cell to attract or accept nutrients is compromised. People in this depleted state often seek professional nutritional counsel and say, "I don't feel well. I need a cleansing program to get rid of toxins." But they are misled by all the diet philosophies that stress cleansing. Instead, they need to BUILD

TISSUE with a full and varied Pro-Vita! Plan, perhaps along with low-potency, natural supplements, homeopathically prepared alfalfa tincture and specific tissue supports. If the body is built up, it can then direct its own natural cleansing mechanisms via the liver as discussed in *Your Liver-Your Lifeline* (Tips, 1990).

LIGHTLY COOKED VEGETABLES
PROVIDE CHROMATIN FACTORS

Lightly cooked vegetables provide inner cell (chromatin) factors rich in DNA and RNA which are the building blocks of body revitalization. These vital factors will be missed, or in short supply, if a person tries to subsist on strictly raw foods, because the inner cell material of raw food is encased in indigestible cellulose, unless it is broken down by light cooking. Few people have enough cellulase enzyme capability to get the chromatin factors from raw foods. Consequently, good nutrition requires both raw and lightly cooked vegetables. A full complement of enzyme support will be missed if raw foods are neglected. But if some lightly cooked foods are not included, then necessary nucleo-protein factors will be missed.

Lightly cooked vegetables are quick-steamed or quickly stir-fried in the Chinese style so that the cooking temperature in the wok or skillet does not exceed 250 degrees F, and the vegetables themselves do not get too hot or exceed 116 degrees F. At about this point of temperature the inherent enzymes start to be destroyed and heat alteration of the molecules occurs. If a vegetable is for a short while in the skillet or pot, heated to 250 degrees, the vegetable itself will not heat up to that temperature. In the Pro-Vita! Plan classes we demonstrate how to quick-cook vegetables so that they are crisp, delicious, tender and still retain their vital nutrients. To simplify this point, learn to cook with lower heat, or to cook more quickly with higher heat.

Notice the word "lightly" when we talk about cooking vegetables. Overcooked vegetables are virtually useless, because they become acid-forming and lose their ability to provide an alkaline mineral reserve. This means that the vegetables lose their ability to heal. But when lightly cooked, as in waterless cookware, by quick steaming, or gentle stir-frying, the indigestible cellulose sack that surrounds the cell nucleus is broken down, and the body can absorb the vegetable's DNA/RNA factors.

Here is an easy demonstration that you can use to verify this process of releasing chromatin factors. Juice a variety of vegetables retaining both the juice and the pulp. Use carrot, celery and maybe a little bit of beet, cabbage, parsley and green beans. Drink the juice. You may feel a little lift based on the sugar content. It is best to dilute the juice so that it is not quite so concentrated.

Next, put the pulp in a blender. Add an equal amount of boiling water. If there is one cup of pulp, add one cup of boiling water. Blend for a minute. The hot water breaks down the cellulose sack surrounding the individual cells, thus releasing the chromatin factors. Strain the fibers from the liquid. Now drink this liquid golden elixir.

What a difference! Vegetable juice is nice, but the inner cell factors are exhilarating to many people. Now you understand how some lightly cooked vegetables contribute greatly to your nutritional requirements. This is why Dirk Pearson and Sandy Shaw recommend using supplemental DNA/RNA in their "life extension through nutrition" research.

In 1930, experiments were conducted to determine at what level of cooking foods become toxic. The research report explains how our recommendation to cook a small portion of vegetables at low temperature follows the implications of this study. The entire report appears in the Appendix as "The Influence of Food Cooking on the Blood Formula of Man," by Paul Kouchakoff (Swiss) M.D., Institute of Clinical Chemistry, Lausanne, Switzerland.

To summarize the contents of Kouchakoff's vital research, always buffer your proteins with raw and some lightly cooked vegetables. This prevents a response by the immune system to the proteins, thus saving wear and tear on the immune system's lymphocytes as well as provides nucleo-proteins needed to replenish enzymes.

From this research we now know how to minimize or eliminate the toxicity problem associated with certain aspects of our nutrition. Through their living enzymes, raw vegetables buffer the effects of proteins, both cooked and raw, if the amount of the protein food is small. The vegetables also provide for safe passage of food through the bowel, thus helping with proper elimination. The minerals and vitamins contained in vegetables help with the assimilation of amino acids. Consequently, vegetables become the determining factor in our diet, whether it is healthful or stressful.

It is a sad fact that the mass-produced vegetables flooding into our supermarkets contain toxic elements, such as herbicides, pesticides, fungicides and synthetic growth stimulants. In addition, because crops are grown in depleted soils and their growth stimulated with chemical fertilizers, vegetables are also depleted of important trace elements. Fortunately, there is a rapidly growing organic produce movement underway so that we can buy truly nutritious vegetables in our supermarkets, if we seek out the organic produce.

Vegetables vary in the amount of carbohydrate (starch) that they contain. With a protein meal, the starchy vegetables should be minimized and the non-starchy vegetables maximized. With a carbohydrate meal this differentiation does not matter. The following is a guide to help focus on vegetables.

VEGETABLE CATEGORIES

Non-starchy vegetables are excellent with protein.

alfalfa sprouts (also a protein)	Lettuce
asparagus	bib lettuce
bamboo shoots	Boston lettuce
beet greens	red leaf lettuce
bell pepper, green,	romaine lettuce
red, yellow	(not iceberg*)
broccoli	
brussel sprouts	onions, green,
cabbage	parsley
green and purple	sea vegetables
cauliflower	scallions
celery	spinach
chard	sprouts, alfalfa
chicory greens	chia
collard greens	mung
cucumber (no skin)	radish
daikon radish	sunflower

dandelion greens
endive
escarole
kale
kohlrabi
garlic

green beans
sweet peppers
Swiss chard
tomatoes
turnip greens
watercress

*NOTE that iceberg lettuce is not recommended because it is depleted of nutrients and contains opiates (opium alkaloids) that retard bowel function.

Medium starchy vegetables are okay with proteins.

artichoke
beets
carrots
egg plant
chayote
corn (lightly cooked)
daikon
jicama
okra
parsnips

peas, English, snow
radish
raw summer squash
rhubarb
squash, (yellow, acorn,
    banana, pumpkin,
    spaghetti)
turnips
water chestnut
zucchini

Starchy vegetables are carbohydrates and should be avoided with proteins.

beans, boiled
cereals
grains
Jerusalem artichoke
potatoes, cooked/baked
pumpkin

rice
rutabaga
split peas
sweet potato
yams

Note that proper cooking of beans at low temperature will allow small amounts to be used with protein meals. Corn, if not cooked too long, can also be used with proteins.

Chestnuts are generally used very little with exception of macrobiotic diets. The health advantages of chestnuts are that they contain less than 2 percent fat content compared with more than 50 percent fat content of other nuts. Most importantly, the protein contained in chestnuts is a high quality vegetarian protein, similar to the protein in eggs. Though mostly carbohydrates in their make-up, a few chestnuts can be included in a protein meal. Recently, "Chestnut Hill," an Austin-based company, is reintroducing the valuable chestnuts to the U. S. Grown by a farming cooperative in the mountains in northwestern Italy, these are another important food resource for the Pro-Vita! Plan. The company not only sells chestnuts, but also is a tree nursery, developing nursery stock to help replant chestnut trees in the U. S. where large stands were destroyed by a blight in the early part of the century.

VEGETABLES AND FIBER

Vegetables are important for good health because they provide dietary fiber which is essential for health, particularly colon health. Vegetables provide an excellent fiber for bowel maintenance. Even vegetarians remark on beginning the Pro-Vita! Plan that they have never eaten so many vegetables before, especially green, leafy vegetables!

The importance of fiber in our diets is well established. When Harvey Kellogg began teaching "fiber for health" 50 years ago, the medical profession ridiculed him, but now doctors agree that fiber is important to good health.

Fiber is the part of foods that our digestive systems cannot digest and absorb, such as cellulose, pectin and gums. It is a component of all plant foods, fruit, vegetables and seaweeds. Tomatoes and strawberries provide excellent fiber. The generous amount of vegetables in the Pro-Vita! Plan provides a full complement of fiber for optimal health.

But what good is fiber, if it is indigestible? Fiber helps to regulate the transit time of foods through the intestine. It lowers the absorption of cholesterols; regulates sugar absorption by slowing it down; absorbs toxins and poisons for removal from the body; adds bulk; and softens the stool. Fiber also spreads out the concentrated foods for better digestion and absorption.

Recently, the medical profession realized that fiber has a great impact on the quality of the bloodstream, because it helps to reduce high cholesterol and triglyceride levels and assists in eliminating toxins. For this reason, for several years people have begun to add fiber to their diets in the form of wheat bran. However, recent research shows that wheat bran is not an ideal fiber, since the bran's phytic acid can deplete mineral absorption by binding important minerals, such as zinc and calcium, so that they are not absorbed. Wheat bran also can cause rapid introduction of sugars into the system, constipation and gas. Consequently, oat bran has become the fiber supplement of choice.

The best fibers are those in whole foods, such as vegetables, seeds and fruits. If people eat a proper diet as outlined by the Pro-Vita! Plan, they automatically eat an abundance of fiber. Should a person need to supplement fiber, flax seeds are an excellent source of protein and oil, providing a fine fiber as well. Guar gum, pectin and psyllium husks are also fine fibers.

People following the Pro-Vita! Plan will find their fiber needs are fully met by the diet itself. Here is a table of fiber found in Pro-Vita! vegetable foods:

Food	Quantity	Fiber (grams)
black beans	1 cup	20
broccoli	1 cup	9.5
carrot	1 medium	4
kale	1 cup	8.5
leaf lettuce	1 cup	.9
peas	1 cup	17.5
potato, red	1 medium	5.2
strawberries	1 cup	2.8

In vegetables we obtain fiber, enzymes, protein buffers, vitamins, minerals and water all in a variety of delicious packages. Ever thought of starting a small garden?

PROTEIN HUMANIZATION
REQUIRES QUALITY OILS

High quality oils enhance amino acid assimilation and utilization. Wheelwright advocated the use of high quality oils with the protein meal. Most often this use occurred as oil in salad dressings and the oils inherent in seeds. In his method of stir-frying, the vegetables were coated by hand with a light film of oil and quickly steamed in a wok. Rather than use heated oil, Wheelwright would use two tablespoons of water in the wok, thus his stir-fry was really a steaming process. He determined that the addition of high quality oil to a protein meal rounded out its nutrition because the liver requires oil to "humanize" the protein.

It is important to remember that high quality oils are essential to health. Currently, an irrational fear of oils is instilled in the American population by people of medical authority and advertisers with products to sell. The ads create fear and then focus on selling a product that puts people's minds at rest. However, the current oil-a-phobia trend will be useful only if people quit eating massive quantities of red meat, poor-quality oily foods, hydrogenated oils, excessive amounts of saturated fats and fried foods. But a trend to avoid all oils is detrimental for good nutrition and counterproductive to optimal health.

Recent research by Dr. Budwig (1988, 1992) shows how protein and oils work together for both assimilation and utilization in the body. Specifically, Budwig notes that the mixture of non-fat cottage cheese and flax seed oil enables the proteins and fatty acids to associate readily for easier digestion and assimilation.

THE WHEELWRIGHT 5 + 5 MEAL

Dr. Wheelwright designed the optimal meal for human nutrition to be a 5 + 5 meal. This meal is explained in detail in the next chapters, but it is important to introduce the concept now.

The 5 + 5 meal means to have 5 vegetables (1 cooked + 4 raw) and 5 protein foods (1 cooked + 4 raw) for the meal. The rationale and effectiveness of such a meal will be discussed further as we rediscover Wheelwright's research.

Practically speaking, a 5 + 5 meal could be as simple as grilled snapper, garden salad and asparagus.

The snapper is the cooked protein; vegetarians could have the grilled tofu. The garden salad provides our raw proteins: sunflower seeds, sesame seeds, feta cheese, alfalfa sprouts on a bed of greens. The asparagus is the cooked vegetable. The garden salad also provides the four raw vegetables, romaine lettuce, celery, carrot, tomato. A simple meal is thus terrific nutrition. We now discuss what makes this meal so special.

PROTEIN ECONOMY: STRENGTH IN VARIETY

OPTIMIZING PROTEINS

Some authorities in the health field teach that it is not necessary to eat complete proteins all in one meal, since incomplete amino acid structures will be completed later by the addition of amino acids from the lymphatic protein pool. To a certain extent this is true, and it certainly makes sense that a person may not have a full complement of protein sources available all at the same time. But this theory, or the body's ability to "make-do," does not solve the problem of amino acid deficiency at the cellular level, nor does it serve to optimize nutrition. Therefore, we now take a new look at a way of optimizing proteins and rebuilding health.

Wheelwright was quite knowledgeable in recent vegetarian research regarding proteins, but he did not agree with the conclusions that it was acceptable to let the body make up protein deficits. He once stated to me, "If it wasn't for the body's tremendous ability to cut and patch to survive, we'd see a lot more heart attacks with protein-deficient people, particularly vegetarians who do not follow my diet. The incomplete vegetable proteins cause the body to have to shift its proteins to the digestive area. If proteins are removed from the heart, or from the extracellular fluid around the heart's cells, then alkalosis results, the heart has a Charley horse, and the person dies. This fact may well be the determining factor in the case of the person who gets a heart attack after eating. Or it can happen to a protein-deficient athlete, that the amino acids can shift from the heart to the legs."

The day after Wheelwright had told me this, a famous vegetarian runner died of a heart attack while jogging. A week later, while we were in Houston, a basketball player had a heart attack after working out at the Houstonian Athletic Club, missing his consultation with Wheelwright. That evening, we went over to the athlete's hospital room where Stu drew a plate on a napkin and illustrated the food groups for an optimal meal. Wheelwright told the athlete that his life depended on it.

To explain such cases of heart attacks, we need to understand that the lymphatic pool consists of humanized amino acid structures in the lymph fluid. When the lymphatic pool has to make up the missing proteins in the intestine because a meal is incomplete, there is an approximate 20% loss of amino acids from the lymphatic pool. The body's mechanism of completing proteins is not a perfect system. The body does not reclaim all the amino acids that it puts into the intestine or combines with the new proteins. There is a surcharge for the transaction which can result in tissue breakdown over time, because the body may claim the proteins that it needs for the amino acid completion from the kidneys, heart and connective tissue. This happens particularly if the lymphatic pool is congested. Some of the borrowed amino acids are lost and may not be replaced right away.

For example, if a meal lacks two essential amino acids, the body will complete this imbalance in the small intestine using amino acids from the lymph pool or tissue. This completion process has been verified by the research of Dr. Royal Lee. The missing amino acids were derived from the lymph pool or tissue, picked up by enzymes and brought to the small intestine to complete the imbalance created there by the meal. In this process more amino acids were delivered than were needed. These extra amino acids pass out with the stool, resulting in an overall loss of available proteins. Although this example is oversimplified, the basic idea is all we need to understand at this point. To achieve the assimilation of protein, the body prefers to work with complete structures and accomplishes this even if the diet is incomplete in proteins.

For another example, let's suppose that a meal lacks an amino acid, such as L-Lysine in rice or L-tryptophan in beans. The body borrows the missing amino acid from the heart tissue matrix to complete the proteins from the meal for assimilation with the intent that the borrowed amino and will soon be replaced. But the person begins jogging and the proteins must supply the leg activity. The end result could be a weaker heart, because the borrowed amino acid was not returned to the heart right away.

The body is able to move proteins around. During exercise such as running, proteins can be stripped from one area of the body (heart, kidneys, etc.) and delivered to another area (legs) that is doing the work. Some researchers think that the high rate of heart attacks among people whose sole form of exercise is jogging, is caused by the body's loss of proteins from the heart because they are put in transit to the legs. Therefore, the concept of whole body exercise is becoming more popular. Exercise with the arms is necessary to balance the leg exercises. Moving the arms works the lymphatics (protein pool) for the organs and systems above the second lumbar (L-2) vertebrae. This way more proteins become available for organs and tissues in the upper body during exercise.

Wheelwright was concerned with this issue of protein completion, because in his research he discovered that the grain combinations, thought to provide complete proteins for vegetarians, were not working. As already explained, he surmised that even though a combination such as beans and rice was complete, the body was not rendering full protein value from the combination due to cooking and poor assimilation.

To assist with better assimilation, Wheelwright developed the herb-based formula PRO to solve the problem of the loss of viable amino acids back into the intestine. The PRO formula provides essential amino acids, minerals and enzymes. Wheelwright was of the opinion that adding PRO to the vegetarian meal would greatly enhance amino acid assimilation. Consequently, the body would be prevented from giving up its valuable amino acids to facilitate absorption of the meal.

THE LAW OF ECONOMY

If complete proteins are eaten at a meal, there is no need for the body to do the costly work of making up deficits of amino acids. Therefore, relying on the protein pool is actually a back-up system, a survival system. Knowing this process of compensation, we now have the ability to "live smart" and create good health, rather than "just making do."

Just because the body has the ability to compensate amino acid imbalances does not mean that we should make it do so. The liver has the important task of humanizing, organizing and restructuring proteins. If the liver is sluggish, a person will have more difficulty working with proteins. But when complete protein structures are readily available, the liver does not have to work as hard.

Making complete proteins available for the body is a law of economy which means longer life.

From another perspective, if amino acid proteins from a meal are not balanced, the body will use the given protein only to the level of its amino acid in shortest supply. When the essential amino acid in shortest supply runs out, the rest of the amino acids are extraneous and are excreted as waste (urea), stored as fat or converted to glucose for energy. As a result, it is easy to waste a million amino acids for want of a single essential amino acid. An analogy is trying to play Scrabble® with the vowels missing. Providing complete sources of amino acids maximizes what the body can do with its raw materials.

Another important point is that incomplete or unbalanced proteins tax the liver. If the liver is healthy, it can convert the essential amino acids into most of what the body needs to be healthy. If the liver is toxic, swollen, alkaline, sluggish, over-oxidized or congested, it is best to provide a small and complete supply of low-stress amino acids. Then the liver does not have to work so hard and can cleanse and repair itself as well as perform its myriad other functions. Thus, the Pro-Vita! Plan automatically assists the liver.

The liver has other functions besides organizing proteins and cleansing poor protein by-products. One important function is recycling hormones so that the glands do not become fatigued. The liver functions are explained in more detail in the book *Your Liver-Your Lifeline!* (Tips, 1990). We often forget that it is not what we eat that nourishes the body, but what the liver processes.

Proteins from different sources will have different digestive qualities and will yield different amino acid structures. It is highly unlikely that one source of protein can supply all of the essential amino acids, particularly if the liver is not functioning well. Although meat provides a complete protein, it is not an optimal food overall, because meat is cooked or altered by heat, and most meats contain the residue of antibiotics, growth hormones and pesticides. Consequently, selecting proteins from varied sources can provide far greater nutritional value. The fact that a variety of foods is a key to health and longevity also applies to protein sources.

Another important fact is that proteins help each other synergistically, because they assist each other to become more complete and assimilable. This is particularly true of seeds, because they help assimilation of other protein structures. Therefore, seeds—soaked overnight in pineapple juice or water—are a vital protein source.

There is much discussion regarding the body's ability to digest different proteins in the same meal amongst food combiners—people who follow the hygienic philosophy of combining or not combining certain foods in an exclusively raw food diet. Since the Pro-Vita! Plan treads in questionable areas as far as the strict hygienist rule of not eating more than one concentrated protein in a meal, we address this issue.

The Pro-Vita! Plan's protein meal consists of 65-75% vegetables, both lightly cooked and raw. The protein portion consists of varied sources, usually five, to provide a wide variety of amino acid structures and protein synergists. Most important is the point that the Pro-Vita! Plan capitalizes on low-stress proteins which are the easiest to digest.

We agree that the food combining rule, "Don't eat two concentrated proteins in one meal," is valid in respect to combining beef and milk, or egg and pork. But this rule is superseded by the Pro-Vita! Plan's use of comparatively large amounts of vegetables with its proteins. Because of this novel vegetable combination rule, the Pro-Vita! Plan's proteins are not concentrated. In any event, high-stress proteins are not considered to be viable for daily use in the Pro-Vita! Plan as discussed earlier. Milk, beef, soybeans (Textured Vegetable Protein), large amounts of raw nuts and pork are high-stress proteins and to be avoided in a low-stress meal. Consequently, low stress proteins, eaten with vegetables, are a completely different nutritional situation than milk together with greasy gravy on roast beef.

Combining a variety of protein sources has the advantage of synergism as well as completeness. "Synergism" means that the total is greater than the sum of the parts. The varied protein sources provide different factors. For example, the proteins from soaked, partially germinated seeds act to transmit protein values to the cells. They help the other protein structures to be more usable. Seeds such as sunflower, sesame, pumpkin, squash, chia and flax are an important part of building protein values at the cellular level. The use of soaked seeds is absolutely essential for a vegetarian diet to succeed.

We summarize an important principle of the Pro-Vita! Plan. Although the body does not have to have complete proteins, that is, all essential amino acids, at one meal; it is optimal nutrition to eat complete proteins. Providing complete and balanced proteins to the body improves assimilation, thus reducing the wear and tear on vital organs and conserving the body's resources. The simple addition of sprouts and seeds to a meal greatly enhances its protein nutritional value. Sprouts and seeds are a consistent part of the Pro-Vita! Plan.

THE OPTIMAL TIME
FOR PROTEIN FOODS

THE VALUE OF BREAKFAST

To know when a food should be eaten, it is important to understand when it is metabolized; how or if it is stored in the body; when its energy is released; and when its by-products are detoxified and eliminated from the body.

From this perspective, there is an optimal time to eat protein, there is an adequate time, and there is a detrimental time. Knowing the times to maximize your protein values provides you the ability to choose and eat wisely. The same holds true for the carbohydrates and fruit. However, vegetables are universal because they can be eaten any time of day.

After years of research, Wheelwright established several forthright rules of the optimal times for the body to eat, digest, assimilate, utilize and discard its nutrition. Wheelwright's discovery of the optimal times for protein consumption represents a major innovation in the traditional food combining plans. Therefore, the concept of the optimal time is a crucial and novel feature of the Pro-Vita! Plan. Here are Wheelwright's time parameters.

6:30 am -	2:00 pm	low-stress protein consumption
12:30 pm -	7:30 pm	protein digestion, assimilation, humanization
7:30 am -	9:00 pm	mild exercise for protein utilization
12:30 pm -	6:30 am	most restful sleep

Another point concerning the optimal time for food consumption and digestion relates to the pH factor. During his research, Wheelwright experimented with a variety of pH norms including a range of 5.5 - 6.4 for several years until further research showed that range to be too acid. Thus, according to his studies, the optimal values rose to 6.4 - 6.8 with daily swings between 5.8 and 6.8, where they remained. Since Wheelwright's studies, many other authorities agree on these pH values, so now 5.8 to 6.8 is a widely accepted optimal range.

Wheelwright also experimented with the best time to have the major meal of the day, and whether it should be breakfast or lunch. For a while, he tried to place the major meal at 11:00 am to coincide with the time the pH completed its morning acid swing and had just begun its alkaline swing. As research continued, the trend for the major meal became earlier and earlier in the day.

However, if we consider his entire research, we can generalize that it is best to eat the major protein meal before 11:00 a.m. Some people are ready for this meal early in the morning or soon after arising. Others, however, are not ready to eat until they get a few hours into the day. Body typing according to glandular dominance can play a role in when the body is ready for the first meal, so each individual should endeavor to eat the first meal early in the day within the parameters of what works well.

Early in the day, the protein digestive enzymes are strongest because they were replenished during the rest and rebuilding time of the night before. Also, at this time the overall digestive processes are at their strongest point. The body is moving into the acid (high-energy) metabolic swing of its pH cycle, and there is time enough during the day for the body to process the protein while still awake and active. You might want to consult the section on the body's pH cycle to understand this important aspect of timing the consumption of proteins.

The point about timing the major meal is quite simple. Protein foods are best introduced to the body early in the day, so they become available when we want to be active and productive. Carbohydrates and alkaline foods are best eaten in the meal preceding sleep, because they are more sedative in their effect. These foods also support the cleansing of the acidic metabolic wastes during sleep.

Breakfast is the crucial meal in the Pro-Vita! Plan. The body heads into its acid swing, which peaks around 9:00 am. Breakfast eaten a couple of hours earlier, takes the edge off that swing, because the digestion process itself causes a slight pull to the alkaline and provides stability to blood sugar. The initial digestion of the vegetables in the meal causes a slight alkaline pull on the system within 30 minutes of eating. Later, the proteins from breakfast will set up a mild acid field in the body and help keep the metabolism stable during its alkaline swing.

However, fruits eaten for breakfast cause severe alkaline swings. One swing derives from the digestive process, and a greater one from the quick digestion and rendering of alkalizing minerals, resulting in an inhibition of the productive acid swing in pH. A stronger swing into alkaline in the afternoon occurs as a further result of eating fruit for breakfast and can cause post-prandial drowsiness and hypoglycemia.

Thus, eating protein properly for breakfast works to stabilize the natural pH swing. Eight hours later, in mid afternoon, the proteins have been digested, assimilated and are being used. At this time, the body pH is swinging into alkaline pH. Then the proteins buffer that swing, preventing alkalosis and low blood sugar, thus preventing fatigue or the need for sweets and coffee.

Consequently, when the natural pH swing is towards the acid side in the morning, eating the Pro-Vita! breakfast helps to prevent a too-acid swing, while still maintaining the productive acid swing. Concurrently, the breakfast supplies the nutrients which will prevent a too-alkaline swing in the afternoon. Obviously, the Pro-Vita! breakfast is a vital meal because it works to balance the pH and blood sugar cycles, thus providing stamina and stability.

It is often the case that when fruit is eaten for breakfast over an extended period of time, the fruit causes less of an acid swing, but then an excessive momentum is given for the alkaline swing. This results in a loss of productive energy and blood sugar stability. Moreover, this situation taxes the body to compensate its pH swing in the afternoon. Complex carbohydrates, which are mildly acid, when eaten for breakfast can support the acid swing, but cause the release of seratonin in the brain resulting in a tranquilizing effect. This may be fine for people with too much energy, but most people require good mental energy for the day's work.

An analogy is the pendulum on a clock. Optimally, we want it to swing a little to the left and an equal amount to the right. The Pro-Vita! breakfast keeps the pH swing moderate and balanced. In contrast, a fruit or carbohydrate breakfast inhibits the acid swing too much and pushes the pendulum the other way resulting in an imbalanced alkaline swing.

When we talk about eating fruit only for breakfast, we do not mean a half of a grapefruit before a regular meal. However, the person who drinks a large glass of orange juice and eats a banana in the car on the way to work is not building good health overall. Of course, the orange juice and banana are far superior to coffee and donuts and certainly don't contribute to a major toxic problem as bacon would! And a fruit breakfast would be beneficial when a large, heavy supper is eaten the night before. The fruit gives the overstressed digestion a rest and helps move the poorly digested food on out.

In the Chinese acupuncture tradition, 7-9 a.m. is the time when the stomach meridian activates and rules the body's energetic system. (Refer to the Meridian Clock in the chapter, "Natural Body Cycles and Nutrition.") Therefore, this is the time for the sustaining meal and the time for consuming the majority of nutrients, calories and the bulk of the diet. The Pro-Vita! Plan follows the Chinese tradition by emphasizing a light but hearty breakfast of vegetables and proteins.

NATURAL pH CYCLE OF
THE BODY AND NUTRITION

Further examination of how diet and the pH cycles can complement or interfere with each other, will help show why a Pro-Vita! breakfast is important to vitality and health. Here is the normal pH chart for reference.

NATURAL pH CYCLE OF THE BODY

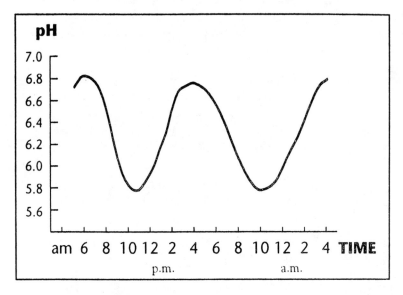

In the chart of the natural pH cycle you can see how a meal eaten between 6:00 and 8:00 am can buffer the acid drop which dips to its lowest point shortly thereafter. Eight hours later, the digested amino acids are available for metabolic activity and stabilize the alkaline swing's peak around 3:30 to 4:00 pm. When this occurs, it is easy for the body to maintain a more optimal pH without the stress of excessive swings.

But proteins eaten late in the day at 7 p.m. can interfere with the restful and regenerative alkaline sleep cycle, which peaks around 3 a.m. eight hours later. They can also interfere with the liver's cleanse cycle.

In effect, proteins eaten later in the day, after 2 or 3 pm, cause many problems. They are not properly digested or completely metabolized during sleep and thus contribute to a toxic overload of the lymph and blood. The lymphatic system sleeps when you sleep and is dependent upon exercise to circulate. The lymphatic system as protein pool transports amino acids and acts as a waste-disposal system. Proteins eaten late in the day can sit in the sleeping lymphatic system and cause congestion, since they are not properly metabolized. This situation holds true especially for people who eat meat at night as well as for people who consume heavy or complex vegetable protein (soy beans, nuts, etc,) at night. Both the meat eater and the vegetarian can end up with congested lymphatics, if proteins are eaten late in the day.

In contrast, proteins eaten for breakfast can signal the protein pool to release amino acids and nutrients for immediate use by the body, because the body knows that more amino acids are on the way. The amino acids released from the protein pool can then be used for energy and to build the tissue integrity. The newly digested amino acids replenish the pool, since the body (and therefore the lymphatic system) is still active eight hours later in the day, when the protein has been digested and processed by the liver.

As the body transits into its building cycle in the afternoon, the proteins from breakfast are digested enough to provide a good preliminary report to the brain as to what amino acids will become available. Therefore, the body can safely begin to use its proteins.

Since most people are active during the day, the lymphatic system is also working. As a result, proteins can be delivered to the cells to renew the life processes during the building cycle, which lasts until around midnight.

However, if proteins are eaten late in the day, the time for their metabolism arrives when the body is sleeping and going into a cleansing mode. These proteins interfere with sleep, are not available to build tissue and become toxic wastes. This situation is a major problem for people trying to follow the hygienically-based "fruit for breakfast, protein for supper" plan as prescribed in "Fit for Life" diets, and explains why such diets lead to poor tissue integrity over time.

The following chart portrays how proteins eaten late in the day not only create toxic stress if they are not digested properly, but do not cooperate with the natural pH cycles.

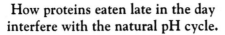

How proteins eaten late in the day
interfere with the natural pH cycle.

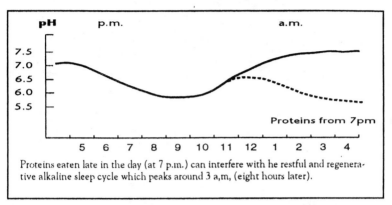

Proteins eaten late in the day (at 7 p.m.) can interfere with he restful and regenerative alkaline sleep cycle which peaks around 3 a,m, (eight hours later).

One of the highly-promoted "fruit for breakfast" diets advises people to cleanse on fruit until noon and eat protein for supper. But this plan is completely backwards. The protein eaten late in the day becomes toxic and actually creates the need to cleanse on fruit in the morning to extend the detoxification time. This type of diet puts people into a pattern of creating toxins and having to spend a lot of time cleansing them. Such a diet is a toxify-detoxify pattern with no time to BUILD the body. Most fruits do not build tissue, instead they cleanse. However, eaten in the afternoon and "in the season thereof," fruits can renew tissues.

OPTIMAL PROTEIN DIGESTION

Looking even deeper into the crucial protein issue, the basic fact is that protein digestion is critical to protein use. Looking back at Wheelwright's seven rules for consumption of low-stress protein, we notice that six of the seven rules deal with digestion: Eat protein 1) early in the day, 2) in small portions, 3) with a variety of vegetables, 4) without carbohydrates, 5) without liquids, and 6) do not snack on protein.

When proteins are eaten early in the day, the body provides its best digestive powers, such as hydrochloric acid, protease enzymes, chymotrypsin. The factors required to construct these enzymes have been recharged or renewed during the fasting/sleep period. Wheelwright commented once that if carbohydrate foods are eaten regularly for breakfast, components of the protein enzymes are not made available and are used for other enzymatic duties, thus weakening the body's ability to handle proteins eaten later in the day.

As discussed in the chapter on "Glorious Vegetables," enzymes play a key role in the process of protein assimilation. Enzymes are constructed, reconstructed and "on demand" where needed most. The protein-digesting enzymes are available in the morning, unless the dietary pattern teaches the body to be prepared for morning carbohydrates. In contrast, the protease enzymes are not so readily available in the evening, if their components have already been used for other body processes. If proteins are eaten late in the day, the enzymes have to be constructed, depriving other enzymatic functions in the body.

Because enzymes are a major factor in longevity, eating protein early in the day conserves and supports the enzymatic functions. The proteins eaten early can then build new enzymes via their amino acids and support all aspects of the body's metabolic processes.

Clearly, protein is one of the most difficult foods to digest. Unless the proper enzymes are provided, the eaten protein will not be made available to the body and will contribute instead to the body's toxic load through indigestion and putrefaction. As any colon hygienist knows, one cannot have good health with toxic fermentation or putrefaction in the bowel.

Unless proteins are eaten properly, a person is better off not eating protein at all. This means that it is probably better to be a little protein-deficient than to be protein-toxic. Both conditions cause ill health. But toxic protein causes degeneration quicker, because the body has the ability to temporarily make up an amino acid deduction by borrowing the missing ones from tissue. Protein toxicity must be cleansed through the bowel, lymphatics, liver and kidneys, causing a lot of stress throughout the body. Protein toxicity is a direct cause of cancer. The point here is that it is probably better to have low energy and low tissue integrity but still have the ability to replinish proteins than it is to have to fight cancer. However, both protein toxicity and deficiencies can be solved by following the nutritional principles of the Pro-Vita! Plan.

It is crucial to note that after the hydrochloric acid in the stomach takes the lead role in digesting protein, the remaining digestion is left up to enzymes. It is important to remember at this point that enzymes are made up of amino acids. Consequently, if a person is low in protein, the ability to digest and assimilate proteins is reduced. Fortunately, nutritionists can help to rebuild the digestive system with dietary recommendations, herbs and enzymes to support the weak organs and glands (pancreas, liver, duodenal stomach, intestine, hypothalamus).

Homeopathy is an effective therapy to rebuild a weak digestive system and strengthen the body's abilities to digest and synthesize proteins. Such therapy can be used to enhance the nutritional results of the Pro-Vita! Plan.

From a pH perspective, proteins generate an acid field in the body. If proteins are eaten late in the day, the body pH becomes acid during sleep, causing poor sleep. But the best sleep and dream state occurs when the body is in a mildly alkaline pH. When in an acid state, the oxygen content is reduced and sleep is fitful, as the body wakes, tosses and turns to get oxygen to the brain.

For these reasons, people bothered by poor sleep should eat proteins early and carbohydrates late in the day. Carbohydrates tranquilize the brain through the release of endorphins. Poor sleepers usually require adrenal gland nutritional support earlier in the day to help the body hold on to its alkaline minerals and electrolytes.

Homeopathy provides excellent results for people troubled by sleep difficulties and who will not solve their sleeping problems with drugs such as sleeping pills. Tranquilizers and sedatives do nothing about the acid pH or the lack of oxygen to the brain. Consequently, these drugs only force the body to sleep in an oxygen-deficient state.

To summarize this information about optimal digestion of proteins, the major, protein meal should be eaten earlier in the day. Having the Pro-Vita! 5 + 5 meal for breakfast is excellent timing for optimal nutrition because it

- maximizes digestive capabilities;

- supports energy metabolism co-operation with natural pH cycles;

- maintains consistent blood sugar;

- supports the body's natural abilities and exercise to distribute and help to utilize amino acids;

- allows proper removal of metabolic waste products.

Wheelwright was quite adamant about his dietary rule, "Don't eat protein after 2 pm." Of course, few people wanted to listen to him, because culturally Americans and many people in the world are accustomed to eating meat for supper. Also, many people like to get together socially with other people for supper.

However, Wheelwright would never modify this important rule, "Eat protein early in the day; do not eat protein after 2 pm." He felt very strongly that protein eaten late in the day was toxic and caused disease. Eaten properly with vegetables, early in the day, protein becomes a sustainer of the body's myriad processes.

Wheelwright was fond of the adage, "Eat like a king for breakfast and like a pauper for supper." Even if you eat like a king for breakfast, a prince for lunch and a pauper for supper, you will be miles ahead of those who starve for breakfast and pig-out for supper!

As a point to clarify the Pro-Vita! perspective, I have cited important differences between hygienic fit-for-life philosophy and Wheelwright's research. I would like to clarify that I agree with much of the information presented by Harvey and Marilyn Diamond in their nutrition classic *Fit For Life* (1985) and am grateful for their pioneering work. The major difference presented here is that proteins are best eaten in the morning, and fruit in the afternoon and evening.

PROTEIN:
A LITTLE GOES A LONG WAY

EAT PROTEIN IN A MEAL—NOT AS A SNACK

Wheelwright taught that snacking on proteins, such as cheese, nuts, peanuts, or meats, depletes the body's digestive powers. Proteins are the most difficult foods to properly digest and require a considerable amount of energy for digestion. Therefore, protein snacks are inadvisable since they require hard digestive labor from the body and thus deplete its digestive powers. Fruit, vegetables and carbohydrates make better snacks.

Since proteins take a long time to digest, it is likely that a snack protein will be overtaken by the next meal. If a person has a proper protein breakfast, then ideally lunch should come four-and-a-half hours later without any snacks in between. The body uses energy for other processes besides digesting food. If a person chooses to snack, things like celery, carrot sticks and popcorn (cooked by hot air rather than in oil) are preferable. Fruit also makes a good afternoon snack item. Some people use frozen organic red grapes as a popsicle-type snack in the summertime.

The Pro-Vita! Plan provides stable blood sugar and full nutritional values. The desire for in-between meal snacks naturally decreases as this takes effect—usually within two to three months.

Unfortunately, most people want to snack on sweets, candy, desserts and other high-stress items. One advantage of the protein-and-vegetable Pro-Vita! breakfast is that the detrimental effect of sweet snacks eaten in the afternoon is minimized due to the strong metabolic pattern established by the breakfast.

The best advice is to avoid snacks altogether, or to use snack time to boost nutrition with a small organic carrot/vegetable juice. But if you do choose to snack, use fruits, vegetables and carbohydrates. If you succumb to the cookie urge, late afternoon is the least detrimental time. But have a glass of vegetable juice with it. No deprivation—just hedging your bet. Adding a couple of raw vegetables, or vegetable juice, to a sweet snack will help prevent activation of the immune system against the high-stress snack, and it will help conserve energy by adding enzymes. Just add a carrot and a celery stick to your cookie snack and you will fare much better.

Keep in mind that a strong craving for sweets is a classic symptom of protein deficiency at the cellular level. Build your protein values as explained in this book and the sugar craving will go away, usually in three to four weeks. If a person is preoccupied with this symptom of craving sweets, homeopathic remedies, such as Lycopodium, Argentum nitricum, Sulphur, Calcarea carbonicum, may be recommended to accelerate the internal changes for a balanced metabolism.

It is interesting to note that many of the homeopathic remedies that help with the sugar craving symptom check out energetically in the protein-enhancing matrix, usually through stimulating the liver. Other remedies seem to balance the hormonal system. Thus, craving sugar is a symptom of metabolic dysfunction. From the bioenergetic perspective, a correction in this disturbance of the vital force results in a balanced carbohydrate metabolism which is a physiological system dependent upon amino acids.

The important point is that with proper nutrition based on the Pro-Vita! Plan, the desire for snacks disappears. A well-nourished system does not keep the "appestat button" (the hypothalamus and pituitary) pushed, calling for more nutrients. Blood sugar becomes stable, and stamina and steadfast energy become new characteristics. Stabilization of the blood sugar takes effect usually within three weeks to three months after beginning a proper Pro-Vita! regime.

Snacking on protein is not a way to cure hypoglycemia as some people are led to believe. Frequent introduction of proteins to the digestive system will ultimately weaken a person. The proteins should come from a balanced, complete meal. And snacks, which are often needed temporarily until health improves, should be complex carbohydrate with raw vegetables.

EAT PROTEIN IN SMALL PORTIONS

Small portions of food is a general rule for good digestion regardless of what the meal may consist. People constantly eat too much food. When the volume is bigger than the digestive system can handle, the result is waste and toxins from fermentation. Eating too much can result in nutritional deficiencies and disease.

Stomachs have a variety of sizes and shapes, but as a general rule, 14 ounces by weight of food is all the human stomach can handle. Many (particularly American) stomachs are expanded and distended due to stuffing them too full time and again. Then, when they are not stuffed too full, they feel hungry. After eating smaller portions for a couple of weeks, the stomach can shrink back to a more normal size and the abnormal hunger impulse will not continue.

Ultimately, smaller meals result in more nutrition, more energy and greater health. The fact is that smaller meals mean longer life!

Earlier we discussed how 22 to 30 grams of Pro-Vita! protein per 100 pounds of body weight could do the work of the current standard endorsed by many nutritionists of approximately 50 grams per 100 pounds of body weight. Here is a table on common protein sources and how many grams are potentially available. Please understand that some of the best protein sources are low in protein, and some high protein sources are mostly unavailable to the body. Often tables like these, derived from biochemistry, are worthless unless we understand that bioenergy and bioavailability must be included when analyzing protein. QUALITY, not quantity, counts when working for optimum health. Pro-Vita! proteins are marked with an asterisk (*).

Dairy Food	Quantity	Gm/Protein
milk, whole (cow)	1 cup	8
milk, skim (cow)	1 cup	9
milk, powdered, whole	1 cup	27
milk, powdered, skim	1 cup	29
yogurt	1 cup	8
ice cream	1 cup	5

Dairy Food	Quantity	Gm/Protein
cottage cheese* (nonfat, low-fat, raw milk)	1 cup	34
feta cheese*	1 cup	4
egg, yard or range*	one	7

Meat and Fish	Quantity	Gm/Protein
chicken, organic*	3 ounces	25
turkey, organic (medium stress food)*	3 ounces	27
beef or veal	3 ounces	23
cod*	3 ounces	27
haddock*	3 ounces	16
halibut*	3 ounces	26
octopus*	3 ounces	19
scallops*	3 ounces	17
squid*	3 ounces	20
shrimp*	3 ounces	21
tuna, fresh*	3 ounces	25

Vegetables	Quantity	Gm/Protein
asparagus	6 stalks	1
beans, sprouted, cooked below 200° F*	1 cup	15
bean sprouts*	1 cup	16
broccoli	1 cup	2
soybeans	1 cup	22
lentils, sprouted, cooked below 200° F*	1 cup	15

Cereals and Grains	Quantity	Gm/Protein
bread, whole wheat	1 slice	2
corn bread	1 piece	3
oatmeal	1 cup	5
rice, brown	1 cup	15
shredded wheat	1 ounce	3

Protein should be consumed in context of the 5 + 5 meal, not as a snack. Small portions are the rule for good protein digestion and to avoid the excesses so prevalent in today's chronic degenerative lifestyles.

PROTECTING PROTEIN DIGESTION

ABOUT HYDROCHLORIC ACID

Drinking liquids while eating proteins dilutes the hydrochloric acid (HCl) needed to digest the proteins. This is a particularly important point for people with candida (yeast overgrowth), since the HCl is also a first-line defense against bacteria and yeast entering the small intestine.

A dog's digestive juices are approximately 4% HCl. For this reason dogs are able to eat garbage and partially rotted, putrid meat and not become sick. The strong HCl takes care of the bacteria.

A human's HCl can be 1% strong, but seldom is. It is generally much lower primarily due to poor eating habits, worry, stress and activities such as smoking tobacco, drinking alcohol and using marijuana. All of these detrimental habits exhaust the parietal cells that manufacture hydrochloric acids. HCl is necessary to activate the enzyme pepsin to continue the digestion of proteins. When liquids are drunk with meals, the already weak HCl is further diluted, perhaps to a point where pepsin is not even activated. As a result, protein digestion is ruined and the ever-present bacteria begin to ferment the mass. This fermentation causes many toxins in the bowel that impact the liver through the portal vein. In this way disease begins.

Nutritionally and bioecologically, prescription medications such as Tagamet can be very detrimental. Often given for ulcers, such drugs inhibit the parietal cells' ability to make hydrochloric acid. Without HCl the body cannot properly digest proteins, and it loses its first-line defense against yeast, fungus, bacteria, virus and parasites entering the body through the gastro-intestinal tract. Fortunately, there are very effective herbal and homeopathic treatments for ulcers that do not inhibit digestion or cause dangerous side effects.

Most people's HCl is too weak. This is particularly true of people on salt-free diets, since the chloride in sodium chloride (salt) can help replenish the hydro**chloric** acid. HCl is an inorganic chemical manufactured by the body. Inorganic salt not processed through plants is perfectly capable of replenishing the HCl. Sea salt that has not been refined by kiln-drying and is therefore not heat-altered is preferable.

For a healthy body, a little salt is valuable. But for an unhealthy body, excessive salt is detrimental. Salt is not detrimental in its intrinsic value because we need sodium chloride ions to live. But the metabolic aspect of salt as an anabolic and alkaline substance can adversely affect people who are too anabolic or alkaline in their metabolism. This fact is discussed in detail in *The Next Step to Greater Energy* (Tips, 1990). Salt should not be blamed for high blood pressure. Instead, we need to examine our excessive use of it.

Dr. Emanuel Revici (1961) discovered how to balance salt so that its effects would not be too anabolic, or excessively alkalizing. He added magnesium thiosulphate (1 part magnesium thiosulphate to 15 parts salt) to salt to bring it to balance and make it a beneficial food and source of electrolytes. But the FDA banned this mixture as a food, claiming that there was no nutritional value in magnesium thiosulphate even though it is widely used in Europe. You can improve the salt you use by adding garlic powder. The sulphur in garlic helps to balance the sodium in salt.

STIMULATING HYDROCHLORIC ACID PRODUCTION

Many cultures have methods of boosting HCl production prior to meals. The Japanese have used salt plum and pickled ginger root as an appetizer. The salt plus the acetic acid in the vinegar are the two precursors which the parietal cells require to make HCl.

In the Near East it is quite common to chew a few fennel or anise seeds to encourage the digestive juices thus avoiding gastritis and acid rebound. In many Mediterranean villages people commonly chew a couple of raisins before eating.

In Mexico and here in Texas the hot salsa serves as an appetizer. It is enzyme-rich if it is fresh. However, the chips usually eaten with the salsa are undesirable due to the high amount of rancid oil they contain. A person is much better off dipping celery and other vegetables in the salsa, or perhaps using the soft tortillas, or the homemade chips described earlier, if the meal is to include a focus on carbohydrate.

People with weak hydrochloric acid can boost their HCl levels and their digestive systems by taking one teaspoon of vinegar such as apple cider vinegar, rice wine vinegar, or umeboshi plum vinegar; plus one teaspoon of sea water in three ounces of pure water 30 minutes before a meal. These products are available in most natural food stores. People with candidiasis can use white distilled vinegar since it does not contain live yeasts as does the recommended vinegars. In this therapy the vinegar is used for its acid, not its other nutrients.

It is always a good idea to add 1/4 teaspoon of cream of tartar to vinegars other than apple cider vinegar to provide potassium so that the vinegar won't cause a mineral depleting action. Apple cider vinegar is already rich in potassium, but is usually aggravating to people with candidiasis because it contains live yeasts. Distilled vinegars do not contain live yeasts. The minerals and the vinegar acids can work together to replenish the parietal cells so that HCl can be produced. Further information on this subject is contained in *Conquer Candida* (Tips, 1989).

PROTEIN POWDERS

Some people try to supplement their protein intake by drinking protein drinks or brewer's yeast drinks. This is not advisable since proteins need to mix with hydrochloric acid in the stomach. If protein is taken in the liquid medium, there is no bulk for the stomach to recognize. Therefore, the proteins quickly pass undi-gested into the intestine where they putrefy and burden the body with large-chain amino acid structures.

If the protein powders contain soy, they are even harder for the body to process. It is not uncommon for people who use "hi-pro" protein powder drinks too long, or too frequently, to develop high toxic levels, weak livers and kidneys, acidosis and eventually allergies.

In summary, it is best not to drink liquids with a protein meal. A good schedule for getting water is to drink 8 oz. of pure water after getting up in the morning. Then eat breakfast 30 minutes later without liquids. A couple of hours later, you can drink more water, if you are thirsty. If a person does not indulge in recreational beverages such as sodas, coffee and teas, the natural thirst of the body will be able to guide when and how much to drink. This method will ensure adequate water intake as well as proper digestion of proteins.

This ends our discussion of Wheelwright's seven rules of proper dietary use of proteins. You will find that by following his advice, your nutritional health dramatically improves. For a quick review, his rules are as follows:

- Eat protein away from carbohydrates.

- Have vegetables with protein.

- Have a little high quality oil with proteins.

- Eat complete protein combinations.

- Eat protein-based meals early in the day.

- Avoid protein snacks. Eat them as meals.

- Avoid excessive liquids with protein meals.

The more you follow these rules, the more you will preserve your digestive power and build your health and vitality. If it is necessary, or a matter of choice, to break these rules, use a digestive supplement such as Wheelwright's formula D (Digestive), for help in the short term.

PART III

HOW TO MANAGE THE PRO-VITA! PLAN

This section provides useful information how to implement the Pro-Vita! Plan from day to day.

HOW TO PREPARE
LOW-STRESS PROTEINS

SOAKED SEEDS

Fresh organic seeds are a wonderful, sustaining protein source, because they enliven other proteins and help with assimilation and utilization of essential amino acids. Seeds act as transistors and synergizers that make other proteins work better. The best way to use seeds is to soak them in water or pineapple juice overnight. This soaking process helps to break down the proteins for easier and more effective digestion.

Put a mixture of organic seeds (one Tbsp. of each), such as hulled sunflower, pumpkin, squash and sesame into an eight ounce glass. Add pineapple juice or water to completely cover the seeds. (Use juice that comes in glass bottles.) Stir briefly so that all the seeds have a chance to sink to the bottom of the glass. Discard any seeds that float since they are rancid. Place the glass into the refrigerator and leave it overnight. In the morning, scoop out the seeds that you need for breakfast. These seeds will be plump and firm. Leave the rest of the seeds for the next meal.

If you like a softer, more gelatinous texture, add flax and chia seeds. These seeds become somewhat slimy like mucilage Many people enjoy the texture and these seeds certainly help the bowels to function with ease.

The pineapple juice prevents molds and fungus spores from forming while the seeds soak and helps break down the proteins. Seeds can also be soaked in pure water that has been treated with a few drops of stabilized oxygen such as Aerobic 07®, because this provides an aerobic environment detrimental to mold or fungus. A teaspoon of 3% hydrogen peroxide can be used to protect the water. But this procedure is not optimal since we want to avoid the oxidation of the oils in the seeds. It is best not to use tap water for soaking because of the chemicals in it. In a pinch, use tap water and only soak an ounce of seeds overnight to eat the next morning. Then obtain water, fit for consumption, to soak the seeds.

Soaked seeds will last several days in the refrigerator. They are firm, chewy and delicious. Their flavor is better than that of dry seeds. Choose a variety of organic seeds and make them a staple of your diet. This vegetarian source of amino acids is essential for good health.

RAW RED POTATO JUICE

According to Dr. Wheelwright, the protein in raw red potatoes is one of the highest quality proteins available. Red potatoes contain only about 2% protein, but it occurs with a copper-bearing vitamin C with the enzyme tyrosenase which is an extremely rare and valuable nutrient.

In naturopathy, the science of healing the body according to the laws of nature, raw red potato juice is given rectally to children with colds and pneumonia. This simple treatment has helped many people and has achieved many "miraculous" recoveries.

The results of using raw red potato juice are so comprehensive that several health clinics in England offer rejuvenating regimens based on drinking the juice daily. The rejuvenating power of the potato juice is due to its nutrients which build strong connective tissue. The raw red potato juice is also an excellent cleanser of the lymphatic system.

Actually, many varieties of potatoes can be used such as red, new, Finnish, white, salad and Urantia. But the RUSSET (baker) CANNOT be used, because it contains an antiproteolytic enzyme under its skin which interferes with protein assimilation. The Russet potato is fine to eat cooked as the enzyme is destroyed by heat. Thus, the Russet makes a good baking potato, but it is not optimal for juicing.

To juice raw potatoes, scrub them and remove any sprouts or green areas since these areas are toxic. Then juice the potatoes and drink the juice immediately. Since potato juice oxidizes very quickly, it must be used immediately after juicing. The Champion and

Norwalk juicers are best to use for this process, because they grind and press the potatoes rather than spinning them at high RPM like other brands of juicers. The spin/centrifugal juicers oxidize the juice and deplete its enzymatic values.

The recommended use of red potato juice is to drink 4 ounces once or twice a day. The foam from juicing potatoes can be applied to the face for a quick enzyme-mask to nourish the skin and keep it youthful. The rare nutrients in raw red potato juice are well worth the effort of juicing.

HOW TO COOK YARD EGGS TO MAXIMIZE PROTEIN VALUES

Always use range or yard eggs, because mass-produced cage eggs are nutritionally and ethically inferior. Caged chickens are subjected to artificial light to stimulate their body clocks to produce more eggs. They get feed which is laced with antibiotics, steroids and chemicals. These chickens are highly-stressed creatures, since they are completely removed from their natural environment. They have no community with other chickens and they can't peck the ground. They can't be chased around by a rooster. Their eggs are so nutrient-depleted that yellow dye is added to the feed to make the pale yolks yellower. In contrast, yard eggs are an excellent protein, if prepared properly.

To prepare yard eggs properly, cook the eggs between 180 and 200 degrees F. If egg whites are eaten raw or cooked below 170 degrees, the avadin—an antiproteolytic, biotin-inhibiting enzyme—is not neutralized and the protein values are jeopardized. If eggs are cooked above 200 degrees F, the sulphur bond is broken, the proteins become heat-altered, high-stress and difficult for the liver to process. Consequently, 180-200 degrees F is the optimal range for cooking eggs. Just cook eggs slowly and lightly; don't worry about the temperature or using a thermometer. Turn the heat down and cook the eggs a bit slower.

Dr. Emanuel Revici discovered that poached eggs are anabolic (alkalizing) to the metabolism, whereas fried, scrambled or overheated eggs are catabolic (acidifying). You can use this information to maintain your pH. Poaching is the optimal way to prepare eggs because the egg heats gradually and is ready to eat when it is firm.

As discussed in the chapter on cholesterol, there is scientific evidence that some of the cholesterols in cage eggs are insoluble. This means that commercial cage eggs are more difficult to digest than yard egg. When used moderately and prepared properly, yard eggs are an excellent food. They are also rich in lecithin and valuable trace minerals.

The cholesterol in a wholesome yard egg does not cause cholesterol in the body. Before it can be assimilated, it is digested into lipids, a valuable nutrient. The liver must reconstruct lipids into cholesterol as needed. If the body does not have enough cholesterol in the diet, the liver will have to make it. In a diet free of all animal products, the liver constructs needed cholesterol from plant oils.

One of the major causes of arterial plaque, often blamed on cholesterol, is the eating of proteins and carbohydrates at the same time. Also, pasteurized, homogenized milk is a major source of arterial plaque. Rancid oils cause great damage but yard eggs do not.

The natural yard egg, used properly, is a highly nutritious food. Most of the value is in the yolk, which is rich in minerals, lipids and lecithin. The yolk makes the chicken's body. The egg white is mostly albumin and turns into feathers.

Cooked properly, yard eggs used a couple of times a week provide a high quality protein and build tissue integrity. People who think they have allergic reactions to eggs sometimes find that properly cooked yard eggs are not allergenic. Perhaps these persons were actually allergic to the chemical pesticides used around commercial egg cages. Once again, cooking eggs over low heat and adding raw vegetables to the meal may prevent the typical immune response and allow eggs to be a useful food.

Once you gain proficiency in preparing a Pro-Vita! meal, you find that with a little preparation the night before, this meal can be served within few minutes. This makes the Pro-Vita! breakfast a practical meal in the morning rush. It is well worth preparing such a breakfast for the sustained energy and productive mental capacity it brings.

After a transition period of two to three weeks on the Pro-Vita! Plan, you should notice several beneficial effects, such as sustained energy, blood sugar remaining steady instead of dropping mid-morning with the urge for coffee and sweet rolls, greater mental clarity and productivity. You will experience many other subtle benefits, such as improved complexion, amelioration of PMS symptoms, fewer allergies and more stable mental attitudes.

SPROUTED COOKED BEANS AS PROTEIN FOOD

We have discussed earlier that cooked beans are carbohydrates, but sprouted and lightly cooked beans are an excellent protein source. The following recipe shows how to quadruple the protein values of beans. Carefully prepared in this manner, beans can rival meat proteins in bioavailability when balanced with seeds and sprouts. Sprouted beans and soaked seeds with liberal use of raw red potato juice, beet tops and soy ferments are the best foods that strict vegetarians can use to increase cellular protein values, IF their liver function is vital and strong. The liver function is dependent on a health history free of drugs, alcohol, caffeine, nicotine, anger, excessive cold proteins such as nuts and excessive use of red meat. Effective liver function also depends on whether a person has had illnesses, such as hepatitis, mononucleosis, cytomegalo virus or Epstein-Barr, the chronic fatigue syndrome.

Here is the recipe for preparing bean protein.

1. Use organic beans, such as black, pink, pinto, ana-sazi, navy, small white, azuki, kidney, brown, lentil or chili beans. To cook properly, they must be fresh—the current season's crop.

2. Wash the beans to clean away dirt. Pick out any rocks, shriveled or damaged beans.

3. Soak beans overnight in a stainless steel container. Use three times their volume of pure water. It is a good idea to add a few drops of stabilized oxygen to the water to minimize bacteria. Some people add a tablespoon of baking soda to take the "pop" out of the beans and reduce the problem with intestinal gas.

4. The following morning pour off the water into another container and refrigerate. Spread the beans on a terry cloth towel or dish towel and cover with an additional

towel. Keep them damp for two days. To avoid molds, you may need to rinse them once or twice.

5. Usually within two days the beans have germinated, as evidenced by approximately 10% of them showing a tiny white nub sprouting out. Do not sprout any further. They are ready to cook. When the beans are cooked, no one will be able to visually tell that they were sprouted. Sprouting increases the beans' nutritional value greatly.

6. Take an appropriate amount of the soak water which has been in the refrigerator and bring it to a boil in a non-aluminum pot, such as a crock pot, glass pot, or stainless steel pot. This boiling will destroy any bacteria that might be growing in the bean water.

7. After 12 minutes of boiling the water, lower the temperature to 190 degrees F. This temperature is just below simmer. The water should not bubble.

8. Add the beans to the water. Season as you like with vegetables, bouillon, garlic, bayleaf, chili, herbs or peppers. Epazote is used by Maya Indians in Central American to make beans easier to digest. The herb is available in health food stores. Cook the beans slowly. Good quality beans (a current crop) will cook in approximately one hour. Keep an eye on them so that they don't overcook.

9. Do not allow the beans to boil. If they do, the proteins will soon be compromised and the beans will become predominantly a carbohydrate food. If the water boils, turn down the heat a little.

Beans cooked in this manner have a wonderful, chewy texture; excellent flavor; are easily digested; and do not cause intestinal gas. As a protein food, they are excellent in small amounts with the Pro-Vita! protein meal plan.

This method of cooking beans comes in handy, because a person could have the famous Texas meal of barbecued chicken (organic, skinless), cole slaw and beans, and render it digestible and properly combined. But omit the beer, chips, bread, pecan pie and watermelon with this meal, if you want the meal to keep its nutritional values.

If this method of cooking beans is too time consuming for you, just boil the beans as usual and use them as complex carbohydrates away from proteins. Add the herb epazote – as the Mayan Indians do – for easier digestion! As carbohydrates, the beans will not build the degree of health that they can as proteins. But boiled beans work well for supper time carbohydrates with tacos, for example.

As a point of interest, Shabda Fresh Foods in Austin, Texas, prepares several foods according to Pro-Vita! cooking guides: Rose's Just Right Fresh Salsa, Fresca Salsa Verde, Mom's Spaghetti Sauce and Sicilian salad dressing. The fresh green onions, garlic, peppers and cilantro get the recommended de-tox soak. Extra-virgin olive oil is used for the fresh salsas, dressing and Mom's spaghetti sauce. The tasty pasta sauce is cooked at a low temperature and is laden with fresh garlic cloves and basil. Products are available by mail order from Shabda Fresh Foods, 2311 Thornton B, Austin, TX 78704-4957. (Note that the author has no vested or financial interest in this company but is pleased that the Pro-Vita! principles can find viable commercial applications.)

HIGH STRESS FOODS

DIGESTIVE DIFFICULTIES

So far, this book has focused on low-stress, high quality foods. In this section we look at the HIGH-STRESS foods. These foods are best avoided, or at least minimized, in our food plan. If you do use them, do so occasionally rather than frequently.

This plan is not intended to be overly restrictive. The rule that calls for a "full and varied diet" supersedes the restrictions engendered by this high-stress category. Occasional and moderate use of high-stress foods will not ruin health when the Pro-Vita! foundation is in place.

Most nuts, except for pine nuts, are high-stress foods. They are difficult to digest and tax the body's energies to process them. Yet, nuts are a natural, wholesome food. In our cooking classes we teach that it is okay to add a couple of almonds, cashews or pecans to the soaked seed mixture. Soaking the nuts helps to predigest and improve them to a medium-stress level. And the nuts are undeniably tasty. When nuts, particularly almonds, are turned into nut milk by soaking and blending them, their amino acid chains become shorter. Nut milks can then become the base for salad dressings.

The Pro-Vita! Plan is a pathway that leaves each individual step up to you. Some people do not digest nuts very well, others do. Red meat is detrimental to most people most of the time. Occasionally, in rare instances, it is a lifesaver. We will attempt not to burden you with too many absolutes because flexibility is a key note of health. Make determinations for yourself and let your body communicate with you. Often, people who eat high-stress foods exercise good judgement and take supplemental digestive support when they use high-stress foods.

The following foods often cause digestive difficulties:

almond	goat	pork
banana*	high gluten	sardines
beef	lamb	soy (unfermented)
Brazil veal	milk	soy flour
cashew	mustard greens	soy milk
crab	nuts:	soy protein
flours	peanuts	powder
	pecan	

* Bananas, unless organically grown, picked and shipped quickly, are high stress. Commercial bananas are picked green before they are ripe and are gassed for ripening and fumigated for pests. In this condition they do not ripen properly and the natural sugars do not mature.

Nutrient-Depleted and Nutrient-Depleting Items

The following foods lack nutritional values. Notice that, with the exception of Jello (protein and sugar), they are all carbohydrates.

angelfood cake (albumen and carbo-hydrate)	crackers	pancakes
	fruit drinks, sweetened	pastries
		pies
bread, "enriched"	ice cream, commercial	preserves
cake		sodas
cereals (processed)	jam	soft drinks
colas	jelly	soups, canned
conserves	macaroni	syrup
cookies	"natural" sodas	waffles
corn starch	noodles	

"Foods" Containing Excessive Toxic Substances

alcohol
ascorbic acid (high milligrams)
bacon
baking powder (aluminum)
carrot tops (unless boiled)
chocolate (caffeine, sugar)
cocoa

coffee
cucumber skin
custard
gravy
ice cream
iceberg (opiates)
liver (commercial)
maraschino cherries
meats (luncheon)
milk products

MSG (Monosodium Glutamate)
oak leaf lettuce (opiates)
potato sprouts(raw, green)
puddings
tea (pekoe, black)
tobacco

Preservatives: BHA/BHT • nitrates/nitrites (additives to processed meat) • sodium bisulfide • sulfites • wax (on fruits and vegetables)

Foods Containing Rancid Oils

brown rice
chicken skin
corn chips (unless baked)
cottonseed oil
crackers
donuts
dumplings
french fries
fried foods

fried pies
lard
lecitin, granular
margarine
mayonnaise
nuts, roasted
potato chips
rice (unless fresh, hulled)

shortening
soy oil, linseed oil
tempura
tortilla chips
wheat germ
whole wheat products

Some of the items listed are detrimental to health at all times, such as cottonseed oil and partially-hydrogenated coconut derivatives. Other items should be used with good judgment such as honey.

Many of the items listed, such as mayonnaise, are detrimental due to commercial processing. Make your own mayonnaise from fresh, organic ingredients and you have a wholesome, better tasting food. Or buy mayonnaise made from organic tofu.

COMMERCIAL MEAT:
NOT A FOOD FOR HUMAN HEALTH

Commercially-raised animals are not a viable food source for people who wish to be healthy. There are many issues involved in the topic of eating dead animals as John Robbins eloquently discussed in his famous book, *Diet for a New America* (1987). Here we will stay focused on commercial production of animals for the table and only address the problem inherent in buying a steak, or chicken, from the local supermarket.

Most animals grown specifically for market exist in an automated world of pens, conveyer belts, artificial light, hormones, antibiotics, and a system that feeds them their own feces. Agricultural research has learned how to mass-produce animals for maximum growth without any regard for nutritional value. The focus has been on how to get the most poundage in the shortest amount of time and still have the meat look like food.

Instead of living on the land, many commercial cows are confined in indoor concrete pens with electric light substituting for sun. An 18-hour light exposure causes more rapid growth. Conveyer belts supply food to one end, while another conveyer belt catches the cow dung at the other end. Since agricultural universities have learned that a cow can eat hay with 25% feces in it, a way to reduce feed costs is to recycle the cow dung back into the cow food.

To speed the growth process of the cows, steroids are added to cattle food. People who eat commercial beef receive these hormones because they are not inactivated by cooking. Thus it is no wonder that obesity is a major problem among people who eat commercial beef.

To prevent disease from occurring in such an unnatural cattle environment, antibiotics are added to the food. These harmful chemicals go into the fat and muscle tissue of the animals and are then passed on to the consumer. Unbelievably high levels of antibiotics are needed to prevent infections because cows grown in such conditions are not fit to live. Their life is maintained on chemicals until an early slaughter puts an end to their existence and disease.

Other chemicals are contained in commercially grown beef. Cows are fed a poor quality hay grown by commercial agriculture with chemical fertilizers and insecticides. Therefore, extra feed additives are used to make the cow grow quickly.

Yet another key point concerns the slaughter of these animals. Commercial slaughtering of animals ignores the validity of Kosher or Islamic meat processing, or treats such practices as religious ritual instead of a social necessity for health. In commercial slaughter no special attention is paid to the draining of the animal's blood. At the time of slaughter, the animal experiences fear and therefore adrenaline is pumped into its body and is concentrated in the blood. Not letting the blood drain properly gives the consumer a dose of adrenaline hormone which is certainly not needed.

Since commercial cattle raising results in nutritionally inferior beef (and certainly an emotionally-inferior life for the cow), the meat is often a cadaverous, pale color. But the industry has a solution for this dilemma. It adds chemical dyes to make the meat more appealing to the consumer. Since meat producers know that commercial raising of meat results in inferior taste, flavoring agents are added to the meat. Finally, to keep the meat from rotting like a dead animal should, preservatives are added.

The meat industry is proud that the U. S. is a world leader in the production of food. From our continental resources, we can feed the world. But what are we feeding our own people in the USA? Something that looks like meat and tastes like meat, but is far removed from what such a food could be.

The same story is true of the chicken industry. The chickens are stacked in cages with artificial light, artificial food, chemicals, antibiotics, hormones, and dyes so the inferior egg yolks look yellow. They are killed before they die a neurotic, disease-ridden death.

The "humane vs. inhumane" practices of raising food animals are issues that have nutritional implications. The inhumane practices of the commercial meat industry are two-fold. First, the animals often have a miserable existence in an unnatural environment. Mass production and mass slaughtering are procedures devoid of any normal animal husbandry. They are devoid of any feeling for the animals and any responsibility for our human role in caring for the animals over which we have dominion. A food-animal's life could be so much better because an animal deserves to roam the earth with its own kind and have a full, natural life. Second, the neurotic, fear-imbued, chemically laced tissues brought to meat-eaters' tables impart an inferior level of nutrition to the people. This practice lowers the national health standards, forming a basis for many social problems including sickness, degenerative disease, learning disabilites and crime.

Our point is that commercial meat is not healthy. The commercial agricultural industry never once asked, "What is best for human health?" Instead they only ask, "What is the cheapest and easiest way to get a product out and a fat animal to market?" Unless human health and nutrition is put first, a food cannot be as good as it should be.

To avoid such commercial meats, there are three options: 1) do not eat meat, 2) buy meat from an organic source, or 3) raise and slaughter your own animals.

Let's address yet another important point. The less commercial meat you buy, and the more organic vegetables and meat products you buy, the quicker American agricultural methods can produce foods that support human health. Although good beginnings exist in this direction of food production, your support is still greatly needed.

For people who need meat to support their current level of health because their biochemistry requires some animal protein at its current level of function, here is a summary of major considerations for a better level of health.

- Buy only organically raised meat. Organic meat
  producers are increasing due to public demand. One
  company, Carabeef, markets organic water buffalo to

health food stores around the country. Buffalo, raised on the range, is also available. If you have to have a hamburger, there are low-fat, improved ways to do it.

- Keep red meat consumption to a minimum, (once a week, preferably less). Use organic range chicken, game meat, or turkey.

- Rely on fresh ocean fish because they have not been raised on hormones and antibiotics. Consult Steinman's book, *Diet for a Poisoned Planet* (1990) for the least toxic fish.

- Eating more than one small portion of meat per day is excessive high-stress protein intake.

I do not adhere to the philosophy that everyone can be a vegetarian because I have seen people whose health has suffered on such a diet. While I believe that people should be vegetarian with the exception of eating fish occasionally, I recognize that some people need the animal proteins to best support their health at particular times. Pro-Vita! is a plan that can be adapted by everyone — vegetarian or not!

As people become more healthy and vital, the need for animal proteins diminishes. People can make the transition to a vegetarian-based diet with improvements in their health. Many situations in life are paradoxical. There are people who cannot improve their health until they eat less meat. There are people who cannot improve their health unless they eat a little meat. Health is dynamic and ever-evolving. The phrase, "One person's meat is another person's poison" is certainly true.

What we are trying to accomplish with The Pro-Vita! Plan is to set the parameters of the basic tenets of health. It is very difficult to have a nutrition plan be all things to all people. However, on this plan, everyone should benefit. Vegetarians learn to work more diligently with seeds, tofu and vegetarian proteins. Some persons definitely need to add some fish to their diets. In contrast, meat eaters learn to cut back and maximize the nutritional value of any meat they eat. Such guidance will improve anyone's health.

Where you fit in is determined by your individual, biological needs; your level of vitality; and your attitudes. The universal rule for this section is that commercially-produced meat is not fit for human consumption.

IRRADIATED FOODS: DO NOT BUY THEM!

As everyone should know by now, modern science has figured out a use for the toxic radioactive wastes being produced by nuclear reactors. Foods can be exposed to radiation and thus be preserved for longer shelf life while at the same time bacteria, fungus, molds and parasites can be controlled. Consequently, rather than having to store deadly radiation in toxic waste sites, the radiation can be used on our food and spread out all over the country.

Battle lines have been drawn on this issue. On one side, we have the government and its scientists claiming that they have a great way to use the toxic radiation, preserve foods, and make them safe from spoilage and possible pathological organisms. On the other side, we have anti-nuclear activists pointing out the dangers of transporting radioactive substances to the irradiation sites and the likelihood that terrorists could take over a site and threaten massive destruction.

We will discuss the issues here that are limited to nutrition. We are concerned with the question of what happens to the nutritional value of irradiated foods. The simple answer is that THE NUTRITIONAL VALUE IS RUINED because the radiation renders the food sterile or dead. A major thrust of this book is to encourage you to eat more raw, living foods. But dead foods do not provide health, do not impart living enzymes, do not provide vitality!

Many spices are already being irradiated to control the little bugs that hatch out. Have you ever had little buggies in your spice jar? You won't any more if you buy commercial spices, because irradiation killed the bugs' eggs as well as the food value (but not the taste value) of the herb.

The irradiation proponents never learned the first law of health that LIFE BEGETS LIFE! The more we eat dead foods, the more we need antibiotics, health insurance, fancy lab tests, expensive drugs and therapies. To provide health, our foods must be alive. When the bread gets moldy, it means that it can support life!

We need to oppose irradiation because it kills the life force in our foods, kills the enzymes and maybe even alters molecules into new chemicals. We all know that radiation affects cells resulting in mutations. If new molecules are created or altered by the irridation process, they will be extremely foreign to the body and present new problems for the immune system. Scientists opposing irradiation of foods are concerned that such new molecules may cause cancer. They are also concerned about alteration of the food's inherent molecular structure making it unable to function as a food in the body.

The government has done no research on the altering of the molecule. However, some scientists employing Kirlian photography, a method to photograph the energetic patterns of a substance, are concerned about the major differences between a fresh strawberry and one that has been irradiated. The fresh strawberry shines with vital energy, radiating out an inch or more in an aura with vibrant patterns. In contrast, the irradiated food has virtually no aura, is flat, dull, and the patterns which can be seen are significantly altered.

Fight the use of irradiated foods at your individual supermarkets. Voice your concerns. Make the store label such foods. Refuse to purchase such foods. The last thing we need, in light of all our diseases, is more dead food. The irradiated foods are another example of science turning out a substance that looks and tastes like food, but has little resemblance to it from a nutritional perspective.

The U.S. government is deliberately trying to sell the public on irradiation of foods. Be informed and aware that the government often acts for its own self-interest at the expense of its people. Most assuredly, there are health risks associated with irradiation of our foods.

GENERAL NUTRITIONAL GUIDANCE

It is important to minimize detrimental foods and maximize beneficial ones. Although this list is captioned "Strive To Avoid," the truly best advice is "Throw Away!"

Strive To Avoid:

- Highly processed foods like sugar, white bread, noodles, cookies, crackers, TV dinners, etc.

- Foods that contain chemical preservatives, dyes, artificial flavors, etc.

- "Foodless" snacks (candy, donuts, etc.)

- Commercial meat that has stilbestrol (DES), steroids, antibiotics, or other chemicals such as pesticides, or from animals that have been inhumanely raised.

- Fruits and vegetables that have been sprayed, fumigated, dyed, or waxed.

- Canned fruits and vegetables. Most canned fruits are oversweetened and canned vegetables are over cooked. Make organic produce your first choice, then make do with commercial produce as needed.

- Commercial eggs produced by hens in small cages, force fattened, treated with chemicals. Use yard eggs or range eggs instead.

- Commercial white bread or other bakery products.

- Hydrogenated shortenings, heat-treated oils and margarine.

- Deep-fat-frying because fatty acids break down into toxic by-products at high temperatures. Avoid fried foods.

- Chocolate because it interferes with mineral assimilation and is highly allergenic and addictive to some people.

- Commercial milk, milk products and ice creams that contain artificial coloring, flavoring, emulsifiers, sweeteners.

- Processed cow's milk: pasteurized, homogenized, dried, or canned. This is a source of toxic growth hormones and homogenized fats. Unless butter comes from a certified, organic, raw milk dairy, it contains the bulk of the toxic steroids, antibiotics and pesticides used in the dairy industry.

- Soft drinks with or without sugar. Avoid stimulating drinks, which exhaust the adrenals and the pancreas.

- Coffee. Use water-processed decaf in transition. Keep in mind that decaf-coffee still contains tars. Pekoe teas (black teas) also have caffeine. Substitute alternative, roasted grain beverages.

- Junk food.

- Sugar in all of its many forms and synthetic sweeteners, such as Nutra-Sweet® or Saccharine. Keep in mind that Nutra-Sweet is a wolf in sheep's clothing and not fit for human consumption. For more information see The Next Step To Greater Energy (Tips, 1990).

- Any product with preservatives, BHA, BHT, nitrates, nitrites, sodium bisulfide.

- Commercial peanut butter.

- Commercial cooking oils (hydrogenated).

- Sulphured, dried fruit.

- Refined, heated, table salt. Use natural evaporated sea salt.

- Salted, roasted nuts.

- Irradiated foods.

BASIC INSTRUCTION FOR NUTRITIONAL IMPROVEMENTS

- Cook only in stainless steel, Corning or porcelainized ware, or glass. Do not use aluminum pots, cast iron pots, or pressure cookers. Cast iron pots are reactive with acids and can reduce the value of foods.

- Use balanced, organic butter instead of substitutes. For a spread high in unsaturated fats stir together one pound organic, raw, sweet cream butter and 1/2 cup organic flax seed oil. Add a little liquid lecithin and vitamin E. Harden this mixture in the refrigerator. Instead of butter and margarines use high quality oils for cooking and tahini as a spread. Olive oil with herbs and garlic makes a healthy and tasty substitute for butter.

• Use pure drinking water liberally. Avoid tap water. Use home-made soups often.

• Use a natural sea salt sparingly or an organic sesame/sea salt seasoning; or get Dr. Revici's balanced salt from Europe.

• Use a variety of herbs and spices in cooking—parsley, basil, thyme, rosemary, sage, nutmeg, cinnamon, dill, etc.—for flavor and for stimulating the appetite and the gastric juices.

• Use vinegars occasionally to maintain good gastric acidity. They do wonders for soups. Try brown rice vinegar and Umeboshi plum vinegar for mild flavor enhancers.

EATING OUT GUIDE

Many people have commented that it is difficult to eat out and follow the Pro-Vita! Plan. But this is actually easier than you might think. Once you understand and have practiced the Pro-Vita principles for a while, you will know how to choose and combine foods in a restaurant to make an acceptable meal. Here are a few examples of how to follow the rule to avoid protein/carbohydrate combinations.

• "I'll have the broiled fish, hold the rice and substitute broccoli and cheese sauce."

• "I'd like the pasta primavera."

• "I'll take the baked potato, garden salad and fresh asparagus."

• "I'll have the shrimp curry, hold the rice and egg roll, and would you add broccoli and snow peas to the shrimp curry? Thanks!"

• "I'll have the vegetable soup and the salad bar." At the salad bar you can either stick with just vegetables

> or add proteins like cottage cheese, sunflower seeds, a
> bit of egg.

One thing to remember about eating out is: YOU DON'T EAT OUT TO GET HEALTHY. When restaurant owners go into business, they do not ask themselves "What can I serve to fully support human health and nutrition?" They are much more likely to ask, "What's the cheapest oil I can get, and how infrequently can I get away with changing it?" So don't plan on eating out to build your health. You're either asking too much or you're kidding yourself. If, however, you are a strong and healthy Pro-Vita! eater, then you will enjoy the fun and unusual foods which occasional eating out can provide.

Here is yet another way to order at a restaurant that fits in with one aspect of the Pro-Vita! Plan's philosophy, the 80% of the time rule:

> "I'll start with the lobster bisque, then have the sweet and
> sour shrimp brochette on rice, a glass of white wine and
> the blueberry cheesecake. I'm following the Pro-Vita!
> Plan and this is my NIGHT OFF!"

PRO-VITAL PLAN

SUPPLEMENTATION:
BENEFICIAL OR DETRIMENTAL

THE ISSUE OF SUPPLEMENTATION

Like the subject of nutrition, supplementation is a broad issue with many variables and opinions. The dietary choice, whether or not taking a supplement is beneficial, is individually based. Let's examine several issues on dietary supplementation including vitamin, mineral, herbal and food supplements to provide insights on possible benefits and potential hazards.

A good place to start with is the philosophy of ideal nutrition and optimal health as the basic blue print for life. Then we examine what undermines our opportunity to experience the best of health, and whether or not a pill or drink can make a beneficial difference.

Ideally, it is only right and natural that the Earth's bounty would fully support human nutrition, particularly for a person living in accord with natural law. Over thousands of years, the human being has adapted to survival and life based on the foods of the Earth. Consequently, the best of health should come from a natural foods diet tempered by prudence and judgment.

Rarely has any culture experienced optimal nutritional health due to limitations of geography or ignorance of natural law. Some cultures have had all the raw materials for a high level of health such as islands abounding in fruit, vegetables and sea foods. But the people only ate favorite foods or engaged in self-aggrandizing activities such as war with neighbors, resulting in poor economic and nutritional conditions.

We now know more than ever before about the components of nutrition for the body. We know about vitamins, minerals, enzymes, fatty acids, amino acids, water, fiber, and some of their roles in supporting the body. When we look only at the factors in biochemistry, it is difficult to construct a model for optimal human nutrition. But when we look at the whole picture via the laws of natural health and allow natural foods to fulfill their innate role, then a model becomes much easier. Finally, when we can build our model on the laws of health and then apply some of the biochemical knowledge, or pieces of the whole picture, then we have the advantage of being able to apply nutrition specifically to compensate for weak areas.

Our optimal blueprint is the following. Innate within every person is the ability to know how to support the body in its best operative condition. With a variety of natural foods available, the body should be able to live well and enjoy a high level of nutritional health. Thus, the optimal picture would be that supplements are not necessary. The food for human beings consists of vegetables, fruit, grains, seeds, sprouts, with possibly a little fish or game as we have already investigated. A good diet would provide all the raw materials for optimal health.

Here we are back to our five-element model. Good food (Earth), plus good air (Air), plus pure water (Water), plus the warmth of the sun (Fire) and a good vital force (Ether) equal good physical health. If a person is blessed with healthy mental and emotional bodies and practices a dynamic spiritual life, then the quality of that life will be exceptional!

Now the question becomes, "How far is a person removed from living an exceptional life?" The further removed an individual is, the more likely the need arises to make up deficits through some form of supplementation.

It does indeed seem difficult to ensure that we get all the nutrients we need to function effectively in today's world. The question is whether we really can obtain what we need to overcome a number of deficits facing us each day. Let's examine the five elements again to see if any of them are balanced in our personal lifestyles.

The Earth is being covered with chemical pollutants from industry, automobiles, chemical fertilizers, poisonous pesticides, radiation from atomic testings and reactor accidents, as well as toxic waste dumps. Where is the integrity of what the Earth bears forth? Where is a vegetable free from poisons? Unless you have a biodynamic garden, or always eat organic produce, your earth element is being undermined.

Generally speaking, people today are not eating enough vegetables and natural foods from the earth. When they do eat vegetables grown in depleted soil boosted with chemical fertilizers and sprayed with pesticides, their nutritional value is not the same as that of the biodynamically grown produce. Commercially grown foods have fewer nutrients and more toxic chemicals than food grown naturally.

The second element, the Air, is affected by chemical pollutants from industry, exhaust from transportation, the person smoking nearby and other pollution. The trees and rain forests that purify and reoxygenate the air are being cut down and burned. Where do we get a clean, vital breath of air?

Water, the third element, is contaminated virtually all over the world from industrial chemical pollutants, improper sewage disposal, industrial wartime pollutants, and the myriad household chemicals that go down the drain. Industrial and war wastes the world over have poisoned the oceans, the cradle of life, to their very depths. What do you do for the clean, pure water the body's blueprint requires?

The Sun's influence as the fourth element has shifted to a more detrimental effect due to the thinning of the ozone layer around the earth. In addition to the warmth the sun provides, sunlight is also a nutrient and activates body chemistry via synthesis with vitamin D and hormones from the pineal gland. How do we get safe sun? Blocking it with chemicals such as sun-block is not the answer. Small doses of sun exposure provide immunity to the harmful effects of the sun. But getting sufficient and safe sunlight is more difficult now.

What about the fifth, the more enigmatic Ether element? Our planet is now covered with electromagnetic radiations from power lines, radio waves, microwave communication devices. In fact, doctors are currently telling pregnant women to not sleep under electric blankets or on heated water beds because of the electrical circuit's electromagnetic radiation which can cause birth defects and leukemia. Computer terminals, appliances with transformers and electric motors, such as hair dryers and electric shavers, televisions and fluorescent lights, all emit a harmful magnetic fields to which most people are subject to daily (Becker, 1990).

As the natural magnetic frequencies of the earth are being disrupted, people become estranged from the natural energetic field we live in. This disassociation, or estrangement, from the Earth's magnetic field has resulted in a clearly identifiable environmental illness characterized by symptoms of chronic fatigue and hypersensitivity.

How do we take control of these vital five elements to form the basis for a healthy life? Already the market is flooded with water purifiers, air purifiers, food-purifying systems, no-rad shields for TV's and computers, diodes to protect a person from extra low frequency (ELF) magnetic fields and other devices. It now seems that having such equipment is becoming a fundamental part of everyday life.

Since the body is mostly water, a good place to start your supplement program is with pure water. Avoiding tap water has become a necessity. Municipal waters contain as many as 300 toxic chemicals including chlorine, fluoride and by-products of industrial pollutants. See the section on "Water: Your Foundation of Life" in this book.

Another way to supplement your diet and life is to buy organic produce whenever possible. First, pick what you've grown in your organic garden. Then supplement that food by shopping at the organic department of your health food store or local supermarkets. Then, when necessary, buy commercial produce and treat it to rid toxins as outlined in this book. Increasing the quality and quantity of your vegetable intake is the best way to increase your vitamins and minerals. Then you do not have to buy so many supplements. Nobody has improved on the quality of vitamins and minerals as found in whole, raw, living foods.

From time to time a supplement appears on the market making a claim that a computer has analyzed all the nutrients the human body needs and the manufacturer has put them all in this supplement. Nutritionists often joke about this type of supplement because it is so contrary to valid nutritional thought. Our bodies, our health and our foods are all more than the sum total of their ingredients one natural food provides 100% of everything that is neede optimal nutritional health. Instead, health and nutrition are a process. Thus, nutrients enter the body in a process, not all in a pill. Further, science has not identified all the nutrients the body requires, so variety is a key to nutritional health.

Westerners may laugh, but in Japan and other places oxygen is sold by the dose. It is a novelty item in some airports. You can put some coins in a slot and get a breath of pure, oxygen-rich air. Electrostatic air filters and air purifiers are becoming more commonplace in people's homes. Many people cannot sleep well with open windows, but they would benefit from having cleaner air available during sleep. Having plants in the home can improve the quality of air also since they provide additional oxygen.

It is difficult to supplement the sun, but human beings do need exposure to sunlight. Precautions are needed, not so much because of the sun's ultraviolet rays but because of the saturated fatty acids and hydrogenated oils contained in most people's diets. The sun reacts with these substances under the skin and can cause abnormal cell development. It is not so much the sun's fault as it is the poor quality foods we eat that can predispose a person to skin cancer. A little exposure on a regular basis provides immunity to the effects of the sun. A small dose of sunlight in the morning or evening serves as a "homeopathic" or a "like-cures-like" immunization to detrimental effects of sunlight. The secret to surviving in the sun is a little dose repeated frequently. Sunlight has been a part of many naturopathic cures. Have you had a few minutes in the morning sun?

Environmentally safe homes are being built that do not enclose the house in an electrical field. The wiring does not run into all four walls, or all four sides, leaving an opening to minimize the effect of the resulting electromagnetic field generated by the cycling current in the wires. Shields and blocking devices are now entering the market to clean up electromagnetic radiation from televisions and computers. However, such protective devices are not really supplements.

The issue with supplementing the ether element pertains to the esoteric sciences. Energy from the earth can be obtained from a tree.

The American Indians knew how to press their backs against the trunk of a tree, extend their hands and receive energy from the earth to increase their stamina. Acupuncture is known to balance etheric energies. The needles serve as antennas for energy from the earth and possibly from the practitioner. Meditation and contemplation attract energy into a person's orbit. Selfless acts of giving often result in an increase of subtle energy to a person. Supplement your life with a selfless act every day. Unconditional love is a powerful magnetic field of energy and love in return.

VITAMIN, MINERAL AND HERBAL SUPPLEMENTATION

In the section above, universal supplements for the benefit of all people have been listed. They included pure water, fresh air, whole foods, especially raw fruits and vegetables, giving love and brief sun baths in the morning. Few authorities, if any, would object to this common sense advice.

Now we get to the more difficult topic of vitamins, minerals and herbal supplements. This topic is difficult is because adding synthetic or unnaturally potent substances to our bodies is actually a therapy. However, therapies must be based on a need, used for a limited period of time, then abandoned when proper health is restored. We must never confuse a therapy with our foundational nutritional plan.

The body does not have a requirement for vitamin supplements. It has a requirement for vitamins as found in fresh, raw fruits and vegetables. The body does not have a requirement for concentrated minerals, but it has a requirement for foods rich in minerals. The body does not have a requirement for medicinal herbs, but it does have a requirement for pot-herbs, such as ordinary vegetables.

It is not natural to think that a manufactured vitamin supplement is part of a balanced meal. A pill is a therapy, not a food, though officially food supplements are considered dietary. First, let's get our diets and nutritional intake straight. Then, if a therapy is needed, a person can consider an extensive array of therapies including vitamin/mineral/herbal supplements, acupuncture, chiropractic, massage, allopathic (drug) and homeopathic therapies.

The basic question is whether diet alone can provide what the body needs to overcome the environment and maintain an optimal level of health. The honest answer is that this is probably not possible, unless a concentrated effort is made, including organic gardening and avoiding eating out.

The crux of the problem is that it is difficult to live in today's world and maintain good nutritional health. An obvious solution to turn to are food supplements to make up the nutritional deficit. When this happens, a person enters a controversial and risky world of opinions and conflicts, such as natural vs. synthetic, low-potency vs. mega potency, common nutritional substances vs. rare ingredients, and varied high quality vs. inexpensive nutrients. Entire books have been written to provide guidance on which nutritional supplements to take and how. Most often these books just become another part of the problem.

There is no doubt that natural food supplements work, and that many synthetic supplements work. We take a brief look at how these substances work so we can decide if we want to use them.

Vitamins are catalysts which stir minerals into action. They make things happen. Enzymes are formed and chemical reactions occur. If a person has a vitamin deficiency, then a set of symptoms occurs because the body is unable to perform necessary functions. If a person has too much of a vitamin, then symptoms also occur because the body is overactive in a particular chemical reaction.

Most people are aware of the fact that sailors used to get scurvy on long voyages due to a lack of fresh fruit to provide vitamin C. The solution to the problem is fresh fruit. If that is not available, then a vitamin C supplement is the next obvious choice.

The effects of too much of a vitamin are not well known. The body is able to work with vitamins and minimize their impact if too much is taken. The liver will synthesize them into something else or seek to neutralize or excrete them. Thus vitamin toxicity is not a major concern. More of a concern is the alteration, but not cure, of symptoms. When illnesses are masked by symptom-alleviating vitamin therapy, the true nature of the illness is not known.

Few people today base their supplementation on any sound reasoning. They take a vitamin or mineral because someone said it was good. But this is contrary to good sense. A supplement must be based on a need for it, or it will create an imbalance. If a vitamin is a catalyst and that catalyst is not needed, then it only stirs up the body's responses needlessly and detrimentally. Although the body creates a buffer to control natural substances and maintain its homeostasis, to supplement with a high-potency vitamin without any biochemical basis could well be called "drug therapy!"

Before taking supplemental vitamins or minerals, it is best to have a basis for doing so. If the basis is to make up deficits due to poor diet and environmental concerns, then the best approach is to find a natural, low potency, multi-vitamin/multi-mineral supplement. The idea here is just to provide the body with a balance of nutrients in a gentle, non-demanding form. Such a supplement would mimic a food and be rich in vitamins, minerals and enzymes. The key to effective dietary supplementation is to ease the nutrients into the body and make them available for the body to use as it directs. This cannot be done with a high potency formula because it will inevitably make biochemical demands on the body. If there is not basis or need for those demands, then the supplement will ultimately be a stress to the body and therefore harmful.

People who take a mega vitamin B complex often do so for energy. Although they feel more energy, B vitamins are not the proper energy source for the body. They are only feeling the stirring up from the vitamin and not a genuine energy. Such use of B vitamins can result in greater fatigue later on.

To supplement safely means to buy supplements that are actually derived from foods. For example, flax seed oil provides essential fatty acids lacking in most people's diets. Taking the oil improves health and does not make a strong demand on the body.

Rather than taking a single amino acid which could imbalance other amino acids, a low-milligram multiple supplement of all the amino acids could be used with food without making a strong demand on the body.

To supplement enzymes, a green drink, or barley-green t
product, could be used in moderation. Powdered grasses pr
chlorophyll, enzymes, vitamins, minerals in a fairly non-intr
form and enter the body as a food for the body to direct. But even
here there can be problems if a person were anabolic (alkaline), as
is often the case with environmentally sensitive people. For these
persons the addition of a healthful green drink could be
quite detrimental because this would further imbalance their biochemistry. Once again, there should be a nutritional basis for adding
a supplement.

As for vitamin supplements, these are the most risky because
they are often synthetic or concentrated beyond the abilities of any
natural food. As catalyst, they are risky because their job is not so
much that of a food but that of an initiator of chemical reactions.

Most people are misinformed about vitamins and think that
vitamins are "good" for them. This is a myth. Vitamins are neither
good nor bad. They are unbiased catalysts for specific chemical
reactions. If someone is deficient, or not sufficient, in a vitamin,
then getting the vitamin is good. If someone is sufficient in a
vitamin, then taking a vitamin pill is only needless stress to the
body's homeostasis. The best source of vitamins is organic fruit and
vegetables. All the vitamins your body can possibly use in a year can
be contained in a thimble. Yet, it is hard to dispute that most people
do not have the vitamin nutrients to experience optimal
body function.

Dr. Wheelwright spent much of his life dealing with just this
problem. His research yielded many breakthroughs as he perfected
a prenatal vitamin formula by using low potency, natural sources for
vitamins and then reintroducing them to plant materials so they
would be reincorporated into the plant kingdom. Thus, he created
what he hoped would be a food supplement that the body would
accept to use as a super-food without the supplement making
demands on the metabolism. He sought a way to concentrate
nutrition and deliver it so the body could direct its use as it would a
good food. This supplement, "AZV", became his premier nutritional
supplement. It was approved by the Japanese government for impor-
tation and public use because of its non-invasive, non-drug

approach to nutrition. This approval came at a time when the Japanese government rejected 95% of the supplements from the United States.

Wheelwright was also concerned that many vitamin and mineral supplements taxed the liver. As you know, it is not what we eat but what the liver processes that sets the standard of our nutritional health. Wheelwright felt that his process of combining the vitamins with plants created pro-enzymes and thus significantly reduced the liver's work in processing the supplement. His AZV formula became one of the numerous crowning achievements in his life.

Minerals are yet another supplemental concern. Clinical evidence to this point in nutritional research suggests that a body, rich and balanced in minerals, is a healthy, happy one. Again, the best sources of minerals for human nutritional health come from fruits, vegetables and sea vegetables, such as dulse and other seaweeds popular in macrobiotic fare. To supplement minerals without a clinical basis is to flirt with creating imbalances. Too much of one mineral and a dearth of another will cause problems. Fortunately, the body excretes, or tries to excrete, what it cannot use. Thus, people do not cause too much damage with individual mineral supplements.

Wheelwright applied his keen insights to mineral supplementation as well. It took him over thirty years to perfect his mineral supplement formula. Basically, he first had to discover the plants to match various supplemental minerals to them so the plants would be the carriers of the more concentrated chelated minerals. Kelp, Irish moss, and numerous other plants were painstakingly keyed to inland sea minerals to make a supplement that would be balanced, gentle and nutritional rather than force nutrients on the body. He named his formula MIN and sought to provide all the mineral elements that operate the forty-four electrical processes in the body.

SUPPLEMENTS AND
THE HOMEOPATHIC PERSPECTIVE

Generally, homeopathic prescribers do not allow many, if any, supplements to be used. Knowing the reasons for this helps us understand what Hahnemann meant by a "rapid, gentle cure." It will also help us determine if and when we need to supplement our diets and with what.

Homeopaths are concerned about factors that alter health, mask symptoms, fail to restore health and effect cure. Their primary focus is on understanding the CAUSE of a person's discomfort, or dis-ease, as portrayed by the unique expression of the symptoms of the vital force.

I recently had a brief "trouble-shoot" consultation with a person displaying allergies localized in the eyes. He experienced swelling, redness, hot tears and inflammation with a discharge upon awakening. He also appeared restless. With a good degree of certainty I recommended the remedy *Apis mellifica*. Several days later, the man came back with no improvement. His restlessness was even more pronounced.

Puzzled, I asked him about more of his symptoms and the restlessness. He explained that he had been taking mega-doses of Vitamin B-6 for over a year which kept him a little "wired."

I then had to ask why he felt it necessary to supplement that way. He replied that he had carpal tunnel syndrome causing a hot, swollen wrist with much pain. He had not thought to mention this before, because he kept the pain under control with vitamin B-6 and a stretching exercise he did every morning. It was certainly a manageable condition in light of the irritation occurring in the eyes.

Knowing that *Apis* was not an effective remedy for him, I asked him a few more questions and learned that he was frequently thirsty. Since the *Apis* state is often characterized by a lack of thirst, I soon realized that I had not chosen that remedy on the "totality of his symptom state" and needed to select another remedy.

Other facts and symptoms soon emerged during further questioning. He desired milk, had occasional herpetic eruptions, and had experienced sciatica pains seven times over the last year. He did not like cold or damp weather.

Keying on the fact that the carpal tunnel syndrome was improved by the motion of his self-developed exercise, the remedy *Rhus toxicodendron* was recommended in the LM-1 potency, twice daily. I took him off all supplements (gradually over a six day period) much to his distress.

Two days later, his eyes were completely well as he reported in his phone call. I then saw him twelve days later when his supply of the homeopathic remedy ran out. The change in him was quite noticeable because he was able to sit still. Further, except for some twinges, the carpal tunnel syndrome had not recurred and by all appearances was on the mend.

Over the next five months, this client continued taking ascending potencies of *Rhus tox* up to LM 6, during which time the sciatica and herpes were resolved, and his mental state improved, including symptoms of paranoia and depression.

This is a case where the vitamin supplementation had palliated the wrist problem, but had not effected a cure. It also altered the symptoms produced by the vital force in such a way that I did not receive a clear picture at the first appointment, resulting in an ineffectual remedy. In the beginning, I was unable to see the correct remedy picture because of the vitamin B supplementation. Then, a telling fundamental *Rhus tox* state emerged, and the client was able to reap benefits to his health on the mental, emotional and physical levels. He even had relief from painful sciatica and genital herpes outbreaks. Although the client came initially for his eye allergies, we fortunately did not miss the wonderful opportunity for improving his overall health.

The high doses of vitamin B-6 had certainly imbalanced his body chemistry because his therapy became a way of life. But the B-6 was all he had found to help with the pain. In his case, the vitamin supplement functioned just like an allopathic drug, masking a symptom and causing other problems. It certainly did not heal.

In a case of scurvy, vitamin C is an appropriate therapy because it is a disease, or set of symptoms, that is cured by the use of a vitamin. However, scurvy can also be cured by a homeopathic remedy. But most health concerns are not this simple. Vitamins have an impact and can help, but we must always seek the complete, gentle and rapid cure.

For the homeopathic system to accomplish its goals of cure, the true symptoms of the vital force must be examined. Anything that alters or changes symptoms without effecting a cure only clouds the case and makes it more difficult to apply the correct remedy that will elicit a complete healing response by the vital force.

RID YOUR FOOD OF TOXINS

POISONS IN OUR FOOD

As we know, most of our produce is laced with insecticides and chemical fertilizers, gassed to induce ripening and chemically treated to preserve shelf-life. Furthermore, industrial wastes are turning up in agricultural water and getting into our crops. Steinman's (1990) research indicates how massive and pervasive the toxins in our food supply are. In addition, produce often has molds, fungi and parasites, or parasite eggs, on it. Therefore, it is important to treat foods to help rid them of poisonous sprays, bacteria, fungus and heavy metals.

THE CLOROX® SOAK

A simple procedure protects yourself and your family from this contamination. Called the CLOROX SOAK or the HYDROGEN PEROXIDE (H₂O₂) SOAK, it should be used before any produce goes into your refrigerator. Basically this cleansing process entails soaking fruits, vegetables, eggs and meats in a Clorox or hydrogen peroxide solution for a few minutes. Frozen meats may be soaked, but ground meat does not have a suitable texture.

The Clorox soak has been used in the natural health field for over thirty years and has been discussed in various publications. Such articles claim that this simple soaking procedure removes pesticides and toxic chemical fertilizer residues from produce. Stu Wheelwright also favored this soak, having taught the procedure in his nutrition courses for years. In 1986, Wheelwright added hydrogen peroxide as an alternative soaking agent for people who were environmentally sensitive or reactive to chlorine, a component of Clorox. Supported by his personal experiments and testing, Wheelwright claimed that the Clorox soak was effective in reducing toxic, cancer-causing pesticide residues from produce.

There are many other advantages to this treatment. Fruits and vegetables will keep much longer before molding or wilting, flavors are improved, color is improved, nutritional value will not be compromised, and you will not end up eating chlorine or peroxide.

For the soak use only the regular Clorox bleach, not any other brand and not the Lemon Scent Clorox or Clorox II. Only Clorox is made in stainless steel containers and bottled without the chance for oxidation in the plastic bottle. Upon opening the bottle, it is best to transfer the Clorox to a glass container. This avoids an oxidative reaction with the plastic container after it is opened.

Use one teaspoon of Clorox to one half sink full of cool water. Tap water is acceptable, but not preferable. However, since it comes out of the faucet at the sink, most people use tap water for the soak. Using more Clorox is NOT better. In fact, too much Clorox can cause oxidative damage to tender vegetables like sprouts, so measure accurately.

The goal of the soak is to make a precise dilution of Clorox. The strength of the soak is actually in its dilution, not in the Clorox per se. People who are familiar with the homeopathic principle of gaining power of the substance by dilution will understand that this bath uses the energy of the electrons freed by dilution, not the concentrated Clorox, to accomplish its goal. This solution makes something similar to a homeopathic solution of the Clorox, except that it is not succussed. The action of the Clorox is said to be magnetic, which means that its strong negative charge will pull the toxins, which are positively charged molecules, out of the produce.

For people who are environmentally sensitive to chlorine, a solution of hydrogen peroxide (H_2O_2) will accomplish much the same as the Clorox solution. People who prefer the hydrogen peroxide soak usually use the 35% food grade H_2O_2 and dilute it to .01% with the water in the sink. The measure is about one tablespoon to a half sink of water.

The general time of soaking is about 10 minutes. Leafy vegetables and thinly skinned fruits will require up to 10 minutes; roots and eggs will need 15 minutes; meats will need up to 20 minutes of soaking. Do not soak anything longer than 20 minutes.

Some people separate their produce into four categories and soak them separately. The categories are:

1) leafy vegetables (lettuce, sprouts, etc.), vegetables (squash, peppers, eggplant, tomatoes, etc.), apples, peaches, bananas, citrus; 2) roots and tubers (carrots, potatoes, etc.); 3) eggs; and 4) meats and fish. Each group gets a fresh soaking solution.

The length of soaking time differs for the different categories. Soaking times increase from 7 minutes for category 1 items; to 10 minutes for category 2 items; to 15 minutes for category 3 items; and to 20 minutes for category 4.

People often forget to soak their eggs. However, eggs rate very high as an allergy-causing food due to the pesticide sprays used around the pens. Since eggshell is actually very porous, eggs can absorb many of the toxic sprays from their environment. Salmonella bacteria is also usually present in the egg. By soaking eggs in the Clorox bath for 20 minutes they have a better flavor, and when cooked properly at 180 to 200 degrees F, they lose their tendency to create allergies. Keep in mind that for eggs this procedure is also a soak, not a scrub. The viscid coating on eggs, provided by the hen, protects the eggs and should not be scrubbed off. Eggs should just be soaked and then left to dry.

The Pro-Vita! Plan only recommends the use of yard eggs, fertile or not, as a suitable food. We base our recommendation upon research published in the *New England Journal of Medicine* (Simopoulos & Salem, 1989) which investigated the differences between cage eggs and range chickens in Greece. Cage chickens are raised in inhumane circumstances and are subjected to hormones, antibiotics and artificial additives to their feed.

After the produce soaks in the Clorox or H2O2 solution, it needs to be soaked in plain water for 10 minutes to remove any traces of Clorox or H2O2. Then, rinse the produce and spread it out on a clean terry cloth towel to dry. When it is dry, put the food into storage containers, preferably glass containers, and store it in the refrigerator.

People have inquired whether they can cut the ends off celery and lettuce before soaking so that each stalk and leaf can soak and be cleaned prior to putting them into the refrigerator. It is best to wait with this until the produce is soaked in the rinse water, because cutting into the vegetables results in an oxidative loss of vitamins during the soak. Preparing the vegetables for storage after the rinse creates a ready supply of salad and snack materials for an instant salad.

Meats need to soak the longest time, because they are carriers of many toxic materials, including antibiotics, steroids, drugs, sprays and ingested toxins. Fish can also have a high mercury content. Soaking helps remove some of these toxic substances. The magnetic action of the Clorox pulls some of the heavy metals out of the produce. Of course, it is best not to purchase such toxic-laden foods.

The soaking of all produce in Clorox should become a standard procedure in your home. It is accomplished the easiest way if you soak food items directly from the grocery bag as soon as you get home from the store.

This cleansing technique is an important part of the Pro-Vita! Plan. There are seemingly incurable conditions affecting people today caused by the massive accumulation of environmental poisons. The Clorox or H_2O_2 soak is one way to minimize the danger that sprays, metallics, insecticides, as well as bacteria and fungus, represent to you and your family. Another way to minimize the impact of toxins is to do the "Liver Triad Program" so that your body can better process toxins. This program is an herbal regime designed by Wheelwright to break the "toxic stress cycle" and build health. For further information on this program, see the book *Your Liver-Your Lifeline* (Tips, 1990).

THE GRAPEFRUIT SEED EXTRACT SOAK

Since 1988, several products have appeared on the market with the claim to rid produce of toxins. Their active ingredient is hydroxy quinaline sulfate acid which is a derivative of fermented grapefruit seeds. Wheelwright had been a manufacturer of this natural substance for over twenty years. Therefore, I inquired about its effectiveness and why he did not recommend a few drops of his XL formula for the cleansing soak.

Wheelwright replied that he had experimented with the grapefruit seed extract internally for parasites and fungus conditions with good results. He had also had good success with this substance as a topical bactericide and fungicide. Moreover, he had experimented with it as a preservative for various topical skin products and had found it effective.

In fact, Wheelwright had also experimented with the extract for produce soaking. He discovered that the substance works well for cleaning bacteria and fungus. It also works fairly well for removing some pesticides, but not for all of them. From his experience he felt that Clorox was best for the soak because it was more effective in removing toxins in shorter time. Wheelwright also was of the opinion that Clorox covered radiation toxicity. Also, it is inexpensive and readily available. His basic attitude was, "There is no perfect system for undoing our sins committed against our food. The chemicals and poisons should not be put on the food in the first place."

If produce is grown organically, then the hydroxy quinaline sulfate acid is the best soak because no chlorine is added to the environment. Also, oxidation of the produce is thus minimized. The soak consists of 10 drops of Systemic XL formula per half a sink full of water to rid organic produce of molds, fungus or parasites. If other products with grapefruit seed extracts are used, their instructions should be followed.

The issues and concerns regarding the clean-up of commercial produce are far from being resolved. However, we are fortunate to have three valuable cleansing methods which help to reduce the negative aspects of living on foods that are not grown in our own backyard gardens.

BUY ORGANIC PRODUCE!

Fortunately, more people and businesses are becoming aware of the dangers of our toxic food chain and are taking some action. At one of the Wheelwright lectures in Dallas, when he explained the Clorox soak, a lady in the audience explained that she was a waitress at Kip's Restaurant and that Kip's always soaked their lettuce in a Clorox bath to make the lettuce last longer. Therefore, she had started doing the same thing at home and found that the soak extended the freshness of her leaf lettuce by two days.

Today, many large chain supermarkets dedicate a corner of their stores to organic produce. One day, I asked the produce manager at the Tom Thumb store in Austin how well the organic produce sold. He replied that most of it was thrown out after it wilted on the shelf. He thought that the organic produce did not sell well, because people did not want to pay $1.09 for organic lettuce when the commercial kind was only $.79.

Because of such situations we issue a plea to support the brave efforts of our supermarkets and organic food growers by buying the organic produce. The old saying of "being penny-wise and pound-foolish" certainly gets a new application in these shopping situations when people buy pesticide-laced food to save pennies a pound. Increasing consumer demand for organic produce opens the door to the availability and lower pricing of more organic and biodynamic produce and foods free of chemical pollutants which are known to cause cancer, chronic fatigue, birth defects and allergies.

We must rethink our entire shopping mentality. The undeniable bargain is organic produce, because it provides more nutrients than the nutritionally impoverished, commercial produce. Most importantly, organically produced food is not tainted by as many environmental toxins and therefore protects our health.

To change traditional shopping habits is a big adjustment for people who spend hours clipping and filing coupons, and roaming from store to store to save 6 cents per item of food. But the change can be made. Understanding the principles of healthy nutrition and organic food production principles can help us to shop more effectively.

As a hint, shop the organic produce and food items first, getting all that you can eat in a week. Then buy the commercial items that "will have to do."

We look forward to the day in the near future when commercial produce wilts, or petrifies, on the shelf because organic produce occupies the majority of the shelf space. We can make this happen by increased consumer demand. Support the organic farming movement and take home organic apples, grapes, oranges, broccoli, beans and cucumbers to demonstrate to the stores that we want clean foods for ourselves, our children and our grandchildren. Support human health and reject toxic, impoverished foods whether grown in the USA or abroad. You will help to save the lives of the farm workers, as well.

As a final thought, be wary of out-of-season produce imported from Mexico, Central and South America. When DDT was banned in the USA, it was then sold to countries south of the border. Now, the DDT returns to us in the imported vegetables, fruits and other foods.

20

THE WHEELWRIGHT
5 + 5 MEAL CONCEPT

THE OPTIMAL MEAL

Since we know how to maximize proteins and minimize stress and toxins, let's see what a well-though-out meal might be. To design an optimal meal, we use five sources of protein (one cooked, four raw) and five vegetables (one cooked, four raw). The volume on the plate will be 65-75% vegetables and 25-35% low-stress protein foods.

This combination will provide maximum nutrition. The five protein sources guarantee that the amino acids will be complete. Four protein sources will have a completeness probability factor of 90%; three will only have a 58% likelihood of being complete. However, with five low-stress proteins the completeness of amino acids is assured.

The five vegetables provide a variety of enzymes, chlorophyll, fiber and chromatin factors (DNA/RNA) to buffer the protein acids and assist with digestion and assimilation. They also provide a small amount of carbohydrate for an easily accessible energy supply.

A bit of balanced, organic butter on the cooked vegetables, a little flax seed oil on a salad, a few olives, or simply the oils found in the seeds, will provide the lipid factors that will be used by the liver to humanize the protein so that it will not be "foreign" or toxic.

DO NOT EAT CARBOHYDRATES with this protein meal. This includes sugars, potatoes, rice, breads, crackers, cereals and grains. Combining carbohydrates with protein causes mucoid matter and can form insoluble cholesterols and thus disease. In fact, many people's sinus problems and allergies are caused by this poor food combination. Save carbohydrates for another meal.

THIS IS HOW THE MEAL COULD WORK:

1 cooked protein = fresh fish (cod, halibut, herring, mackerel, mahi-mahi, mullet, snapper, octopus, scallops, shrimp, squid), eggs (soft boiled, poached, scrambled), or, for the vegetarian, tofu burger.

4 raw proteins = soaked organic seeds (sunflower, sesame, pumpkin, squash, flax, chia, etc.) sunflower sprouts, alfalfa sprouts, low fat or nonfat cottage cheese, French feta cheese, tahini. Avoid molds on sprouts by washing in Clorox®, hydrogen peroxide, or preferably grapefruit seeded extract; see section on treating produce to rid it of molds.

1 cooked vegetable = broccoli, bok choy, artichoke, cauliflower, kale, collards, green beans, asparagus, cabbage, celery, green and red bell pepper, and most any of the other "pot herb" vegetables available, or a green leafy vegetable.

4 raw vegetables = salad of leaf lettuce (not iceberg), endive, spinach, arrugula, cress, dandelion, celery, tomato, cauliflower, carrot, beet, radish, jicama, parsley, cabbage, cucumber, collards, beet greens, kale, cucumber (without the skin), sprouts (they do double duty as vegetable and protein).

YOUR MEAL MIGHT LOOK LIKE THE ONE PORTRAYED IN THIS DRAWING:

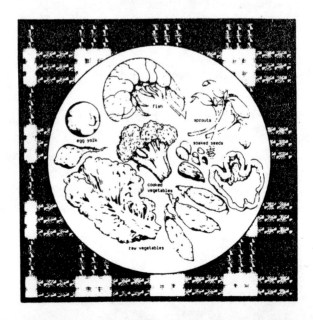

PRO-VITA! PLAN MENU SAMPLE

Now that we have examined the foundation of the Pro-Vita! Plan, we take a look at a sample menu to see what it is like.

Upon Arising: Drink 6 ounces of pure, room temperature water to flush out toxins and meet water requirements. A little fresh vegetable juice (green drink) may be used in addition to water, if you like. Exercise lightly to raise basal metabolism.

Breakfast: The plan is to have 60% of the day's total calories and nutritional value.

- Small yard egg omelet with broccoli or spinach, cooked above 180º F but below 200º F to retain protein and enzyme values.

- 1 tablespoon soaked seeds mix (sesame, sunflower, pumpkin, flax, chia, etc.)

- 1 cup sauteed vegetables and leafy greens mix (beet greens, bok choy, chard, collard greens, kale, etc.)

- 1 tablespoon low or nonfat fat cottage cheese or organic feta cheese (optional)

- Raw cabbage salad, or raw sauerkraut, and a large portion of sprouts (pre-soaked to get rid of molds)

- A few celery and carrot sticks, perhaps with tahini

NOTE: Do not eat carbohydrates with this meal. Restrict your water intake during and one hour after the meal, because water and fluids dilute the digestive enzymes. Nutritional supplements can be taken with this meal.

Mid-morning: 2 and 1/2 hours after breakfast.

Drink a glass of pure water if you are thirsty or some raw vegetable juice. The raw red potato juice is particularly beneficial. This is a good time to check the urinary pH and make an adjustment: If too acid, use lemon or lime juice in water; if too alkaline, use a little cranberry juice in water.

Lunch: Another example of a Pro-Vita! 5+5 meal, representing 25% to 30% of the day's total calories and nutritive value.

- Small piece of sauteed ocean fish, shrimp, curried organic chicken, or for vegetarians a tofu patty, sprouted grain patty, or miso soup.

- Lightly steamed asparagus or other green vegetable

- 1 tablespoon soaked seed mix

- 1 tablespoon organic feta cheese, crumbled on salad

- Large fresh salad (lettuce, cabbage, spinach, lentil and sunflower sprouts, olives), with homemade salad dressing

NOTE: Do not eat foods high in carbohydrates with this meal. Again, restrict water and fluids. It is optimal to have lunch 4 and 1/2 hours after breakfast. This period gives the digestive system time to recover from breakfast. This second Pro-Vita! meal is for people who wish to build their cellular protein values, recover from illness, loose weight, or balance blood sugar. Otherwise, this meal could be a complex carbohydrate meal for people who wish to gain weight or who will be engaging in strenuous physical exercise that afternoon.

Mid-afternoon: Drink a glass of pure water if thirsty, or drink fresh vegetable juice if you wish to build your nutritional values. Adjust pH if you need to. This is an excellent time (4-6 pm) for strenuous, aerobic exercise as the breakfast nutrients are becoming available to the metabolism.

Supper: This meal is optional and best if it is light, i.e., soups, salads, fruit salads, or popcorn (cooked with hot air, not with oil). People who want to lose weight should skip this meal. After all, breakfast is just around the corner. Some persons may want to eat fruit salad only at this time. People who want to gain or maintain weight may have complex carbohydrates (potatoes, pasta, rice, boiled beans, grains, oatmeal and cereals) with vegetables as follows:

- Baked potato with condiments (salsa, herbs)

- Stir-fried or steamed vegetables (snow peas, celery, bell pepper, carrot, peppers, garlic, onion, asparagus, Brussels sprouts, cauliflower, sweet potato, green beans, cabbage, corn, etc.)

- Fresh garden salad with sprouts which are excellent with both carbohydrate and protein meals

- Vegetable soup

NOTE: Do not eat protein with this meal. It is okay to drink a little water or other fluid.

30 Minutes Before Bed: Herb tea, juice, or a glass of water if desired.

This diet matrix allows a great deal of improvisation depending on what you want to accomplish. Athletes who are working on endurance and pushing their bodies to new limits should have protein plus vegetables for breakfast, complex carbohydrate plus vegetables for three or four lunches a week, and complex carbohydrate plus vegetables for supper. The additional complex carbohydrate meals provide the needed energy for a body system undergoing the stress of athletic training and performing. Also, a less active person might want to switch to two low-stress protein meals a day to maintain a desired weight once it is reached.

To lose weight, use two Pro-Vita! 5+5 meals a day and limit supper to a light salad or, preferably, just herb tea or a little fruit.

The following table presents an ideal arrangement of meal types for different people. We use the following abbreviations for the meal types:

PV = Pro-Vita! 5+5 meal; CC = Complex Carbohydrates + Vegetables Meal; LF = Light Foods (fruit, soup broth, small salad); When two meals are listed, alternate them.

Person	Breakfast	Lunch	Supper
Athletes	PV	CC	CC
Children	PV	CC/PV	CC
Overweight	PV	PV	LF
Underweight	PV	CC	CC
Normal Weight	PV	CC/PV	CC/LF
Pregnant	PV	PV	CC
Convalescent	PV	PV	LF
Immune Deficient	PV	PV/CC	CC/LF
Highly Stressed	PV	PV	LF
Hypoglycemic	PV/CC snack	PV/CC snack	CC
Menopausal	PV	PV	CC/LF
Infants	Breast-feed		
Nursing Mothers	PV	PV/CC	CC

One key point about the PRO-VITA! PLAN is that it DOES NOT RESTRICT YOUR FOOD INTAKE beyond what common sense dictates. Instead, it reorganizes the food planning. You can still have eggs and toast, but preferably not at the same meal. Instead, have sprouts and vegetables with the eggs and thereby quadruple your nutrition intake.

Inevitably, there is a transition period when you change your dietary pattern. Give yourself some time to accomplish the new planning. Cut yourself some slack. Be sure to break the diet plan once a week and do everything wrong! This will keep you from developing restrictive attitudes and also be a lesson in how you feel when you do not follow the body's natural laws. This break in the routine might include pancakes for breakfast on a Saturday morning or pizza for supper Saturday night. Enjoy fun foods in moderation. When you dine out, order what pleases you. Afterwards, return to building your health with the Pro-Vita! Plan the following day.

Over the course of several months, you will experience a more sustained energy level, and this method of eating will become more and more comfortable for you. You will also be experienced, by this time, how to order low-stress meals in restaurants when you want to.

Remember: What you do 80% OF THE TIME sets the tone for your metabolism. You do not have to follow the Pro-Vita! Plan perfectly all at once.

TWO WEEKS OF PRO-VITA! BREAKFAST PLANS

Just as your parents told you, breakfast is the most important meal of the day. Try to make sure that all of the needed nutritional elements are included to get the day off to a great start. First, here are some suggestions that can help to make breakfast a complete, delicious and easy meal. Following that is a week's worth of wonderful breakfasts for you and your family to enjoy.

For people who are adverse to having breakfast early in the day, attempt to have a light Pro-Vita! meal as early as possible. Avoid skipping breakfast and relying on your reserves until lunch. It would be better to have a Pro-Vita! breakfast at 10 am than to run on coffee and donuts.

Try to have a variety of soaked seeds on hand in jars in the refrigerator. You can mix and match them for variety. It is also a good idea to have a nice variety of sprouts ready for daily use. If soybean sprouts are used, they should be cooked with stir-fried vegetables because cooking breaks down their anti-proteolytic enzymes. Raw soy sprouts can inhibit the assimilation of dietary proteins.

Develop the practice to clean all foods as soon as you bring them home from the store and before you put them into the refrigerator. Use the Clorox®, hydrogen peroxide or grapefruit seed extract soak described in this book.

Arrange your refrigerator in accordance with the Pro-Vita! Plan. One shelf can be dedicated to proteins, such as soaked seeds; sprouts; yard eggs; seafood; organic chicken; raw milk, low fat or nonfat cottage cheese; organic feta cheese; nut butters; tahini; tofu; pine nuts; miso; tempeh and beet leaf. Add condiments such as capers and olives, served with proteins. Another shelf can be used to store carbohydrates, such as breads, corn bread, tortillas, boiled beans or rice. Still another shelf, or maybe a drawer, can hold fruits, and another two shelves or drawers can contain the vegetables. In this arrangement you group foods which makes for easier Pro-Vita! meal planning.

SAMPLE BREAKFASTS FOR TWO WEEKS

The focus here is not on vegetarian dishes. Vegetarians should substitute vegetarian proteins where needed.

1. Cole slaw (organic green and purple cabbage, cottage cheese, fennel)
   Yard egg omelet with sliced, fresh broccoli stalks (peel the stalks), seeds, fresh herbs
   Soaked seeds mix (1 tbsp.)
   Feta cheese (1 tbsp.)
   Fresh sunflower and chia sprouts
   Carrot, celery, jicama slices

2. Asparagus, lightly steamed
   4 oz. orange roughy or other ocean fish, broiled or pan-fried in a bit of grape seed oil
   Soaked seeds
   Large, fresh garden salad with sprout mixture (alfalfa, radish, lentil)

Natural salad dressing or flax seed oil and
umeboshi vinegar

3. Medley of fresh vegetables, lightly steamed
   Four large shrimp grilled lightly with garlic,
   thyme and basil
   Sprouts, soaked seeds and finger vegetables
   complemented with tahini or a dip

4. Garden salad (variety of fresh vegetables),
   Avocado slices
   Chicken Omelet Ranchero; a few pieces of
   previously grilled organic chicken can be
   added to a yard egg omelet along with some
   jalapenos and ranchero or picante sauce
   Complement with lightly grilled bell peppers
   Soaked seeds and sprouts

5. On the run! (It's easy to travel with this meal.)
   Tahini vegetables. (Sprout mix with assort
   ment of raw vegetables such as celery, car
   rot, jicama, broccoli, cauliflower)
   Two deviled eggs (medium boiled rather than
   hard- boiled) with a dollop of raw milk or low
   fat/nonfat cottage cheese and herb seasoning
   A few olives, capers, a pickle
   Cole slaw with sunflower seeds
   Baby corn

6. Steamed broccoli with herb-seasoned organic,
   balanced butter sauce
   Marinated fish/haddie/ceviche, calamari
   Bib lettuce salad with artichoke hearts,
   palm hearts, etc.
   Blend soaked seeds with a little flax seed oil and
   herbs for salad dressing

As you can see, there are many possible combinations for a nutritious Pro-Vita! breakfast. Use your imagination to work with the foods available to you.

And in case you wondered, "a week's worth" of Pro-Vita! 5+5 breakfasts adds up to SIX meals. This brings us to an important health tip for those of you who want to go the extra step for optimal health. It's the one day a week "fast" or abstinence from food. This is discussed in a subsequent chapter.

Before going further with our discussion, we present another week's worth of Pro-Vita! Plan breakfasts. These two weeks of non-repetitive meals are really only a start on all the possibilities! Let' start with a vegetarian meal which is recommended for the vegetarian and non-vegetarian alike.

7. Tofu, scrambled like eggs, including sesame seeds
   (see recipe)
   Red & white salad (raw beet & turnip)
   Steamed vegetable (kale)
   Soaked seeds, sprouts

8. Caesar salad, large
   Grilled or steamed organic chicken breast
   Sprouts, seeds, olives,
   Steamed vegetables (green beans)

9. 3-Lettuce salad with array of sprouts
   Calamari, sauteed with garlic, or grilled like scampi
   Garnish with seeds, feta cheese, sweet peppers,
   olives

10. Avocado omelet (yard egg folded over avocado
   slices, grated carrot and sunflower seeds, garnished
   with crumbled feta cheese)
   Finger vegetables (carrot, celery, cauliflower,
   jicama)
   Dressing or tahini on assortment of sprouts

11. Artichoke, steamed
   Cottage cheese (raw milk or low fat/nonfat) dip
   with assorted dipping vegetables
   A cup of steamed vegetable greens (kale) with
   tahini/ginger sauce
   A few sprouts and seeds

12. Spinach, lettuce and greens (kale, endive) salad
   with sprouts, seeds, walnuts and dressing
   Grilled, organic chicken hot dog, or organic
   turkey patty
   Sprouts and soaked seeds

These are just a few suggestions, some with a non-vegetarian focus, which is where most people will start. Vegetarians will use miso with tofu more frequently for breakfast, as the Japanese people do, to provide low-stress protein early in the day.

21

PRO-VITA! FOR CHILDREN

A SUCCESSFUL SCENARIO

The Pro-Vita! Plan orientation is excellent for children. In fact, children naturally take to the plan when it is properly implemented.

It is my experience that children in a household with a Pro-Vita! kitchen have fewer allergies, fewer colds and are less susceptible to flus. These children grow well, heal well and experience a higher quality of health in general.

In my household, my children help with the meal preparation. They choose which vegetables to put in the salad, set the table and open jars. My four-year-old daughter chooses foods to garnish her plate, such as olives, baby corn, carrot sticks, celery sticks, capers and sprouts.

I would like to draw upon my personal experience with children who are involved in a Pro-Vita! nutrition plan. I will idealize it a bit and give you a successful, nutritional children's scenario. Then we will look at a case where implementing the new nutrition plan did not work well. Finally, we will discuss easy transitions to the new plan so that you, too, can be successful in introducing positive changes to your family.

Imagine four-year-old Lauren, putting vegetable finger foods on the plates for lunch. The fact that a few olives and carrots go into her mouth along the way is fine, because our first course is salad.

Actually, salad is not the children's favorite food. But they have to eat it to get to the main course which, at this meal, is spaghetti made from spelt grain. The spaghetti is cooking and the wonderful smell of the marinera sauce (without meat) leads the children on. Their salad is small and contains plenty of the vegetables they like.

But the salad also has the vegetables that I choose. I have added a sliver of bell pepper, red beet or raw cauliflower. Just a bite of these vegetables fills out the salad and gives exposure to a wide variety of vegetables, not just those which the children like.

Colin, the ten-year-old, wolfs down his salad to get it over with quick. Lauren adds salad dressing and picks around for a few minutes, until she realizes that Colin is already getting his spaghetti. Then, her salad disappears and she is ready for spaghetti, too.

Along with the spaghetti, a bit of lightly steamed broccoli is served. The portion of spaghetti is a bit smaller than the children would like. But they can have "seconds" whenever their plates are clean. This means that they eat the broccoli before they get seconds of spaghetti.

Lauren gets too full along the way, and I remind her to take a bite of her broccoli so that she can be excused from the table or qualify for a whole-grain cookie a little later. Gulp, the broccoli is gone. Colin has thirds, since spaghetti is his favorite meal.

This is how this successful nutrition scenario happened. There has been no trauma, no threats of having to "eat vegetables...or else." In this way, little by little, day after day, the children are eating many more vegetables than the average kid. And they don't even know it! Because the portions of vegetables are small, and there are incentives to eat them, everything runs smoothly. Consequently, the nutrition plan is very easy and the children enjoy the meal.

Some people are blessed with children who love vegetables, but most of us have children who would rather avoid them. This happens because their young taste buds are exposed to highly seasoned foods like pizza early on, and they encounter massive amounts of sugar in sodas, ice cream, breakfast cereals, bubble gum and candies.

The more "sugar and spice" warped the children's taste and appetite become, the fewer vegetables they desire. Not desiring vegetables, or becoming intolerant of eating vegetables, is a SYMPTOM of a perverted appetite usually due to the use of sugar. Conversely, as sugar is reduced in the nutrition plan, the desire for fruits returns. Then, the desire for vegetables also returns, and there is no struggle to have children eat more well-balanced meals.

AN UNSUCCESSFUL SCENARIO

Now for the unsuccessful attempt to include children in the Pro-Vita! nutrition. It often happens that a person reads information such as in this book, becomes excited about the potentials that improved health can bring, and then inflicts the dietary philosophy on family and children, making the new diet THE WAY of life. Such an occurrence is usually a mistake, even though it is prompted by the best of intentions to safeguard health and improve the quality of life.

Forcing a change can cause family quarrels, uncooperative behaviors, and do more damage in the long run than the benefits of the new nutrition plan could bring. For example, an uncooperative teen was denied her long-standing breakfast of Cream of Wheat® by her mother, who wanted to implement the Pro-Vita! breakfast menu, simply started stopping off at a convenience store on her way to school to eat donuts, candy and drink Coca-cola®. Her mother insisted that she eat eggs for breakfast, so the daughter dropped them into her napkin and headed for junk food.

At the time this particular incident occurred, this girl was taking the homeopathic remedy *Ferrum metalicum* for her symptoms which included headaches, anemia and heart palpitations. Unknown to the mother, a keynote of this remedy picture is "that the person is adverse to eggs, and eggs aggravate." Thus, there was a strong predisposition for the daughter to dislike and avoid eggs. The daughter's lack of progress on the remedy as well as the development of hypoglycemic symptoms were puzzling to me and caused delay of her improvement. I ended up recommending other remedies for two months, until the whole picture came into perspective through an emotional encounter between mother and daughter in my office.

In this unsuccessful scenario to switch to the Pro-Vita! plan, the mother decided, carte blanche, that breakfast would change from carbohydrate Cream of Wheat to protein omelets. She had read and implemented the Pro-Vita! Plan, and it was working well for her. However, I immediately reinstated Cream of Wheat for breakfast for the daughter. Then, I returned to the original homeopathic remedy and the case progressed to a happy conclusion.

This is an example where a little finesse and cooperation would have paid a big dividend. Step one might have been to add some vegetables to the less-than-optimal Cream of Wheat breakfast. Since the daughter was anemic, Cream of Wheat may not have been the best food, if her system was allowing the phytates in wheat to bind up iron and make it unassimilable. But rather than implementing a radical change, adding a carrot or celery stick to the cereal meal would have been an improvement that the daughter would have enjoyed.

Subsequently, instead of serving Cream of Wheat every day, the mother could attempt to serve breakfasts, such as oatmeal, grits, cream of rye, buckwheat groats and other grains without making a new rule or law for a teenager. After attaining some flexibility, the leap to a protein-based breakfast could be attempted. The vegetables would be the same as before, but now other additional foods could be tried with the daughter's cooperation. Miso soup, tofu dishes, left-over chicken breast— whatever was agreeable—could be served. Just because the Pro-Vita! was working well at that time for the mother did not ensure that the plan would instantly work well for the daughter. As the daughter's health improved, there was a good chance that the daughter's aversion to eggs would drop away. Then she might consider making omelets together with her mom.

SUGGESTIONS FOR SUCCESS

Another way to approach dietary changes with children is to plan meals for the week so that they know there are days for their favorite foods. Saturday morning, for example, is pancake day with my children. The pancakes are made from organic, whole grain spelt mix without milk; the maple syrup is organic grade C, or honey is used; and there are finger vegetables to eat between each helping of pancakes. I just make sure that the children have a Pro-Vita! 5+5 lunch later that day.

We need to keep in mind that generally children's bodies burn more carbohydrate energy than adults. Thus, they do better with carbohydrates than adults. Consequently, children might have an extra oatmeal day while the parent has a Pro-Vita! 5+5 breakfast.

Too much restriction in a nutritional plan is not good. Junk foods are not all bad. We have to keep our perspective and move for improvement. The simple addition of one celery stick to a "meat-

and-potatoes" breakfast is an improvement as the first step. Most of the time, it is not good to make dietary changes too fast because the change becomes stressful to the body. The change can also be stressful to relationships.

Anytime you make alterations in your diet, you should let your homeopathic or naturopathic physician know. This is very important to his or her evaluation of how your treatment is progressing. For example, if constipation is a chronic problem, this fact is a consideration in the selection of your treatment program. If you suddenly start eating three teaspoons of flax seeds and start having better bowel movements, your practitioner needs to know that this is the result of a dietary change and may or may not be a healing of your internal predisposition to constipation.

The homeopath is primarily concerned with your complete and lasting cure which, in this example, would be your body's ability to adapt to varied diets and not express constipation as a symptom. Flax seeds are good for nutrition and overall health, but you should not be satisfied with the homeopathic treatment until you have no constipation whether you eat flax seeds or not.

Another perspective to keep in mind when involving children in the Pro-Vita! Plan is the concept that with children "it all comes out in the wash." This means that a parent who goes with the flow and does not force diet on children, will probably be more successful in the long run. As parents, we should look at nutrition as it adds up over a year rather than at one meal.

If I feel that there has been a let-down in good nutrition with my children due to travel, parties, spending the night with a friend, or other events, I just add a little kelp powder to the spaghetti sauce and no one knows. I encourage fruit for a snack and plan dinner a little later. My focus is on boosting nutrition whenever I can, while letting the children live life. With a good foundation of nutrition, the ice cream and cake at a birthday party should not ruin their nutrition.

Some people force their children to eat a lot of vegetables. If children are adverse to eating a vegetable, let them get away with just one bite and make up the difference with something they like to eat like a carrot, for example. Everyone has preferences. Keeping the children's systems exposed to varied foods, and not allowing them to completely abstain from the food, keeps the door of experience open and prevents intolerance from developing. Too many people decide at age six that they don't like Lima beans and then never try them again. Thus, they miss a food which could well contribute to their health later in life. It is not uncommon for a child who hates Lima beans at age six to enjoy them at age fourteen.

If children are not overdosed with sugar in their diets, their instinctive abilities can help guide them to the appropriate foods at any one time. There may be a phase of eating a food that is needed by the body and avoiding some foods that are not needed. As the body's needs change, the child will gravitate to different foods, provided the parents keep them exposed to a variety of foods. This is the reason for presenting children with varieties of foods and allowing them some slack if they are adverse to a food.

Exposure to a wide variety of foods, even just one bite, keeps the instinctive system open. Letting children eat exclusively from their favorites is limiting to their overall health and ability to detect when they should eat more of a nutrient source. The major point here is that one bite can make a difference in the child's health, adaptability and instinctive ability to eat for health.

The general guidelines for the children's Pro-Vita! Plan are to take an easy approach to it attitudinally; promote fruits and vegetables for snacks; encourage children to grow food such as sprouts, tomatoes, or have a small garden; strive for variety so that they have adventures in differing tastes; include vegetables with every meal; and teach them the role of living foods for their bodies.

TRANSITION TO THE PRO-VITA! FOOD PLAN

SUMMARY OF PRINCIPLES

Throughout this book we have discussed guidelines for working with food to create better health. The primary focus, after a foundation of vegetables is established, is on effective use of proteins: How to maximize their digestion, assimilation and use at the cellular level, as well as how to avoid protein toxicity. Achieving maximum effect is accomplished through a rational approach based on biochemistry and bioenergy. For most people this plan will mean reducing the quantity of protein consumed. For some it will mean increasing protein consumption. For everyone it means using protein properly.

The first step for the individual who wants to use this nutritional plan is to separate consumption of protein and carbohydrate and to have one or two protein meals a day prepared correctly. Eggs (properly cooked) with sprouts, celery, soaked seeds and vegetables work very well for a Pro-Vita! 5+5 breakfast. This meal is not too out-of-the-ordinary for most families.

Some people find the Pro-Vita! Plan a little restrictive at first, because they have to reorganize their dietary patterns. But to anyone who is or already has been involved with diet philosophies, Pro-Vita! will, thankfully, open the way to more variety. In either case, the Pro-Vita! Plan is just a matter of mapping out a menu that fits your lifestyle.

At the end of this section is a worksheet that you can use to help rearrange your menu to work for your health.

BREAKFAST IS THE MOST IMPORTANT MEAL and should be the focus for transition to this diet plan. The first goal should be to have six Pro-Vita! 5+5 breakfasts per week for a month. Then work on other refinements.

In regards to your other meals, just exercise your good sense. These meals can capitalize on carbohydrates and center around baked potatoes, fresh-milled basmati rice dishes, spelt spaghetti or soup. Or perhaps you may want to include a fruit meal of sliced apple, grapes, strawberries, or other fruit. Meals of assorted steamed vegetables over rice are popular. Just forego having proteins with the carbohydrates and fruits.

It is not a good practice to make a lot of dietary changes all at once because to do so is stressful for your body. Initially, focus on having one Pro-Vita! 5 + 5 meal a day which means a little protein for breakfast, organized according to this book's instructions, and a lot of vegetables. Some people may need to focus on lunch at first since the Pro-Vita! breakfast so often resembles a high-quality lunch.

Usually, the most difficult dietary habits to overcome are eating sandwiches with cheese or meat, and using milk with breakfast cereals. Both of these practices combine concentrated proteins with concentrated carbohydrates. And both of these food combinations make up a large part of the American diet "philosophy" as sold to us by television ads. By only a little stretch of logic we could say that such dietary principles are involved in the massive constipation, food allergy and degenerative disease trends found in this country.

Sometimes it is difficult to uproot dietary patterns and embark on new dietary adventures. Therefore, transitions are important and the best way to make a transition to a new diet is by having some substitutions which allow us to become accustomed to a new diet without too radical a change.

Substitutions for meat or cheese and bread sandwiches can be found in avocado sandwiches (without cheese) and in vegetable patties made from the mixes available at health food stores. These patties (a vege-mix) are delicious and resemble meat. Be sure to avoid the vegetarian mixes made from soy bean proteins. A sandwich can be constructed to resemble any ordinary meat and carbohydrate sandwich, yet be strictly carbohydrate and stay within the low-stress guidelines.

Milk on cereal is harder to substitute. Some people use hot cereals for supper, such as oatmeal, rye meal or bear mush with just a little maple syrup and balanced, organic butter. Processed breakfast cereals are not a good food source anyway, and the cost is very high for the amount of food received. Only 5% of the total cost of a package of cereal is actually for the food; most of the price is paid for packaging, advertising and marketing. This is reason enough for letting go of these foods. The manufacturers obviously take the public to be idiots, so not buying processed cereals helps break that attitude. Ironically, many cereal makers advertise their products to be healthy due to the high-fiber content and then lace it with BHA and BHT, substances outlawed in several European countries.

Do not worry too much about which food combines with what other food. Your body will tell you what is working for you and what is not. Tummy aches, tiredness, gas, sleepiness after eating, or hard bowel movements give clues how we are handling our diets. Learn to listen to your body.

THE 18% RULE

Please remember that our food planning rules are not hard and fast. A person can have, as a general rule, up to 18% carbohydrate in a protein meal and the body will still recognize it as a protein meal and process it accordingly. Recall that most of that 18% carbohydrates derives from the large amount of vegetables recommended, but it does leave a little extra room for other carbohydrates. For instance, a chicken or tofu fajita can be served on a corn tortilla vs. a flour tortilla and still fall within the 18% rule. Sprouts can go with either a protein meal or a carbohydrate meal.

A good nutritional plan does not mean that life is miserable because all the "good" things are "not allowed." Good diet is characterized by variety, moderation and a focus on whole, living foods, deliciously prepared according to a few sensible rules, in addition to a spirit of gratitude for the life-sustaining processes.

You can see that this food plan is not too restrictive. It simply reorganizes the way we eat. However, people often ask, "Well, when can I have apple pie?" The best time to enjoy sweets and non-protein snacks is in the mid-afternoon. But do include a few raw vegetables with your snack. This way the body can deal with snacks without upsetting the digestion of the food that it needs every day. In most cases, health-conscious people can continue eating many of the same foods they have been eating; just the order of eating them may need to be changed.

SIX STEPS TO A PRO-VITA! KITCHEN

Just as with so many other new things, the first step to start this nutrition program is the most challenging. The following are specifics to get started on the Pro-Vita! Plan.

STEP ONE

Clean out your refrigerator. Make room in your life and kitchen for healthy foods. Throw away the high-stress, empty "foods" listed in the "Strive to Avoid" tables. Make a grocery list. For every item thrown away, replace it with a wholesome substitute. For example:

THROW AWAY	REPLACE WITH
white bread	whole grain bread
frozen pizza with chemicals	pizza with whole grain crust, no preservatives
sugar cookies	whole grain, fruit juice cookies
canned fruit	fresh fruit
commercial eggs	fertile yard eggs
soft drinks	bottled juices (organic) lemonade, hibiscus cooler
shortening	grape seed, canola
potato chips	baked chips, toasted pita
ice cream	organic fruit sorbet,
processed cheese	organic feta, low-fat goat cheese, raw milk cheese
peanut butter	tahini (sesame butter)

THROW AWAY	REPLACE WITH
coffee	herbal teas
boxed breakfast cereals	organic, whole grain cereals
bacon	non-pork, no-nitrate bacon
roasted, salted nuts	sunflower & pumpkin seeds
raisins*	organic raisins

* Steinman identifies commercial raisins as a red light food, that is, they are quite laden with toxins and chemicals. Raisins are a major food for children at home as well as in preschool and school lunches.

This exercise in substitution and replacement keeps you from doing without food and makes the transition easier. It is an essential step, particularly if you have a family. In time, you will think of other items that you want to replace.

STEP TWO

Plan a week's menu. Avoid repetition.

STEP THREE

Go shopping. Buy the items that you need to replace those you have thrown out. Also buy a week's worth of Pro-Vita! 5+5 meals.

Proteins for non-vegetarians may include several kinds of fresh fish, shrimp, squid, organic chicken, game birds, buffalo burgers, several varieties of seeds, several varieties of sprouts, yard eggs, a few raw nuts (almonds), organic turkey roast, organic feta cheese, organic goat cheeses, low fat cottage cheese, tahini, miso, tofu and tempeh.

If possible, buy only organic vegetables. A second consideration is to buy vegetables in season rather than those imported from abroad. The same principles apply to fruit.

Vegetables may include a little of everything from the fresh produce department. Carrots, celery, bok choy, romaine lettuce, bib lettuce, red leaf lettuce, cucumber, tomato, onion, garlic, parsley, green beans, green and red cabbage, green and red bell peppers, asparagus, beets with tops, chard, Brussels sprouts, kale, collards or spinach. Since salads are included with each meal, you want to make a variety, such as Caesar salad, grated carrot salad, garden salad, finger food salad, red and white salad (grated beets and turnips).

Buy a variety of fresh, organic, in-season fruit.

Variety in vegetables and fruits is important for two reasons. If you rotate the vegetables, you will have varied nutrient sources and avoid food allergies. Perhaps most importantly, you will avoid boredom.

Carbohydrates are easy to come by. Take a few organic potatoes, some corn, rice, a loaf of bread, pitas, baked chips or spaghetti.

Buy condiments like capers, olives, seaweed seasonings, ginger, garlic, unprocessed sea salt, organic sesame shake seasoning, dressing made with good oil, organic tofu mayonnaise for special flavors.

STEP FOUR

Soak your newly bought produce before you put it away in the refrigerator. See the instructions for ridding your food of toxins.

STEP FIVE

Put foods away by category, i.e., proteins on the second shelf, carbohydrates on the third shelf, and vegetables in the crisper, etc.

STEP SIX

Prepare your next day's breakfast now. Marinate a small piece of fresh fish in ginger, garlic, sherry and soy sauce. Soak a variety of seeds in water with a few drops of stabilized oxygen or pineapple juice. Prepare some salad in a bowl and cover. Save some of supper's steamed vegetables. With these preparations you will be able to fix a nutritious breakfast in a few minutes!

THE PRO-VITA! PLANNING SHEET

In Appendix D are the Pro-Vita! Planning Sheets. Write down what you normally eat on the left side. Then take those foods and rearrange them into appropriate Pro-Vita! categories on the right side. This way you will see which foods stay, which ones go, and what you need to obtain to have a Pro-Vita! day. Additional Planning Sheets are provided in Appendix D.

WATER, EXERCISE AND FASTING

WATER, OUR FOUNDATION OF LIFE

Water is critical to nutrition because it helps digest, absorb and transport nutrients throughout the body. The chemical reactions in the body occur in a salt water solution. Also, water carries colloidal minerals that are used for cellular function. Both the adage that you should "drink eight glasses a day," and the fact that three-quarters of the body is water should give you the message that it is crucial to drink enough pure water every day.

Unfortunately, most of the water on this water planet is now contaminated with chemicals, pesticides, radiation, bacteria, Giardia, amoebas and other pollutants. Tap water is unfit for drinking and is not conducive to good health. Spring waters are often contaminated, too. Distilled waters, while usually clean, are considered dead because their bioavailability is low due to the heat-altered shape of the molecule and its estrangement from the earth. Volatile gases can be concentrated in distilled water from the distillation process. Consequently, it is vitally necessary to provide yourself and your family with pure, bioavailable, soft, clean and living water.

I am most familiar with Austin's municipal water since I live here, so let's take a look at some considerations regarding what is in hundreds of thousands of people's water pipes. Keep in mind that Austin's water is less polluted than many other places in this country and the world.

Austin's water is of poor quality for drinking, bathing and cooking. Furthermore, Austin's water contains, as all city waters do, unknown elements since there are over 200 trace chemicals in it ranging from small amounts of industrial and agricultural pollutants to overt addition of chlorine, ammonia and fluoride.

Austin's water is alkaline, almost to the point of unsuitability for life. With a pH that stays above 8.5 and often goes as high as 10, the water disrupts the pH values of skin and hair. Skin prefers a pH of 5.5. - 6.5 which is often referred to as the "acid mantle" that protects the body from the external environment. The acid skin is a first-line defense against infectious bacteria such as streptococcus, staphylococcus and fungus. A water pH of 7 (neutral) is ideal because it cleans without disrupting the pH as much as alkaline water does.

Most infectious organisms require an alkaline environment (like the water supply) to survive. Unless tap water is buffered by the addition of a cup of apple cider vinegar, bathing in it can leave a person more susceptible to infections and skin conditions. Impetigo, eczema, barber's rash, acne and infections have all been linked to the overly alkaline quality of water as a contributing factor.

The elasticity of the skin's proteins is maintained in an acid pH. Hard alkaline water ages the skin and contributes to dry skin. Cosmetics, if they contain mineral oil, further damage the skin.

Many people spend considerable sums of money on their hair and for hair products. Washing hair in alkaline, chemical-laden water inhibits proper cleansing of the hair and scalp. The hair's delicate protein sheath is also acidic. Hard, alkaline water leaves hair stringy, lackluster and stiff. To protect the pH of the hair, many people rinse their hair with two tablespoons of apple cider vinegar in a cup of pure water after contact with tap water.

Drinking and cooking with tap water should be considered unthinkable, or thinkable only in emergencies, because it is clearly in the "detrimental to health" rather than the "beneficial to life" category where water must be. Here are four reasons to avoid getting tap water inside your body:

1. Traces of 200-300 unnatural chemicals, some of which may lead to cancer, inhibited immune systems and allergies.

2. Chemical additives such as chlorine and fluoride inhibit the action of vitamin E in our bodies, resulting in free radical damage to the arteries. Chlorinated water has

been linked to cancer of the bladder and rectum by Robert Morris who headed the study at the Medical College of Wisconsin, published in the *American Journal of Public Health* (July, 1992) According to his study, chorine reacts with other organic matter and chemicals in water to form carcinogenic compounds.

Our bodies should not be the receptacle of the aluminum industry's poisonous by-product fluoride. Due to specious reasoning and spurious dental research, our water supply is deliberately contaminated with the unchelated halogen— fluoride—which has been linked to increased urinary tract infections, retarded and abnormal bone development, and carcinoma.

3. The high pH of hard waters inhibits protein digestion. Vegetarians using tap water to boil beans and rice further inhibit the possibility of getting useable amino acids from the meal.

4. The inorganic calcium ions in many water supplies are the form of calcium that deposits in joints (arthritis, rheumatism) and contribute to heart disease. Here in Texas, we often see stiff old cowboys who appear to have become cemented inside. Hard water and hard livin' have calcified their veins.

THERE ARE THREE WAYS TO HAVE PURE WATER FOR HEALTH:

1. Use a high quality, well-maintained reverse osmosis water purification system.

2. Use distilled water that has been enlivened with 1 teaspoon of sea water per gallon, plus 10 drops of stabilized oxygen, plus six hours of sitting in the sunlight.

3. Use expensive bottled waters, such as Volvic or Evian, when dining in restaurants, or verify that the restaurant has a purification system.

HOW MUCH WATER DO YOU NEED?

In a natural state, a person's water intake would be set by the body itself via thirst. Thus, a thirsty person would drink, stop drinking when satisfied, and abstain when not thirsty.

However, few people can be found who express a natural state. Instead, most people are incapable of being in touch with their "thirst" center, because of the extremes in their diets. The salty popcorn, the sugar-laden sodas, coffee and allopathic medications all warp the innate ability to regulate the body's water through thirst.

General recommendations such as "drink 8 glasses of water a day" can help, but for some people this is entirely wrong. Like all dietary matters, the amount of water a person requires is individual. The more fruit and raw vegetables included in the diet, the less supplemental water is needed. Though most people do not get enough pure water, a few get too much and stress their kidneys. People who force water down their throats because they think they need it are usually getting too much.

Most people need to focus on a slight increase in their daily pure water intake. It seems to be correct to say that over the course of a day, a person should have four glasses of pure water. There is no substitute for pure water. No tea, coffee, soda or other beverage can replace the need for pure water. Four glasses is often more than many people get, yet it does not run the risk of being more than is necessary. Beyond the four glass compromise, a person would require more water if there was a lack of raw fruit and vegetables in the diet; or if a person were engaging in strenuous labor or exercise. With consistent use of pure water, the desire for sodas and pasteurized juices, coffee and recreational beverages diminishes.

When practical, have children drink six ounces of pure water before giving them a natural soda. This practice pays respect to the fact that their thirst was asking for water, not soda or bottled fruit juice, and dilutes the impact of the recreational beverage. If they do not finish their sodas or juices due to being too full, that's fine! This way children can often split a recreational juice or soda, thus reducing the expense and improving health.

Since the Pro-Vita! Plan emphasizes vegetables, people following this plan automatically increase their water intake with the wonderful, nutrient-rich water in raw vegetables and fruit.

WATER AND WEIGHT LOSS. Water is a healing and rejuvenating therapy, particularly for people who do not drink enough. The balance of body fluids depends on having a consistent supply of pure water.

One of the first steps in a number of popular weight loss programs is to increase water intake to at least three quarts a day. Keep in mind that this is a therapy, not the normal amount of water. With proper water intake—not too little but not too much—kidney function improves and many waste products are flushed out. This relieves the liver so that it can metabolize the stored fats into energy. As toxins and excessive salt are flushed out, the body no longer needs to hold onto water to dilute the toxins. Thus, drinking the additional amount of water relieves water retention. Also, drinking the right amount of water prevents water retention.

The bowels work better with additional water, because the body does not need to extract water from the colon for its metabolic needs. Constipation is relieved. This also relieves the liver from having to deal with the bowel toxins so that it can work on metabolizing fat instead.

When the liver is relieved by increased pure water consumption, its function is improved. Then the liver is better able to humanize some of the airborne proteins (pollens), such as cedar and ragweed, that cause allergies. Many allergies are caused by the inability of the liver to disarm unusual proteins.

Drinking pure water is vitally important. Make it a high priority for your health. Remember, we have just discussed a popular therapy, not a plan for optimal water intake for day to day balance.

USING THE PRO-VITA! DIET TO LOSE WEIGHT. The book, *Your Liver-Your Lifeline* (Tips, 1990) presents Stu Wheelwright's insights into weight reduction. Here is a brief summary.

Along with the reduction in calories, it is important for most people to release the retained toxins. To do this, the following specific plan is recommended:

- Increase liver function and metabolism.

- Draw out toxins from the tissues.

- Neutralize and expel the toxins.

- Clean out toxin-producing bacteria.

- Speed up the elimination systems.

- Build strong tissues to replace fat.

- Exercise to stimulate the lymphatics.

- Get deep, relaxed rest to de-stress tissues.

- Develop a happy attitude toward life.

Your Liver-Your Lifeline (Tips 1990) discusses how to accomplish these steps, but the Pro-Vita! Plan can assist you with all nine steps. To lose weight correctly little by little with full nutritional support simply have a 5+5 breakfast, a 5+5 lunch, skip supper and drink lots of water. It is that simple! Two wonderful meals early in the day not only help you lose weight, but you should also improve your health!

EXERCISE

Although this is primarily a diet book, the importance of exercise cannot be ignored. As a matter of fact, in many ways, diet and exercise are inseparable as we will discuss. Let's look briefly at how the Pro-Vita! Plan can increase the benefits of exercise and vice versa.

In a primitive or agrarian society, exercise probably was not a problem. People just got their daily exercise naturally, mainly in their daily work. Our sedentary life-styles with automobiles, elevators and desk jobs make some sort of exercise routine vital for health.

Muscles are made to be exercised. In this way they receive new nutrients and discard waste products. Exercise is essential to move proteins out of the lymphatic system into the cells where they can rebuild and renew life at the cellular level. The temporary increase in body temperature caused by exercise kills (pasteurizes) viruses and bacteria, making exercise an important immune system support.

With the Pro-Vita! Plan's 5+5 protein and vegetable meal eaten early in the day, late afternoon to early evening becomes the most productive time for strenuous exercise. By then, the proteins eaten early in the day are already assimilated and ready to build and rebuild tissues.

Remember that upper-body exercise is as important as lower-body. The arms move the lymphatics and work the internal organs. Therefore, swimming and moving the arms through water is a particularly good form of exercise that works both the upper and lower body. Tai Chi also exercises the whole body and is a particularly beneficial exercise as it builds vitality.

Brisk walking and stretching shortly after awakening raises the basal metabolism and makes for an alert, energetic day. However, strenuous workouts and thorough exercise programs are best undertaken eight to ten hours after a Pro-Vita breakfast. It takes approximately eight hours for proteins to be digested, assimilated, humanized by the liver and made available to the cells, provided that the liver is in good working order. Do your exercise then.

The schedule of the Pro-Vita! Plan also takes advantage of the body's pH cycles to have amino acids available when the cells are best able to burn fuel and dispose of cellular, metabolic wastes.

THE ONE DAY FAST

It is a good idea to NOT eat one day a week. This allows the body the chance to rest and cleanse itself. Some people drink only water on their fast day. Others dedicate the day to only drinking herb teas and juices. Some eat only fruit. Water only is the best one-day fast, but not everyone can stick to that at first.

Some people, such as diabetics and hypoglycemics, may have difficulty with fasting and should tailor their fast to their individual circumstances. Light foods, soups and vegetable juices may be just the nutrition to keep such people active and healthy while accomplishing some of what the fast, or day of digestive rest, is to accomplish.

The idea of fasting one day a week has profound implications. In the Biblical account of creation, God rested on the seventh day. Our bodies run on seven-day cycles. For women, four seven-day cycles make up the menstrual cycle, bringing a time of cleansing and renewal. Millions of people are admonished to fast one day a week by their religions. Some donate their day's food to the needy people of their community.

A one-day-a-week fast adds up to 52 days a year—a significant rest for the digestive system, a significant savings for the food budget and a significant gain in health and longevity.

Those who fast one day a week live more in accord with the body's natural cycles. There are always blessings in store for those who live in accord with nature. Such a fasting practice eliminates the need for prolonged therapeutic fasts unless a person just wishes to fast at length for some special reason.

Should you want to participate in the one-day fast, it is recommended that you allow yourself a full 24-hour period. This means that you have your supper one evening, begin fasting as you awaken the next morning, fast all day, and do not break your fast until the following morning. Drink pure water throughout your fast. In the natural life rhythms, Friday is the optimal fast day, but from a nutritional health perspective any day will do.

Do not be discouraged if your body tells you to stop the fast by presenting symptoms of a headache or fatigue. This is either the inability to maintain proper blood sugar, or it is toxins being released. Just switch to fresh juices and continue, or just eat fruit. With time, it will become very easy to fast the one day.

People who fast one day a week usually notice a balancing trend in their health—weight normalizes, allergies clear up, constipation is relieved, and the immune system strengthens.

Most people have a tendency to overeat if food is readily available. This is particularly a problem in Western countries where the food focus has shifted to convenience and fast foods. People who eat too much take years off their lives. Their health suffers under the weight of the toxic debris in their bodies. The one-day-a-week fast allows the body to accomplish both rest and house cleaning simultaneously.

24

QUESTIONS AND ANSWERS

Q: *I am what is known as a slow oxidizer (based on my hair/tissue mineral analysis) and my husband is a fast oxidizer. Shouldn't there be a different nutritional approach for each of us?* —K.G., Madison, WI

A: The foods each of you eat can play an important role in normalizing both of your oxidation rates. In transition, each of you can focus on the foods that will assist optimal metabolism and still follow the tenets of the Pro-Vita! plan. Since Pro-Vita! provides a balanced and flexible foundation, a little finesse tailors it to each person's individual requirements. The slow oxidizer should focus on two 5+5 meals a day with moderate complex carbohydrates (whole grains) for supper. Oils and dairy products should be minimized. The fast oxidizer will thrive on oils and dairy, so the proteins chosen for his 5+5 meal could focus more on the feta cheese, salad dressings, avocado. Carbohydrates should be minimized for the fast oxidizer, so two 5+5 meals and soup for supper is a better plan. Since the Pro-Vita! Diet lets you pick and choose the accompanying foods to the basic protein plus vegetable combination, your and your husband's meals will have many similar ingredients with a different focus or quantity.

Slow oxidizers do well with low-fat proteins (fish, tofu, chicken, game birds, eggs, and bean/rice combinations). They should minimize fatty foods such as liver, avocado, coconut oil, dairy and all fried foods.

Fast oxidizers should focus on proteins such as fish, duck, goose, feta cheese, sour cream, cottage cheese, seed and nut butters, tahini, as well as stir-fried vegetables, avocado, coconut and salad dressings. Minimize carbohydrates, fruits, and unsprouted grains.

After a few months, as the transition to a more balanced metabolic rate is achieved, less concern can be placed on the foods and a well-rounded Pro-Vita! Diet can be enjoyed.

(To find out if you are a fast, mixed, slow, or normal oxidizer, consult with your holistic health professional or write to Apple-A-Day Press for how-to information.)

Q: *According to Ayurvedic medicine, I need to support the water elements in my constitution and I do this by eating fruit for breakfast. How could I tailor this diet, which makes a lot of sense to me, to my particular body type?* —Dr. B.B., Santa Fe, NM

A: The first step on your Pro-Vita! plan is to drink 8 to 12 ounces of pure water upon arising. This serves to flush out the toxins cleansed from the cells during sleep, as well as replace what the bladder empties, so proper body fluid levels are maintained. Pro-Vita! provides the water you need throughout the day, both as drinking water and through the vegetables. If you thrive on fruit, have a fruit salad for supper. This will promote better sleep and cleansing during the natural cleansing cycle.

Q: *Fish seems to be an important part of this diet, and I don't like fish. I grew up in the Midwest. The thought of eggs and tofu for breakfast everyday is frankly unappealing. As much as I like the idea of this diet, and want to cut back on red meat, it won't work for me without fish, will it?* —R.J., Dallas, TX

A: I've only recently learned that many people who don't know what properly prepared fish tastes like. It's not the greasy fast-food fried fish, and it's not the "fishy" baked stuff at the cafeteria. We're talking about a small piece of swordfish or red snapper or salmon, broiled or cooked in the skillet with herbs such as basil, thyme, and Cajun seasoning. Fish may not be your favorite, but, properly prepared, a little bit a couple of times a week should be tolerable. Also, there are people following the Pro-Vita! plan who rely more on the soaked seeds, feta cheese, and chlorella, as well as people who rotate different animal protein sources, such as chicken, pheasant, dove, turkey sausage, duck, water buffalo, deer, quail eggs, Cornish game hen, etc. Flexibility is inherent in the diet and, with a little creativity, it can be innovative and exciting.

Q: *Can I expect to lose weight by following the Pro-Vita! Plan? How much and how fast?* —C.D., Austin, TX

A: If your body is overweight, you'll gradually adjust to a more optimal weight as the body readjusts its metabolism and energy system. This is a gradual, natural weight reduction, not a crash program. People often lose inches before actual pounds are lost. This shows that tissue integrity is maintained while the fat is gradually used and lost. The body will no longer have to be in a mode of turning carbohydrate into fat and storing it for energy, since the proper protein matrix is present with the Pro-Vita! Plan. [When the liver is low in glycogen, the body works to store fats by turning carbohydrates into fats for use at a later time.]

To use the Pro-Vita! Plan to focus on PROPER WEIGHT REDUCTION without exhausting the adrenal glands (as weight-loss pills do), or depleting nutrients (as many calorie-reduction plans, drink powders, and crash diets do), or loss of tissue integrity (as fat-burner plans do), a person can have a 5+5 breakfast and lunch. Skip supper or simply have a broth. This is a high nutrition, low carbohydrate (but not a NO carbohydrate, since the vegetables provide carbohydrate) approach.

The book, *Your Liver...Your Lifeline* (Tips, 1990) gives the nine steps to weight loss. See "Using the Pro-Vita! Plan to Lose Weight" section for a summary.

By the way, underweight people often fill out with the Pro-Vita! Plan. They do this by having a 5+5 breakfast, three carbohydrate-based lunches a week, and a carbohydrate-based supper.

Q: *After nearly two years of fighting candida* [Editor's note: Candida is a yeast/fungus infection, a symptom of a weakened immune system, that further weakens the immune system] *and spending a fortune on both medical and alternative approaches, I found your book,* Conquer Candida, *and followed its advice 100%. I literally felt that if that approach didn't work I would just give up and die, because I had tried everything and was at the end of my rope.*

Within three days I felt better (more clear-headed and energetic). Then on day four I felt terrible, which I attributed to a die-off reaction. By day 10 I was coming out of it again and ever since I have truly conquered

candida. It took me three months to regain the health I had forgotten I could have. My gratitude cannot be measured. Now that I've gotten rid of candida and feel human again, will the Pro-Vita! Diet keep me from getting it again?
                                                                    —C.R., Lubbock, TX

A: Thanks for your letter. It's one of the many we've received, and that's what makes our research worthwhile. The Pro-Vita! Plan is the foundation upon which to build your new-found health. Since you were a person in candidiasis level four, you must pay attention to your health for at least another year while your immune system reestablishes its proper role in controlling yeast/fungus. Pro-Vita! with minimal refined carbohydrates, as well as the recommended therapy will put you on the road to profound recovery in the shortest period of time. We commend you for your work and for once again proving the viability of nutrition as a healing science.

Q: *I do not like the idea of using Clorox on my produce as chlorine makes me react. I'm sensitive to many odors. I prefer to use hydrogen peroxide, as you mentioned. Where do I get the 35% food grade variety? What brand do you recommend? My drug store only sells the 3% kind.*
                                                                —C.B., Palm Beach, FL

A: The 35% food grade hydrogen peroxide is available from chemical supply houses. Brands vary, but the label will say "35% food grade" or "35% reagent grade." Since this is used as a bath for produce, either kind will work just fine. In Texas it sells wholesale for $7.00 a gallon plus shipping. A word of caution is needed: 35% hydrogen peroxide is a caustic oxidizer. If spilled on your clothes it will ruin them. If it comes in contact with your skin it will burn. The advantage is you only need a little bit to soak produce, whereas you need a half bottle of the 3%. Some private individuals sell it as a cure-all for virus and arthritis and recommend drinking a few drops in water. A word of caution is needed here as well: Not only do they charge high prices (up to $128 per gallon), but our clinical research indicates that, although the internal use of hydrogen peroxide rids the bloodstream of rod-form bacteria, it also kills beneficial bacteria, damages red blood cells, and stresses the kidneys. So if you use 35% food grade hydrogen peroxide, we recommend you keep it in the sink and use the stabilized oxygen products in your body if you want an oxygen therapy. This is covered in greater detail in the 1988 edition of *Conquer Candida.*

Q: *I am Chinese and use a lot of sesame oil in my diet. How can I tell if an oil is rancid?* —W.L., Austin, TX

A: Usually by the smell. Sesame oil resists rancidity, but still should be used fresh, and stored properly. Perhaps you might be interested in learning kinesiology (a muscle-testing technique) whereby you could determine for yourself if a substance is good for you or not.

Q: *How can a person tell if he is deficient in protein at the cellular level? (I am a vegetarian.)* —C.M., Lyons, France

A: First of all, most people are low in nucleoproteins because most people eat protein and carbohydrates (meat and bread) simultaneously, and that combination precludes proper protein digestion/ assimilation. Most vegetarians are low in nucleoproteins due to a lack of protein and a reliance on carbohydrate combinations to provide proteins. So the real question is "How low are my nucleoproteins and what is my cellular ability to use the proteins available?"

In 1987 I worked with over 100 vegetarians. Only one showed an excellent level of cellular protein. She was a vegetarian of 7 years, a radiant woman, age 27, who did not rely on grains. Her proteins were based on soy ferments (tofu, miso, etc.), seeds, and vegetables. Grains gave her mucus so she avoided them, and ended up on a self-found Pro-Vita! Plan. It was a thrill for me to meet her as she was a living example of the concepts presented in this book. And because of her beliefs against inhumane treatment of animals, she foreswore meat-eating of any sort. But instead of making herself a martyr and ruining her health with a carbohydrate-based diet, she discovered the value of living foods (seeds, vegetables) and had a very high level of health—one now rapidly approaching "wellness" with the addition of a tiny piece of fish added to miso soup once a week.

There are several ways to determine cellular protein levels. An amino acid profile (based on blood) by a lab such as Tyson can give indicators. Radionic practitioners have settings to measure protein values. The blood from a finger prick reveals protein values by its sphere or lack of sphere. Other indicators of low protein values include fatigue, hypoglycemic tendencies, and a craving for sweets.

Stu Wheelwright taught that the lines in the stems of the toes reflect amino acid deficiencies. People with amino acid deficiencies or amino acid imbalances have lines on each foot's four little toe stems like this:

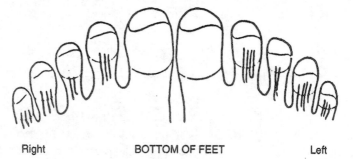

Right   BOTTOM OF FEET   Left

The lowest cellular protein values are seen in heavy red-meat eaters, followed by heavy soy protein powder users, followed by carbotarians, followed by the standard American diet eaters. People with adequate protein values do not have such lines. As the protein values improve, the lines go away. We have documented these changes clinically with people following the Pro-Vita! Diet. The lines lighten and then fade away within two to eight months and overall health improves each step of the way.

Q: *Would you comment on macrobiotics? I have a friend who cured her cancer with that diet. Can the Pro-Vita! Plan do as much?*
—TCF, Orlando, FL

A: First of all, diets do not cure cancer. Herbs do not cure cancer. Drugs do not cure cancer. Homeopathy does not cure cancer. Only the body itself cures its diseases with the adjustment of its resonance to some degree of compatibility with the vital force that animates the body.

Our files contain anecdotes from people who follow the Pro-Vita! Plan and have gotten well from cancers, but they also did other things, such as herbs, counseling, chiropractic, homeopathy, Bio-Energetic Synchronization Technique, and so forth.

Macrobiotics wisely recognizes different kinds of cancers—those caused by too many yin foods, too many yang foods, and too many extreme yin and yang foods. However, the diet itself is very alkalizing or anabolic. By capitalizing on the right foods, a person can reduce the stresses placed on the body and assist its efforts to balance itself.

This is why the Pro-Vita! Plan is so important. It is a balanced hub. Using the Pro-Vita! principles, a person can build a macrobiotic orientation around it. (This is basically what I do, because I love the seaweeds, miso soup, and so forth. I use some grain combinations in the evening.)

Pro-Vita! gives you the chemistry and energy factors, so you can eat however you think best. With Pro-Vita!, high school athletes have a 5+5 breakfast, a school cafeteria lunch, and carbohydrate supper. Vegetarians focus on vegetables and soaked seeds. Macrobiotics use the umeboshi plums and seaweeds. Meat and potato people learn to eat them at different times.

As I said earlier, I've never seen a person who's locked into someone else's diet philosophy have good health. Pro-Vita! will make you work a bit and think a bit as you tailor its principles to your individual life-style. But, good health requires a little effort in our fast-paced and polluted world.

I have some regard for macrobiotics. I have followed the plan and found it to be a helpful. But clinically I see where macrobiotic patients improve even more once the Pro-Vita! Plan is used. Clinically, I have worked with over 80 people following a strict macrobiotic diet. In reviewing my files from 1990, only 16 of them were benefitting from the diet. I think Pro-Vita! is the next step.

Best wishes in your dietary adventures!

Q: *"I'm following the Pro-Vita! Plan and feel at last my dietary needs are being met. I was formerly very attracted to Macrobiotics, but recognized that it wasn't for everyone and also that it left questions unanswered for me. Being a longtime student of Paul Twitchell's herb book I could never quite reconcile Macrobiotic's approach to raw food and enzymes until I read your book on "The Pro-Vita! Plan." My sincere thanks!*

One question: The practice of eating heavier protein-rich foods first in a meal seems like a good one (Yang before Yin, taking advantage of HCL when it's strongest, etc.) I also understand the need to buffer with vegetables. Is the rule "always eat vegetables with protein," referring to each meal or each mouthful? Perhaps a bit nit-picky, but I'm curious.

—J. B., Palo Alto, CA

A: The chemistry between the protein and vegetables does not take place in the mouth. So, simply have vegetables and proteins in the same meal. The same bite is fine, but if the meal is well-chewed, combining at the bite level offers no additional benefit.

LETTERS

"I just wanted to pass this tip along. At first my husband resisted the diet and made it difficult for us all. It seemed he liked poached eggs on toast and was not willing to give up the toast with that meal. One morning I served him the poached egg on a thin piece of turkey sausage and surrounded it with alfalfa sprouts and finger vegetables. This went over well.

One other point: Since cutting back on bread, our allergies are better. Or is it the diet? Anyway, I know some people have a little difficulty changing their diet and I just wanted to pass along (the tip) that persistence and experimentation bring success. Thank you."

—Mrs. A.R., Jr., Kansas City, KS

"For the first time in years I FEEL GOOD about what I am serving my children. We have the Pro-Vita! 5+5 breakfast and everyone gets off to a terrific start. Now I don't worry much about what my two daughters eat at school. For supper we have the fun foods—often the things we used to have for breakfast—oatmeal, rye meal, Oatios, pancakes, as well as fresh salad and soups. Instead of my feeling guilty knowing they had dry cereal for breakfast and sweets at school and trying to ease my conscience at supper by forcing them to eat their vegetables, breakfast is a joy and supper is a joy. The Pro-Vita! 5+5 diet has actually brought our family closer together." — V.St.J., Toronto, Canada

"What a joy breakfast has become for our whole family, particularly our children (ages 6 and 8). We decorate each plate with a variety of

foods—something everyone likes. Each plate gets a black olive, a green olive, a dollop of cottage of cheese, a sprig of parsley, some carrot and celery sticks with tahini, various soaked seeds and nuts. Each person chooses which cooked protein they want. Everyone gets a little salad with some dressing, and a cooked vegetable such as sauteed artichoke hearts or steamed cabbage. Portions and selections vary with appetite. And everyone is feeling so much better—fewer sniffles, less tiredness, less hyperactivity! Thank you."   —L.L.B., Houston, TX

"As a Registered Dietician, I was somewhat skeptical when I first read your book. You were not saying the same things I learned in school. In fact, you were directly contradicting many of the pat-answers my nutritional beliefs were based on. I guess I'd have to say that I was offended by your challenging these beliefs.

So I read up on your references. I read Howell's book on Enzyme Nutrition, I read Dr. Lee's old newsletters. I read Pottenger's research. Now I realize that what I was taught in school was not the whole picture. Actually, I suspect a lot of it was wrong.

Your book has been a humbling experience for me—something I desperately needed—and it has taught me to think for myself a lot more. The Pro-Vita! has caused some significant personal growth and I thank you for it.

It is with pride and satisfaction that I now recommend your book to my clients and watch them gain in health so much more than ever before!"   —Mrs. MMW, Atlanta, GA

25

COMIC RELIEF:
THE HIGH ENERGY DIET

While consulting in Manhattan several years ago, I was the dinner guest of Dr. Russell Jaffe, the eminent medical spokesman for natural health. At the restaurant I ordered a Pro-Vita! meal even though it was a bit late in the day for perfect adherence to "The Plan." I mean, to go to one of New York's premier fish restaurants and order a baked potato is just a bit too austere, don't you agree?

Just to show how easily a restaurant meal can be adapted to the Pro-Vita! philosophy, I'll elaborate on my choices. My cocktail was cranberry juice with a dash of club soda and was accompanied by a plate of garnish foods: celery sticks, carrot sticks, sweet peppers, scallions and radishes. Next came a wonderful salad of garden vegetables which included sprouts, crumbled feta cheese and dressing. The entré was ocean snapper with asparagus. I ate very sparingly of the new potatoes and dinner roll (as they seemed to fit within the 18% rule), and opted to not have dessert because the meal was completely satisfying without it.

During the course of the meal, we discussed the Pro-Vita! Plan in detail and had many lively discussions regarding natural health. Dr. Jaffe was a wonderful host and, on parting, he handed me the following "Dieting Under Stress" program.

So, if you have made it this far with all of the Pro-Vita! information, here's a note of comic relief to help you keep your perspective.

DIETING UNDER STRESS

This diet is designed to help you cope with the stress that builds up during the day.

Breakfast

1 grapefruit
1 slice whole wheat toast, dry
8 ounces skim milk

Lunch

4 ounces lean broiled chicken breast
1 cup steamed spinach
1 cup herb tea
1 Oreo cookie

Mid-Afternoon Snack

Rest of the Oreos in the package
2 pints rocky road ice cream
1 jar hot fudge sauce
Nuts, cherries, whipped cream

Dinner

2 loaves garlic bread with cheese
Large sausage, mushroom and cheese pizza
4 cans or 1 large bottle of soda pop
3 Milky Way candy bars

Late Evening Snack

Entire frozen cheesecake eaten directly from the freezer

Rules For This Diet

1. If you eat something and no one sees you eat it, it has no calories.

2. If you drink a diet soda with a candy bar, the calories in the candy bar are cancelled out by the diet soda.

3. When you eat with someone else, calories don't count if you don't eat more than they do.

4. Food used for medicinal purposes NEVER counts, such as hot chocolate, toast and Sara Lee Cheesecake.

5. If you fatten up everyone else around you, then you look thinner.

6. Movie-related foods such as Milk Duds, buttered popcorn, Junior Mints, Red Hots and Tootsie Rolls do not have additional calories because they are a part of the entire entertainment package and not part of one's personal fuel.

7. Cookie pieces contain NO calories. The process of breaking causes calorie leakage.

8. Things licked off knives and spoons have NO calories if you are in the process of preparing something. Examples are peanut butter on a knife making a sandwich and ice cream on a spoon making a sundae.

9. Foods that have the same color have the same number of calories. Examples are spinach and pistachio ice cream, mushrooms and white chocolate. NOTE—chocolate is a universal color and may be substituted for any other food color.

We hope that you too were able to laugh at this.

Best wishes to you in your GENUINE health endeavors.

PART IV

MANAGING THE PRO-VITA! KITCHEN AND RECIPES

This section provides practical advice on how to operate a healthful kitchen with a minimal amount of time.

Wonderful recipes are included to stimulate culinary creativity.

26

TWO WEEK PRO-VITA! MENU

The following two-week plan of Pro-Vita! menus will help you get started and demonstrate that it is easy to follow. A food plan should be expansive in its variety to offer a broad range of enzymes, vitamins, minerals and amino acids. Many wonderful new foods are just waiting for you to discover them.

While you study this menu, check Chapters 27 and 28 on Pro-Vita! Kitchen and Recipes. In both chapters you will find valuable suggestions for easy preparation of vegetables, salads and protein dishes. Let these meal suggestions stimulate your creativity.

FOR SNACKS between meals or in the evening you can choose from fresh organic fruit; fresh organic vegetable or fruit juices; celery with tahini and organic all-fruit jam w/vegetable juice in the afternoon; organic all-fruit sorbet and fruit salad for evening; and herbal teas.

FIRST WEEK

BREAKFAST	LUNCH	SUPPER

MONDAY

steamed broccoli w/sautéed chicken topped w/parmesan; salad w/sprouts & soaked seeds, feta, olives

steamed asparagus w/shrimp sautéed in garlic; salad w/cottage cheese & soaked seeds

baked sweet potato w/sautéed Chinese greens; salad

TUESDAY

spinach omelet w/fresh salsa & grated raw milk cheddar; salad w/sprouts, soaked seeds, raisins

steamed green beans w/fish topped w/parmesan; salad w/ sprouts; veggie sticks w/tahini

spelt pasta w/meatless sauce, topped w/ parsley or cilantro

WEDNESDAY

snowpeas w/squid or fish; salad w/sprouts, seeds, feta, veggie sticks & salsa

sautéed cabbage & herb seasoned tofu; salad w/ sprouts, seeds, cottage cheese

corn soup w/green garnish; salad; baked cornchips w/salsa

THURSDAY

steamed cauliflower & Chinese peas w/fish & capers; salad w/ sprouts & seeds

chicken taco w/salsa & grated raw milk cheddar; green salad w/sprouts & seeds

veggie patty in pita w/ tofu mayo; sprouts; salsa; green salad

FIRST WEEK

BREAKFAST	LUNCH	SUPPER

FRIDAY

lettuce, sprouts, cottage cheese topped w/poached egg, salsa, veggie sticks & tahini	sautéed green & yellow squash w/buffalo burger; salad w/sprouts, seeds & feta	baked potato w/onion, sprouts, cilantro & flax oil; salad

SATURDAY

steamed broccoli w/garlic shrimp; salad w/sprouts, seeds, feta, olives	steamed artichoke w/ sautéed chicken salad w/ sprouts, seeds, veggie sticks & tahini	rice pilaf w/green vegetable; salad; baked chips & salsa

SUNDAY

broccoli omelet w/salsa & grated raw milk cheddar; veggie sticks & tahini	steamed asparagus w/roasted turkey breast; salad w/sprouts, seeds, cottage cheese	spelt pasta salad on mixed greens; or fruit plate

Snack in pm. As a reward for first week of Pro-Vita! meals: Home-made apple pie with glaze of carrrot juice.

SECOND WEEK

BREAKFAST   LUNCH   SUPPER

MONDAY

steamed broccoli & cauliflower w/ fish or shrimp topped w/parmesan salad w/sprouts, seeds; veggie sticks & tahini

sautéed carrots & snow peas w/precooked chicken strips w/hot oil; salad w/ sprouts, seeds, cottage cheese

rice/lentil pilaf w/ sautéed greens; salad; chips & salsa

TUESDAY

scrambled eggs w/sprouts in taco w/salsa & feta cheese; olives; veggie sticks & salsa

miso-fish soup; salad w/ sprouts, seeds, cottage cheese

pita sandwiches w/ mayo, avocado, tomato, sprouts, onion

WEDNESDAY

steamed green beans w/scrambled herbed tofu; salad w/sprouts, seeds, feta, olives

steamed asparagus & shrimp w/BBQ sauce; salad w/seeds, sprouts, cottage cheese

baked spaghetti squash w/pasta sauce; salad; breadsticks & salsa

THURSDAY

sautéed cabbage & steamed chicken breast w/grated raw milk cheddar; salad w/seeds, sprouts, raisins

garlic sautéed squid or fish w/parmesan; sautéed Chinese greens; salad w/seeds, sprouts, feta

spelt pasta salad on greens; veggie sticks & salsa OR fruit salad

SECOND WEEK

BREAKFAST	LUNCH	SUPPER
FRIDAY		
steamed broccoli w/herbed fish; veggie sticks w/ cottage cheese dip	seafood stew; salad w/ sprouts, seeds, feta	baked sweet potato w/ red cabbage & apple sauce; salad
SATURDAY		
sautéed snow peas; chicken taco w/sprouts, salsa, grated cheese; veggie sticks w/tahini	steamed green beans or greens w/garlic shrimp w/parmesan; salad w/sprouts, seeds, feta	vegetable soup; baked corn chips & black bean dip; salad
SUNDAY		
spinach/herb omelet w/salsa & grated raw milk cheddar; salad w/ seeds, sprouts, raisins	medley of sautéed vegetables w/roasted chicken breast topped w/ parmesan; salad w/sprouts	grain pilaf w/sautéed boc choy or green peas; salad

Snack in pm. As a reward for two weeks on the Pro-Vita! plan: All-fruit (organic) sorbet.

MANAGING THE PRO-VITA! KITCHEN

A summary of Pro-Vita! principles

Here is some practical advice to make the Pro-Vita! cooking a joyful experience and bring health and vitality to yourself and your family. You don't have to stay at home and cook all day to be successful in the Pro-Vita! Plan.

GENERAL SUGGESTIONS:

• Make a shopping list for a weekly trip to the natural foods store. Set aside a couple of hours time to manage the food after you get home.

• Buy only top quality, **organic** vegetables, fruits, chicken, grains, bread, chips, salsa, pasta sauce, herbs, etc. Be frugal but obtain the best foods possible—you'd never dream of putting inferior gas into your car's engine. Your body is much more precious than your car!

• Buy only **high quality oils**: For flax seed oil, buy Barleans, New Dimensions or Sisu because poor imitations—processed under higher heat conditions—are on the market; extra virgin olive oil for use on salads; grape seed oil for cooking; and sesame seed oil. Read the chapter on oils to understand the importance of essential fatty acids in your diet.

• Keep on hand a variety of **seasonings**: Herbs (fresh and dried); miso (keep a small glass container of miso softened with water in refrigerator for quick use); tahini; tofu mayonnaise; umeboshi vinegar (not a true vinegar but the salt pickling solution for umeboshi plums); rice vinegar; hot sesame oil; mirin (traditional Japanese seasoning); balsamic vinegar; capers; olives; kelp; dulse flakes; garlic salt; organic BBQ sauce.

● Buy organic, **raw milk cheese**, or organic goat cheese (cheddar); French feta cheese or organic Greek feta cheese (the fetas have lots of enzymatic factors); raw milk cottage cheese if allowed in your state, or else get low fat or nonfat cottage cheese.

● Keep a jar of mixed **soaked seeds** in refrigerator. Mix together whatever you have of sunflower seeds, pumpkin seeds, sesame seeds, flax seeds, chia seeds, pine nuts, a few almonds in a glass jar, add pineapple juice (try to get this juice in a glass bottle), leaving a bit of space at the top for expansion. You've got ready-made proteins to supplement your cooked protein of fish, shrimp, organic chicken, tofu. This seed mix is great on salads, and you won't need much dressing with it, just a touch of flax seed oil.

● **Salad dressings** are very simple; the easiest, and probably healthiest, dressing is to drizzle a spoon full of flax seed or olive oil onto the salad and sprinkle a bit of umeboshi vinegar or rice vinegar (to your taste) on the salad. You can make easy combinations of olive oil w/balsamic vinegar adding a few finely chopped herbs of your choice and garlic and onions. If you buy salad dressing, read closely for ingredients, especially oils—stay away from soybean oils! Read the chapter on oils to remind yourself about the importance of good oil management.

● Use lots of **fresh salsa** which is rich in enzymes and currently enjoys national fame as topping for fish, chicken, vegetables and baked potatoes. Eat salsa with baked corn chips at supper time or for snacks with veggie sticks. The salsa won't keep too long so you need to eat it within 5-7 days.

● Buy **good bread**. There are several fine organic, yeast-free, frozen breads available; check the Essene breads, Rudolph's bread or the new Spelt breads. Also, various types of pitas made from organic flours are available, as well as nourishing bagels, all in the freezer department. And check for frozen flour and blue corn tacos all made from organic grains.

• Use caution regarding the **vegetarian patties** that you buy. Many brands are made with unfermented soybean products such as textured vegetable protein. Look instead for patties made from vegetables only, which are usually in the freezer department. These also make great sandwich or pita fillings w/sprouts and a bit of onion or salsa. Vegetable patties are a great way to have a sandwich without using meat and thus avoiding a high protein, high carbohydrate combination.

• Other **carbohydrate sandwich fillings** can easily be made by using tahini, tofu mayonnaise or avocado as spread, then adding a combination of the following ingredients: sliced cucumbers; sliced avocado; a variety of sprouts; a variety of lettuces; sliced onion; tender leaves of borage (an herb), kale, collards or spinach; grated carrots, beets, jicama (don't buy the Mexican product because it's full of chemicals!) or radish; sprinkle on dulse (a seaweed) for flavoring.

• Investigate the many fine **prepackaged organic grain** and rice dishes at your natural foods store. Buy spelt pasta, flour and pancake/ cupcake mix; read the information about spelt in chapter 8.

• There are also good **mixes for hummus** and brown bean dip which make easy supper appetizers or snacks with baked corn chips. You can enhance the flavor of these mixes by adding chopped fresh cilantro.

• Invest in a **good juicer.** The Champion brand remains in our opinion the best buy. You need it to make fresh potato juice, it contains a small amount of a wonderful protein; or fresh vegetable juice or carrot juice. The small containers of frozen vegetable or carrot juice, currently available at health food stores, are excellent to take for lunch or a snack away from home.

• **Steam** your vegetables or fish, shrimp, chicken in good clean water and preserve the steam juice for soups or just to drink.

• **Leftovers** are a vital factor for running a time-efficient Pro-Vita! kitchen. So cook sufficient vegetables and low-stress protein dishes to have leftovers for further fast meal combinations. Also, when cooking soup, cook extra to serve on another day or to freeze.

• **Compost** all vegetable and fruit peelings to return nourishment to the earth.

COOKING SUGGESTIONS

• Use only **stainless steel or glass** cooking and baking pots. Do not use aluminum or cast iron pots and pans.

• Store fresh and cooked food only in **glass containers**—throw out your plastic containers because vegetables stay much fresher in glass containers and plastics are suspect of toxins.

• After shopping, **immediately clean** all produce, fish, chicken, shrimp, eggs according to cleansing procedure and store lettuces, sprouts, veggies in glass containers. Use towels to dry the vegetables, especially salad greens and sprouts, thoroughly before storage.

• You can **immediately sauté** fish, shrimp, squid, chicken after cleaning; sauté chopped garlic in a bit of oil at low medium heat before adding fish or chicken; sauté at low heat until done; store in glass containers for easy addition of proteins to vegetables for fast meals.

• You can also **immediately steam** some vegetables right after cleaning—keep them crisp. Store in glass containers for fast meals!

• You make a **fast Pro-Vita! meal** by having prepared vegetables and protein foods as well as clean, crisp salad ingredients in the refrigerator. This comes in handy especially for preparing breakfast and lunch to take with you. You can even put together your next day's breakfast and lunch the evening before. You can fix individual small glass/pyrex containers to be heated in the morning and even fix salad bowls to add only the wet ingredients in the morning. You can prepare the veggie sticks in the evening also. These procedures enable you to have very fast breakfast and lunch service!

QUICK AND DELICIOUS SALADS

The **secret to making quickly the variety of salads** suggested in your Pro-Vita! menus is to keep a variety of cleansed salad greens and sprouts in several glass containers in your refrigerator. Then, all you have to do is combine a few greens, some sprouts, add a few other items like tomato, cucumber, radish, cauliflower buds, broccoli bits, onion, carrot, beet or boc choy to your taste and top off your creation with olives, raisins, feta cheese or cottage cheese, a couple of spoonfuls of soaked seeds, flax seed oil and a bit of umeboshi or rice vinegar to taste, and you have a great Pro-Vita! salad. In fact, in the summer you can easily make an entire 5+5 Pro-Vita! meal by adding to your salad a bit of cooked tofu, chicken, shrimp or fish, topped with capers, as well as a few cooked veggies and have a nourishing repast! By the way, this combination of foods makes a superb take-out lunch all year round.

Lettuce Greens: There is a vast variety! Use all lettuces with exception of iceberg and oak leaf lettuce (they contain opiates and can contribute to constipation); spinach; endives; chicory; dandelion; watercress; arrugula; mache (or corn salad); thinly sliced green and red cabbage; thinly sliced collards, kale, beet leaves, chard, boc choy. It's easy to grow arrugula and mache in a big container outside; they are cold weather crops.

Sprouts: Focus on sunflower because they are not legumes. Alfalfa, lentil, radish, pea, adzuki and others will provide variety; but use soy beans sprouts only sauted! Having a small sprout farm in your kitchen yields a terrific supply of fresh, highly nutritious vegetables.

Making the salad: Create base of salad greens, add sprouts, then add chopped broccoli, cauliflower, zuchini; summer squash; celery; cucumbers; snow peas; chard; tomatoes, onions; or carrots. A colorful and tasty salad is created by grating carrots, beets, squash, daikon (or turnip) on top of the bed of greens and sprouts; add purple onion slices. Use the ingredients you like but venture into new flavors and colors.

Add olives or feta or cottage cheese, some of the soaked seeds and a few organic raisins.

Use fresh herbs: Finely chop basil leaves but not the stems; parsley; organic herbs also give a special flavor to your salad. Just sprinkle on top. Add a couple of chopped sun dried tomatoes!

Edible flowers make a first class salad out of your creation! Use organic pansies; nasturtium; hibiscus, clover, rose petals; violets; sage blossoms, especially the wild sages. It's great to have a little kitchen garden where you can grow your own select greens, herbs and flowers.

Salad dressing: Your own dressing is the most nutritious and least expensive one. Top off your salad with a bit of grated parmesan, romano or dry herb cheese; drizzle a tablespoon of flax seed or olive oil on top; add a few shakes of umeboshi, rice or balsamic vinegar. Although you may be used to commercial dressings, give your own dressing a try. Beware of commercial dressings with bad oils! Almonds (nut milk), yoghurt and avocado can form the base of delicious salad dressings.

Your creativity will enable you to make countless great and fast varieties of Pro-Vita! salads!

HOW TO COOK TASTY, NUTRITIOUS VEGETABLES

The fastest way to prepare vegetables is to **steam** them—always use good water and conserve the steam juice for soups or just to drink!

To **sauté** vegetables, try the Japanese method called *nitsuke*. Heat a couple of tablespoons of grapeseed oil to low medium heat; saute chopped garlic until transparent (do not brown); slice onion thinly, add to garlic and saute briefly; stir and add 3-4 cups of sliced vegetables (thinly sliced cabbage or greens, or carrots, snowpeas, squashes, broccoli, cauliflower, etc.); stir carefully a few minutes until veggies are lightly coated with oil; add 1/4 - 1/2 cup of steam juice or good water; close pot with lid; bring to slow simmer; DO NOT BOIL!; cook slowly, stir sometimes; cook 5-10 minutes depending on the type of vegetable or until vegetable is done but STILL CRISP. This is a great way to cook greens which are traditionally cooked for hours and their vital nutritional factors get completely destroyed. In fact, thinly chopped greens cook very quickly the *nitsuke* way in just a few minutes, and their great cancer-preventing factors are preserved when cooked this way.

Season vegetables according to your taste with shoyu sauce, hot sesame oil (careful, it's quite spicy!), mirin (a wonderfully subtle Japanese flavor), a bit of softened miso, a bit of tahini stirred into the juice of the vegetable, a touch of umeboshi vinegar. Since the greens are such a vital source of cancer-fighting factors, eat them often! They are also less expensive than other green vegetables!

Frozen Vegetables: Recently, some frozen organic vegetables have become available. These are wonderful to have in your freezer in case you are out of fresh cleansed vegetables. They are also relatively inexpensive considering that they have no waste. Cascade farm products (in the natural food store freezer section) is a great source of such vegetables and currently available are tasty green beans; wonderful asparagus; superb small green peas; carrots and peas; and corn. Saute these vegetables only barely in a bit of water to retain their freshness. The frozen veggies also make great snacks when they are barely defrosted or when cooked.

Veggie sticks: You can include a lot of these raw veggie sticks in your menus or use them as snacks. Make a big plate full of them in the evening or early in the morning for the entire day. If the plate of veggie sticks is sitting right in the front of the refrigerator you can bet that the quick-snack seekers will switch to them quickly and munch on them all throughout the day. Use the following vegetables to slice into sticks or rounds: Carrots, celery, boc choy, daikon, radishes, snow peas (they are fine as they are), green beans (also ok in their natural shape), cauliflower, broccoli, sweet onion, apple and pear. Put a small glass dish with organic tahini in the center of the plate for a dip. People who used to love chocolate, now thrive on veggie sticks and apple slices dipped in tahini.

PRO-VITA! PLAN

RECIPES

PROTEIN DISHES

DEVILED EGGS

1 dozen medium boiled eggs (190-200 degrees F)
dry mustard
salt
sesame salt
paprika
mayonnaise (see recipe in section on sauces and dressings)
yogurt
alfalfa sprouts

Cut the eggs in half and remove yolks. Mash the yolks finely with a fork or pastry cutter. Add seasonings and sprouts. Mix with 1/2 cup homemade mayonnaise and 1/2 cup yoghurt. Fill the hollow egg halves with the yolk mixture. Garnish with parsley.

SCRAMBLED EGGS WITH SPROUTS

1/2 cup scallions, chopped fine
1/4 teaspoon sea salt
Dash of red pepper
4 eggs, slightly beaten
2 cups sprouts: alfalfa, sunflower, lentil
1 tablespoon grapeseed oil

Add chopped onion tops, sea salt and pepper to beaten eggs. Let them stand. Wash the sprouts and add them to the eggs. Pour the oil into a skillet and heat it to low/medium heat. Add the egg mixture and cook slowly until done.

GARLIC SOUP (by Cathy Attal)

2 whole garlic bulbs
2 quarts of cold water
6 cloves
1/4 teaspoon sage
1/2 teaspoon thyme
4 teaspoons parsley
3 teaspoons sea salt
1 egg yolk
4 teaspoons organic butter or oil

Cover the garlic with water and blanch it. Remove the skins. Bring 2 quarts of water and the next 6 ingredients to a boil. Reduce heat and simmer for 30 minutes. Separate the egg and beat the yolk. Add 4 teaspoons of melted, balanced, organic butter (or grapeseed oil) to the egg yolk very slowly. Continue to beat the mixture until it is thick and creamy. Turn your mixer to low and add the 2-quart mixture. It's ready to eat! This dish will freeze well, but when you reheat it, do it very slowly so that it won't clabber.

SEAFOOD STEW (by Jessie Keener)

3 tablespoons safflower oil
2 cloves garlic, pressed or minced
1 tablespoon basil, chopped fresh*
1 tablespoon marjoram, chopped fresh*
1 teaspoon each of thyme, sage, cayenne pepper
1/2 bunch of parsley, chopped fine
5-6 scallions, sliced thin—separate tops (greens) from bottoms
2-3 carrots, sliced thin
2 bell peppers, chopped
1 large bunch broccoli, cut
2 1/2 to 3 cups vegetable broth
Pinch of sea salt
4 teaspoons arrowroot
2 cups (or more) distilled water
1 lb. fresh white fish—orange roughy, sole, snapper
1/2 lb. bay scallops

Heat the oil slowly in a large saucepan. Add the garlic and saute it for 1 minute. Add all the herbs, including the parsley. Saute 2-3 minutes. Then add all of the vegetables, except the scallion greens. Simmer the vegetables for 7 minutes, stirring often. Now add the scallion greens. Cook another 6 minutes over medium-low heat. Add all liquids and bring them to a boil. Reduce heat and simmer for 6 minutes. Add the seafood, raising the heat to bring to a low boil. Simmer for 6 minutes. Remove some of the cooking liquid to a measuring cup, let it cool a minute and then add the arrowroot. Stir until the arrowroot dissolves. Add this mixture back to the saucepan, stirring it to thicken the whole dish. Cook for another 2 minutes. Remove from the heat and correct the seasonings. Garnish with a sprig of parsley or basil.

*Dried herbs may be used if fresh are unavailable. Use only half as much.

SCRAMBLED TOFU (by Jessie Keener)

1 lb. tofu with moisture squeezed out
1 large sprig parsley, minced (should equal about 1 tablespoon)
1 teaspoon unrefined sesame oil
Pinch gomasio or sea salt
1/2 teaspoon turmeric
1/2 teaspoon cayenne pepper
2 teaspoons sesame seeds (optional)

Place tofu in mixing bowl, mash well with fork. Add the turmeric and cayenne and mix well. Heat a medium-sized skillet and add the oil. Heat should be moderate—not high. When the oil is hot (test by dropping tiny drop of water into the skillet—it should evaporate immediately), add the parsley and saute for 2 minutes. Add the sesame seeds if desired, and the gomasio seasoning. Stir well and then add the tofu. Scramble (like eggs) for 2 or 3 minutes, until the tofu is heated through. Remove from heat and serve with a complement of fresh vegetables.

Variations:

Saute any of the following vegetables with the parsley: minced scallions, chopped peppers, sliced black olives, soaked and drained hijiki or arame seaweed, minced garlic.

You can also substitute Mexican seasonings, such as minced cilantro, cumin or chile powder for the turmeric. Serve with a picante (hot) sauce.

Substitute curry powder for the turmeric, and for a spicier scramble add a few drops of Eden Hot Sesame Oil to the other oil when you are sauteing.

Try using fresh dill or basil in addition to the parsley.

Before adding the tofu to the cooked vegetables, stir 1 tablespoon of tahini into the skillet and mix well. This makes a richer dish.

Scrambled tofu is quite good cold. Serve it on a salad or like a spread or dip.

MARINATED FISH

1 pound deep sea fish
1/2 cup tamari
1/4 cup sesame oil
1 teaspoon cumin powder or other spice
1/2 teaspoon garlic powder
Grated ginger

Mix tamari, oil, and seasonings. Pour over fish and let stand 2 to 3 hours for slight flavoring or overnight for a more pungent flavor. Broiling is suggested for cooking procedure. This same marinade may be used for organic chicken.

BIRD'S NEST EGGS

Arrange alfalfa sprouts on romaine or red leaf lettuce leaf in the shape of a bird's nest. In a blender, mix 1/4 cup flax seed oil, 1/2 teaspoon lecithin, 1/2 cup cottage cheese and 1/2 cup yogurt. Flavor with Tabasco-like sauce. Blend. Place this creamy mixture in the bird's nest. Lightly poach 2 yard eggs and place them on top of the bird's nest. Sprinkle 1/2 cup finely chopped celery and minced onion with seasonings to taste on top of the whole dish.

STIR-FRIED VEGGIES AND TOFU

In a stainless steel wok or skillet, saute 1 chopped onion, 2 minced garlic cloves and 2 tablespoons freshly grated ginger root for 3 minutes. Add 1/2 pound drained, cubed tofu. Cook 6 minutes, stirring occasionally. Add 3 cups chopped vegetables (carrots, broccoli, celery, cauliflower, snow peas, cabbage, green beans, etc.). Cook 4 minutes more, stirring constantly. Serve with green salad.

FISH WITH HERBS

3 medium, ripe (pink) tomatoes, chopped
3 scallions, finely chopped
1/4 cup minced fresh parsley
2 tablespoons water
2 tablespoons lemon juice
2 cloves garlic, crushed
1 tablespoon olive oil
1 tablespoon sesame seeds
1/2 teaspoon dried thyme or basil
3/4 pound fish fillets, such as orange roughy or snapper

Place all ingredients, except fish, in a medium skillet. Stir together and bring to a light simmer. Reduce heat, place the fish over top of vegetable mixture and cover the skillet. Steam the fish over the simmering mixture about 10 minutes, or until the fish is opaque throughout, but not cooked dry. Carefully remove the fish and keep it warm on a serving platter. Simmer the vegetable mixture in the skillet until it is thick. Pour over the fish and serve.

SAUTEED FISH FILLET

2 small fish fillets
4 cloves garlic, crushed
1 bell pepper, sliced into thin strips
Juice of 1 lemon
1/4 cup pure water
1 tablespoon white wine (optional)
1/2 teaspoon thyme

1/2 teaspoon marjoram
1/4 teaspoon sea salt
1 tablespoon sesame oil

In medium-sized frying pan, gently heat the sesame oil. Add garlic and herbs and saute 1 minute, stirring frequently. Add fillets, vegetables and liquids. Bring liquid to simmer, cover, reduce heat to low and cook 10-12 minutes. Remove fish and vegetables and arrange on a platter. Pour liquid over both and serve with lemon wedges.

SHRIMP KABOB

1 dozen large shrimp
1 onion
1 red bell pepper
1 zucchini
8 cherry tomatoes
salad dressing (see recipes) with 1 tablespoon tamari and
1 teaspoon ginger added
Use bamboo skewers

Clean, devein and peel shrimp. Cut vegetables into bite-sized pieces. Arrange on bamboo skewers. Place on a hot grill, basting with salad dressing or with Herb Butter recipe and turning frequently for 8 minutes. Serves 4.

QUICK SEAFOOD MISO SOUP

Heat water or broth to boiling point; add shrimp, squid, fish, garlic, onion, cilantro. **Simmer slowly** a few minutes until fish is done. Add asparagus or other veggies during the last minute. Take soup off the stove, add tahini, miso and a few drops of toasted sesame hot oil and a bit of mirin to taste.

VEGETARIAN CHILI

1 medium onion, chopped
6 cloves garlic, minced
2 tablespoons sesame oil
1 cup black beans, soaked and sprouted
1/2 cup kidney beans, soaked and sprouted
1/2 cup millet, soaked and sprouted
1 green pepper, chopped
2 carrots, chopped
1/4 cup sunflower seeds
2 cups cauliflower, chopped
3-4 tomatoes, chopped
1 bay leaf
2 tablespoons chili powder
2 tablespoons powdered cumin
1 teaspoon each basil and oregano
1/4 teaspoon each marjoram and cayenne
1 teaspoon sea salt
1 fresh jalapeno pepper, chopped, seedless

Saute onion and garlic in oil. Add black beans, 5 cups of water and
the bay leaf. Bring to a boil. Reduce the heat and simmer for 1 hour.
Bring to boil again, add kidney beans and spices, and cook for 1 hour
more. Make sure beans are almost tender, then add uncooked millet,
seeds and vegetables. Cook 1/2 hour. Taste and adjust seasonings.
Add more water to reach desired consistency.

SUPER BEAN LOAF

2 cups Pro-Vita!-cooked beans, mashed
1 onion, chopped
3 cloves garlic, minced
1 tablespoon sesame oil
1/4 cup tahini
1/2 cup cashews
2 medium carrots, grated
2 eggs, beaten
1 teaspoon each basil, oregano, thyme
1/4 teaspoon marjoram
1/8 teaspoon cayenne
1/2 teaspoon sea salt
2 teaspoons tamari

Saute onion and garlic in oil. Combine all ingredients and place into oiled loaf pan, patting gently. Bake at 350 degrees F for 30 minutes. Serve with steamed vegetables.

COTTAGE CHEESE DIP

1 cup raw or low fat/nonfat cottage cheese
1 slice onion
1 strip green pepper
1/4 teaspoon garlic salt
2 tablespoons rice wine vinegar
1/4 teaspoon celery salt
1 teaspoon Worcestershire sauce
1/4 teaspoon sea salt

Put ingredients into blender. Blend for 10 seconds.

MARINATED OCTOPUS

Boil tentacles for 15 minutes. Take out and put into cold water (will turn reddish). This firms up the tentacles. Scrub well. Freeze what you don't use. Slice up what you want to use and add:
1/4 cup oil (grapeseed, if possible)
1 tablespoon vinegar, lime juice, lemon juice

Garlic slivers and onion slices
The secret to this dish is 1 teaspoon of brown sesame oil. It's okay to put some hot pepper in it. Marinate the octopus for 2 hours in the mixture and serve.

AVOCADO RING SALAD

2 tablespoons Greyslake Gelatin or any unflavored gelatin
1/2 cup hot pure water
1 medium avocado, peeled and sliced
1 tablespoon rice wine vinegar
1 cup plain yogurt
1/4 teaspoon sea salt
1/2 teaspoon onion salt
1/2 teaspoon celery salt
1 teaspoon salad herbs
4 dashes Tabasco
1/2 cup mayonnaise (fresh, homemade, see recipe)
Put gelatin and hot water into blender and blend for 15-20 seconds. Add remaining ingredients immediately, so gelatin won't harden, and blend for 20-30 seconds. Don't over-blend. Pour into oiled 3-cup ring mold. Chill until firm. Serves 6.

MANGO CHICKEN

This protein recipe was given to us by Stu Wheelwright who discovered it during his travels in the Philippines. It's a fine example of how a food-combining rule (that is, eat protein without fruit) can be broken and a meal still be nutritious, healthful and delicious. The strong protein digestants in the mango blend well with the chicken, making an easily digestible, exotically delicious entree. This recipe reduces chicken from a medium-stress to a low-stress food. Steam 4 skinned organic chicken breasts, chop to bite size. Sauté briefly in grapeseed oil, add soy sauce. Add fresh ginger. Peel 2 mangoes and slice them into small pieces. Add the mango and the juice to the chicken. Add 1 can green coconut milk— look for the kind that doesn't have added sugar. Simmer the dish until ready to serve. This recipe goes very well with wild rice cooked without boiling.

SPINACH OMELET

For 2 omelets:
Beat 3 eggs.
Add 1 tablespoon water and beat again.
Add 1 teaspoon finely minced fresh marjoram or a pinch of dried marjoram.
Add 2 tablespoons minced onion.
Add 2 tablespoons minced bell pepper.
Heat 1 tablespoon grapeseed oil in omelet skillet to medium heat.
Pour in 1/2 of egg batter.
Cook until almost set.

Add small hand full of finely chopped fresh spinach (pull off touch stems); fold omelet over; cook a few minutes longer. Serve omelet topped with grated cheese and salsa, accompanied with veggie sticks or salad. **Omelet variations**: Fill with chopped broccoli, alfalfa sprouts, or chopped tomato and peppers.

CARBOHYDRATE AND VEGETABLE DISHES

COLESLAW

Shred cabbage (green and purple), onions (optional) and carrots. Sprinkle with sea water—4 tablespoons per quart. Press down and cover with a plate. Place in the refrigerator for 1/2 hour. Before serving, stir in the following ingredients, which have already been mixed:

1 cup cottage cheese (raw milk or nonfat)
1/4 cup rice wine vinegar
1/8 teaspoon anise seed
1/4 teaspoon dill seed

STU'S JIFFY SOUP

Using five vegetables or more:
Fill a blender 3/4 full of diced vegetables.
Add 1 tablespoon raw milk organic butter or oil, 1 tablespoon
of powdered vegetables, and 1 level teaspoon lecithin.
Pour boiling water over the vegetables and let sit for 3 minutes.
Blend for at least 3 minutes and serve immediately.

VEGETABLE SOUP

4 cups green vegetable juice (celery, sprouts, broccoli, asparagus)
3 cups pure water
4-5 chopped vegetables
3 tablespoons butter (not margarine)
3 tablespoons sesame oil
1 cup whole wheat or rye, sprouted for two days
Salt, pepper and herb spices to taste

Cook all of the ingredients in an electric frying pan or crock pot at
125-150 degrees F for approximately 1 hour. If you don't have a
cooker that regulates the temperature, be sure to cook below the
boiling point.

BORSCHT

2 cups beets, cooked under boiling point for 30 minutes
2 cups yogurt
1 teaspoon onion salt
1/2 teaspoon ume plum or rice wine vinegar

Grate beets and cool them in the refrigerator. Place all ingredients
in blender and blend well for 20 seconds. Chill well and serve.

VEGETABLE BROTH

Use vegetable pulp from juicer. Add pure water equal to 2 times the amount of vegetable pulp. Steep for 20 minutes. Add organic raw milk butter or oil and salt to taste. Strain before serving.

VEGE-MILLET BURGERS

1 cup millet
1/8 teaspoon cayenne pepper
3 cups boiling water
1 teaspoon sea salt
1/2 teaspoon curry powder (or more, to taste)
3/4 cup grated carrot
1/4 cup minced garlic
1/2 cup minced parsley
1/2 cup rye flour
1/4 cup soy flour

Add millet and cayenne to buttered pot and stir 2-3 minutes until the millet gives off a nutlike fragrance. Add boiling water and reduce heat to a simmer. Simmer, covered, for 35-40 minutes, adding vegetables and seasonings 5 minutes before done. Turn off heat, add flours, mixing well to avoid lumps. Let mixture sit until cool enough to handle. Form into patties and fry in unrefined safflower or grapeseed oil until brown on both sides. Serve with a green salad and steamed vegetable.

MOCK SPAGHETTI

1 1/2 tablespoon unrefined olive oil
1 onion, chopped
2 cloves garlic, minced
1/2 small green bell pepper, chopped
1 cup cooked millet (cook only 15 minutes)
1 large jar natural-style spaghetti sauce
1 medium spaghetti squash

Cut spaghetti squash in half, remove seeds. Steam in a large pot for 25 minutes, until tender. Meanwhile, in a skillet saute onion and garlic in oil for 3 minutes, add green pepper and cook for 5 minutes, stirring occasionally. Add cooked millet, stir. Add spaghetti sauce, cook 10 minutes more.

To serve: Take a fork and scoop out spaghetti squash onto plate. It will be stringy like pasta. Top with sauce. Serve with a green salad.

INGE'S RED CABBAGE: TRADITIONAL GERMAN RECIPE THE PRO-VITA! WAY

Sauté chopped garlic and grated ginger in 3-4 tablespoons of grapeseed oil over low/medium heat until transparent. Thinly slice medium onion and saute. Thinly slice small to medium head of read cabbage, cutting out the hard core (4-5 cups). Peel and chop finely 1 tart apple. Add cabbage, apple and 1/2 cup of raisins to sauteing oil and stir until coated with oil. Add 1 cup of steam juice or water. Bring to simmer and cook gently 15-20 minutes or until done, stirring occasionally. Season with 3-4 tablespoons of umeboshi vinegar, mirin or shoyu according to your taste. This red cabbage tastes great with baked sweet potatoes, baked potatoes, baked squash or grain dishes.

BAKED POTATO

Remove eyes and spots from clean baking potato; rub with grapeseed oil. Bake 1 hour at 425 degrees F. (Don't use aluminum foil!).

Serve with topping of chopped green onions, cilantro, bell pepper, sunflower sprouts, salsa and 1-2 tablespoons flax seed oil.Sprinkle on dulse flakes.Serve with a salad or on top of a bed of greens and sprouts.Left-over bakers are tasty when slowly warmed in grapeseed oil over low/medium heat and served with salsa and salad.

INGE'S SPELT PASTA SALAD

1 ten-ounce package Vita-Spelt Rotini pasta, cooked according to directions. 1 twelve-ounce package organic garden peas, cooked in 1/4 cup water over low heat for a few minutes to retain crispness; they can also be used raw. Mix pasta and peas while warm, add 1/2 cup

fresh, organic Sicilian dressing (made by Shabda Fresh Foods). If unavailable in your area, look for fresh olive oil based dressing with herbs. Add all or some of the following: chopped onion, olives, radish, green onions, capers, sliced fresh squash, fresh snow peas, minced cilantro, basil or parsley. If you like your salad a bit tangier, add a few shakes of umeboshi vinegar. Sprinkle a little bit of parmesan or romano cheese for flavor on top of each serving and decorate with tomato wedges. Serves 4 and keeps well for left-overs.

SAUCES AND DRESSINGS

HERB SALAD DRESSING

1/2 cup sesame, flax seed, or olive oil
1/2 cup ume plum vinegar
1/2 cup soaked seeds (sunflower, sesame)
1 teaspoon Veg-Base
2 tablespoons sea water
1 teaspoon lecithin liquid

Place all ingredients in blender and blend for 2 minutes. For variations, add egg yolk, cottage cheese, dill pickle, paprika, cayenne, basil, thyme.

BASIC ITALIAN DRESSING

Juice of 1 lemon
1 clove garlic, pressed
1/2 teaspoon each dry mustard, marjoram, thyme
1 teaspoon chopped fresh basil or 1/2 teaspoon dried
1/4 teaspoon sea salt
1/4 teaspoon cayenne pepper
3/4 cup safflower oil or extra virgin olive oil

MEXICAN CHILI SAUCE

Take 6-8 dried California chili pods (anchos). Remove stem and discolored parts. Crush and simmer in 4 cups of water, cooking gently for 12 minutes. Place in blender and blend for a few minutes. Strain. Add 1/8 teaspoon garlic powder, 1 teaspoon celery salt, 1 tablespoon chili powder, and 1/4 cup sesame oil.

HERB BUTTER OR OIL

1 tablespoon chopped parsley
1 tablespoon minced chives
1/2 teaspoon each savory, marjoram, basil and tarragon
1 minced clove garlic
1/4 teaspoon paprika
1/4 lb. organic, balanced butter or 1/4 cup sesame or flax seed oil

Pulverize dried herbs by rubbing between palms of hands or mince fresh herbs before using. Combine with soft butter or oil. Store in covered jar and keep in refrigerator. Serve on fish, potatoes, vegetables. Expensive Italian restaurants serve warm herbed olive oil to dip bread into—try it, it's a real treat!

QUICK MARINADE

Chop garlic
Finely mince 1 tsp basil leaves
Add 1/4 cup balsamic vinegar and stir
Add 1/2 cup sesame oil and stir again
Marinate chicken, fish, squid for 15 minutes (longer is not better!)

THE FOLLOWING DRESSINGS ARE RICH IN PROTEIN

YOGURT SAUCE

1 cup plain yogurt
2 tablespoons rice wine vinegar
1/2 teaspoon organic lemon rind (optional)
1 teaspoon sea salt
1 teaspoon soy sauce
1/2 teaspoon dry mustard
2-4 tablespoons grated onion
2 tablespoons chopped parsley
Dash of cayenne

Combine all ingredients and stir well. Serve with fresh or chilled vegetables.

YOGURT SALAD DRESSING

1 cup plain yogurt
2 tablespoons rice wine vinegar
1/2 teaspoon sea salt
1 teaspoon paprika
1 minced clove garlic
1 finely chopped or grated onion

Mix all of the above ingredients on low speed in blender for 2-3 minutes. Let stand in refrigerator for at least 15 minutes before serving. Will keep 3-5 days refrigerated.

FRENCH DRESSING

1/2 cup sesame oil
1/2 cup raw milk, low fat or nonfat cottage cheese
1/4 teaspoon vege-salt
1/2 cup rice wine vinegar
1/2 cup enchilada sauce
1/4 cup yogurt (optional)

Put all ingredients in blender and blend for 2-3 minutes. Yoghurt may be added for a creamier dressing.

OIL AND VINEGAR DRESSING

1 cup sesame oil
1 tablespoon extra virgin olive oil
1 tablespoon vegetable or herb salt
1 teaspoon Veg-Base
1 cup rice wine vinegar
1 clove garlic
1 egg yolk
1 cup raw milk or nonfat cottage cheese or yogurt

Put all ingredients in blender and blend for 2-3 minutes. Soaked seeds or sprouts may be added along with chopped dill.

MAYONNAISE

1 teaspoon sea salt
1/2 teaspoon dry mustard
1/2 teaspoon paprika
4 tablespoons rice wine vinegar or lemon juice
1 cup sesame or grapeseed oil
4 egg yolks (yard eggs)
2 tablespoons liquid lecithin (LEV formula)

Mix dry ingredients and egg yolks in blender, blend well. Add 2 tablespoons of vinegar and blend. Add oil in small amounts until 1/2 cup has been used. Add 2 tablespoons of lecithin and blend. Blend in remaining vinegar or lemon juice; add remaining oil in light, steady stream. Store mayonnaise covered in refrigerator. Yields 2 cups.

YOGURT SALAD DRESSING

To one cup of plain low-fat yogurt add one of the following:
2 tablespoons of lemon juice, herbs to taste
2 tablespoons of wine vinegar, herbs to taste
Vary by adding:
1 medium garlic clove (crushed) or
2 tablespoons mild onion (minced) or
1/4 teaspoon dill weed, or
1/2 teaspoon paprika, or
1 teaspoon curry powder

SPECIAL TREATS

INGE'S FRUIT SALAD

Use organic fruit whenever possible. Slice 2 green Granny Smith, Pippin or Delicious apples and 1 firm red apple after coring and cutting into quarters. Sprinkle with lemon juice to prevent oxidation, pick out any seeds. Slice 2 green pears after coring and cutting in quarters. Slice 3 or 4 oranges after peeling, pick out the seeds. Slice 2 or 3 bananas after peeling. Add a few raisins and toss gently. Sprinkle a bit more lemon juice over the salad. If needed, add 2 tablespoons of soft honey—but the salad is actually quite sweet enough without it. Let stand in refrigerator for a couple of hours. Decorate with sliced kiwi fruit. Leftovers keep well in the refrigerator for a few days. In the summer, you can substitute fresh organic fruit like peaches, apricots, plums, nectarines and a few pieces of melon.

ENJOY!

APPENDIX A

WHAT IS HOMEOPATHY?

By Maesimund B. Panos, M.D. and Jane Heimlich

Reprinted with permission from Panos & Heimlich, *HOMEOPATHIC MEDICINE AT HOME*. Los Angeles: J. P. Tarcher, Inc., 1980.

Homeopathy is a system of medicine whose principles are even older than Hippocrates. It seeks to cure in accordance with natural laws of healing and uses medicines made from natural substances: animal, vegetable, and mineral.

Homeopathy was "discovered" in the early 1800s by a German physician, Samuel Christian Friedrich Hahnemann. Shortly after setting up practice, he became disillusioned with medicine, and with good reason. Eighteenth- and nineteenth physicians believed that sickness was caused by humors, or fluids, that had to be expelled from the body by every possible means. To achieve this end, patients were cauterized, blistered, purged, and bled. Hahnemann protested against these brutal and senseless methods, and his colleagues quickly denounced him for heresy. He was also opposed to the way doctors prescribed medicines. In those days it was customary to mix great numbers of drugs in one prescription. In his book *Who Is Your Doctor and Why?* Dr. Alonzo J. Shadman mentions having seen, in the *Pharmacopoeia* of 1875, a prescription that contained fifty ingredients. Earlier, Hahnemann's outspoken criticism of this "degrading commerce in prescription" naturally enraged the chemists, who were as powerful as our drug companies today, and they were to hound him all of his life.

Hahnemann gave up the practice of medicine and turned to medical translating as a livelihood. But he persisted in his lifelong goal—to discover "if God had not indeed given some law, whereby the diseases of mankind would be cured." His sense of frustration increased when one of his children became critically ill and he could do nothing for her.

It was while translating Lectures on the *Materia Medica* by William Cullen, a Scottish professor of medicine, that Hahnemann stumbled on the key to curing sick people. In this work, the author claimed that cinchona bark, or quinine, cured intermittent fever (malaria) because of its astringent and bitter qualities. This explanation did not sound plausible to Hahnemann, who knew of other substances equally bitter, so he did a daring thing; he tested the medicine on himself.

> I took by way of experiment, twice a day, four drachms of good China (quinine). My feet, finger ends, etc. at first became cold; I grew languid and drowsy; then my heart began to palpitate, and my pulse grew hard and small; intolerable anxiety, trembling, prostration throughout all my limbs; then pulsation in the head, redness of my cheeks, thirst, and, in short, all these symptoms which are ordinarily characteristic of intermittent fever, made their appearance, one after the other, yet without the peculiar chilly, shivering rigor. Briefly, even those symptoms which are of regular occurrence and especially characteristic—as the stupidity of mind, the kind of rigidity in all the limbs, but above all the numb, disagreeable sensation, which seems to have its seat in the periosteum, over every bone in the body—all these make their appearance. This paroxysm lasted two or three hours each time, and recurred if I repeated this dose, not otherwise; I discontinued it, and was in good health.

This was the first "proving," a testing of medicine on a healthy person. The symptoms Hahnemann developed corresponded exactly to the symptoms of malaria. Thus Hahnemann reasoned that malaria was cured by quinine, not because of its bitter taste but owing to the fact that the drug produces the symptoms of malaria in a healthy person.

After experimenting on himself, Hahnemann enlisted the help of friends and followers and embarked on an extensive program of drug testing. When he died at age eighty-eight in 1843, he had conducted or supervised provings on ninety-nine substances. More than 600 other medicines were added to the homeopathic pharmacopoeia by the end of the century.

PRINCIPLES OF HOMEOPATHY

The Law of Similars

The term homeopathy (sometimes spelled homœopathy) comes from the Greek *homoios* ("*similar*") *and pathos* ("suffering" or "sickness"). The fundamental law upon which homeopathy is based is the *law of similars*, or "Like is cured by like"—in Latin, *similia similibus curentur*. The law of similars states that a remedy can cure a disease if it produces in a healthy person symptoms similar to those of the disease.

Hahnemann did not claim to have discovered the concept. In the tenth century B.C., Hindu sages described the law, as had Hippocrates, who wrote in 400 B.C., "Through the like, disease is produced and through the application of the like, it is cured." Paracelsus, a sixteenth-century German physician, reiterated the law. Hahnemann, as an erudite thinker, was undoubtedly familiar with these writings, but he was the first to test the principle and establish it as the cornerstone of a system of medicine.

The law works thus in practice: A person develops a fever, with flushed face, dilated pupils, rapid heartbeat, and a feeling of restlessness. The homeopathic physician studies all these symptoms, then searches for a remedy that, under scientifically controlled conditions, has produced all these symptoms in a healthy person. Within a short time after taking the remedy, the fever drops to normal and the person feels well. The law of similars enables the physician to select the one medicine (the *simillimum*) that is needed by matching the symptoms of the individual to the symptoms the remedy induces.

The Law of Proving

The second law of homeopathy, *the law of proving*, refers to the method of testing a substance to determine its medicinal effect. To prove a remedy, each of a group of healthy people is given a dose of the substance daily, and each carefully records the symptoms experienced. Conforming to the standard double-blind method used in pharmacological experiments, approximately half of the test groups are used as controls and given an unmedicated tablet or pill (placebo).

When the proving is completed, all the symptoms that the provers consistently experience, such as dizziness, loss of memory, and restlessness, are listed as a characteristic remedy picture in the

Materia Medica, a prescriber's reference. To treat a patient, the physician looks up the remedy picture in the *Materia Medica*, and, when the symptoms fit, applies the law of similars.

In standard medical practice, drugs are first tested on animals because so many drugs have been found to cause dangerous reactions, even cancer. Homeopaths do not use animals as subjects for testing medicines, since they do not react to chemicals as human beings do. Furthermore, we consider subjective symptoms to be important. And we have no concern about testing homeopathic medicines on healthy human beings because homeopathically prepared remedies are not toxic. The first proving was carried out in 1790, and use of the procedure has continued to the present day. There has never been a report of a lasting adverse drug reaction as the result of a proving.

The Law of Potentization (the Minimum Dose)

The third law of homeopathy, *the law of potentization*, refers to the preparation of a homeopathic remedy. Each is prepared by a controlled process of successive dilutions alternating with succussion (shaking), which may be continued to the point where the resulting medicine contains no molecules of the original substance. These small doses are called *potencies*; lesser dilutions are known as low potencies and greater dilutions as high potencies. As strange as it may seem, the higher the dilution, when prepared in this manner, the greater the potency of the medicine.

In 1800, when the process of potentization was devised, the idea that medicine containing an infinitesimal amount of matter could be curative was inconceivable. In this nuclear age, the power of minute quantities is all too well established. The dose of vitamin B12 used to treat certain anemias contains a millionth of a gram of cobalt. Trace elements, present in barely measurable amounts in the body, are essential for its development and functioning. The human body manufactures only fifty to a hundred millionths of a gram of thyroid hormone each day, yet a small excess or deficiency in this already "infinitesimal" amount can seriously affect the health of the individual.

The power of the infinitesimal dose is not clearly understood, but neither is the action of aspirin and many other drugs. The process of potentization makes it possible to use substances such as certain metals, charcoal, and sand, which are inert in their natural state, as medicines. A potentized remedy does not contain sufficient matter to act directly on the tissues, which means that homeopathic medicine is nontoxic and cannot cause side effects. In over 150 years of use, no homeopathic remedy has ever been recalled.

The Single Remedy

Contrary to the current medical practice of frequently prescribing two or more medicines at one time, most homeopaths usually give only one remedy at a time. We are not sure what the effect of two remedies would be, or the interaction between them, but we are sure of the effect of a single remedy. The single remedy has been proved, or tested, on healthy subjects.

The wisdom of the single remedy is pointed up by the ever increasing problem of drug interactions from multiple prescriptions. In an article in *American Druggist* for September 1978, the author writes: "It has been estimated that during a typical hospital stay the patient gets an average of ten drugs—and the number sometimes goes as high as thirty or more. Among the ambulatory, nonhospitalized public, it is common for an individual to be taking as many as six different drugs, prescription and nonprescription, at the same time.

The *Physician's Desk Reference* (PDR) is sprinkled with warnings of potentially dangerous side effects from administration of certain drugs along with others. Taking a random look at my copy of *PDR*, I find a tranquilizer (tranylcypromine sulphate) which carries the warning that use in combination with certain other drugs may result in "hypertension headache and related symptoms...hypertensive crisis or severe convulsive seizures." Such sedative-hypnotics are the most prescribed medications in the world.

Safe, but Why Effective?

Numerous theories have been offered as to why homeopathic remedies work. A 1954 newspaper report describing the research of the late Dr. William E. Boyd of Glasgow contained this explanation: "The power of the solution does not depend solely of the degree of dilution but on a special progressive method in its preparation; the energy latent in the drug is apparently liberated and increased by a forceful shaking of the liquid at each stage of the process."

Dr. F.K. Bellokossy of Denver compares the process of potentizing a homeopathic drug—shaking a dilution or grinding powdered dry materials—to magnetizing a glass rod by rubbing it. "We thus produce electric fields around every particle of the powdered drug; and the more we triturate [grind], the stronger electric fields we produce, and the more potentized becomes the triturated material."

At present, there is no widely accepted theory to explain why homeopathic medicine works, but with physicists taking an active interest in homeopathy, such an explanation seems imminent. One of these physicists is Dr. William A Tillier, professor in the Department of Materials Science and Engineering, Stanford University. In a letter to one of the authors, he writes:

> As humankind evolves, the individual becomes a more integrated and finely tuned system and more sensitive with respect to changes in subtle energies. Our future medicine will proceed towards the development of techniques and treatments that use successively finer and finer energies....In my modeling, homeopathic remedies treat at the etheric level of substance. ["Etheric" means not directly observable via our physical senses or instruments.] Since this method of treatment is already in use, it is easy to practice, I expect it to flourish in the near future while allopathic (standard) medicine declines.

A COMPARISON OF HOMEOPATHY AND STANDARD MEDICINE (ALLOPATHY)

Meaning of Symptoms

The homeopath believes that the body is always striving to keep itself healthy, or in balance, just as a keel boat attempts to right itself in the water. The force that acts in this protective manner is called the vital force. When the body is threatened by harmful external forces, the vital force, or defense mechanism, produces symptoms such as pain, fever, mucus, cough. These symptoms, although unpleasant for the patient, have a purpose: to restore harmony or balance. Pain is a warning that something is wrong. Fever inactivates many viruses that attack the body. Mucus is produced in the respiratory tract to surround and carry off irritating material. A cough expels the mucus that would otherwise hinder breathing.

A homeopathic physician regards symptoms as a healthy reaction of the body's defense mechanism to harmful forces: such symptoms need to be supported rather than interfered with. Standard medicine takes a different view; it regards symptoms as manifestations of the disease, to be oppose or suppressed. Aspirin or other antifever drugs are given to lower fever, antihistamine to dry up nasal secretions, dough syrup to suppress a cough.

Meaning of Disease

Because symptoms that reflect the body's condition are constantly changing, homeopaths regard disease, or disharmony of the body, as a dynamic condition. We treat the patient according to the symptoms, not according to the "disease." This is contrary to the standard view of disease as and entity unto itself. The allopathic doctor elicits the patient's symptoms and attempts to group them under a known diagnosis. He or she then prescribes the treatment established for that disease.

The Body, Not the Germs

We're always surrounded by germs, inside our body, in our food, in the air we breathe. In the battle raging between the body and invading forces, the homeopath is not primarily concerned with identifying the enemy—the type of bacteria. Our aim is to strengthen the body so it can resist these harmful organisms. In standard medicine, on the other hand, the goal is to identify the invader and select a powerful drug to destroy the specific germ.

Holistic Approach Versus Specialization

We believe that all parts of the body are interdependent, and therefore we treat the patient as a whole person, rather than concentrating on one organ or one part of the body. We do not attempt to separate mental from physical illness; all are symptoms of the individual. Homeopathy is truly holistic, and has been since its inception 180 years ago.

For centuries, standard medicine has taken a different approach; it treats a patient's mind and body as separate entities. A speaker at a holistic health conference recently quipped that in modern medicine the general practitioner treats the body, sends the head to a shrink and the soul to a clergyman.

HOMEOPATHY SUPPRESSED

If homeopathy is such an advanced system of medicine, why is it not more widely practiced?

Many people today do not realize that Homeopathy was widely practiced in the latter half of the nineteenth century. In 1890, there were 14,000 homeopaths as compared to 100,000 conventional physicians. In some areas—New England, the Middle Atlantic States, and the Midwest—one out of four or five physicians was a homeopath. There were twenty-two homeopathic medical schools and over a hundred homeopathic hospitals. The elite of every social community—the social, intellectual, political, and business leaders—patronized the homeopaths.

Homeopathy was first introduced in America as a result of its success in treating the victims of the cholera epidemic of 1832 in Europe. Our country was ripe for a new and humane system of medicine. The regular physician had two standard methods of treatment. One was to administer huge, or "heroic," doses of mercurous chloride, known as "calomel," to purge patients. This frequently caused the patient continuous salivation accompanied by swelling of the tongue. Patients also frequently lost all their teeth and, in extreme cases of mercurial poisoning, were unable to open their mouths. The other treatment that the physician used for every disease was bloodletting. The eminent Dr. Benjamin Rush (for whom a hospital in Philadelphia was named, as well as the Rush Medical College in Chicago) advised: "Bleeding should be continued...until four fifths of the blood contained in the body are drawn away." Children, including newborns, were also bled routinely.

So it is understandable why the homeopaths immediately attracted patients. In place of these barbaric methods, they had dozens of different remedies, none of which caused any disagreeable side effects. As proof that the homeopath's sweet-tasting white granules, often called "little sugar pills," were effective, a large number of homeopathic remedies were adopted by the allopaths and some are still being used today. One of the best known is nitroglycerine, used in certain heart ailments.

The medical establishment was hostile to homeopathy from the time it was introduced into the United States. In the 1830s and 40s when the public was dissatisfied with the harsh practices of regular medicine, homeopathy was not the only "alternative therapy;" botanical medicine and Thomsonian naturopathy were also popular. But homeopathy posed the greatest threat to orthodox medicine because its practitioners were licensed medical doctors. It was galling to the establishment that these homeopathic physicians, well trained in orthodox medicine, were critical of the system and had "defected" to homeopathy.

The establishment promptly took strong measures to suppress this upstart discipline. The American Medical Association (AMA) was formed in 1846 as a direct response to the founding of the American Institute of Homeopathy two years earlier. Homeopaths were denied admittance to standard medical societies. A member of such a society who consulted with a homeopath was punished by ostracism and expulsion. (In 1878, a physician was expelled from a medical society in Connecticut for consulting with a homeopath—his wife!) The hostility increased as "the best people" flocked to the homeopaths, and the regular physicians felt the pinch in their pocketbooks.

What killed, or almost killed, homeopathy? One reason for its decline was the changing life-style in America. The homeopathic physician was the quintessence of the family doctor who knew patients and their families intimately and could afford to devote a good deal of time to them, since most would remain patients for life. The shift to a mobile urban society as well as the rise of specialization changed that pattern. Homeopathic prescribing, which demands both time and intellectual effort, became increasingly out of step with the tempo of the times.

The rise of the drug industry after the Civil War further changed the practice of medicine. The allopath could now buy a proprietary, or compound, drug that saved time and effort, while the homeopath opposed to any mixing of medicines, continued prescribing medicines in the same "old-fashioned" way. As medical historian Harris L. Coulter points out, "The pharmaceutical industry...in the 1890s and earlier 1900s allied with the American Medical Association in its [the medical association's] final campaign against homeopathy."

A further severe blow to homeopathy was the Flexner Report in 1910, an evaluation of medical schools by the AMA. In view of the

AMA's traditional opposition to "sectarian medicine," it is not surprising that the examiners gave a low rating to homeopathic medical schools, among others, thus denying them a share in the millions of dollars, principally the Rockefeller grants, that were being given to allopathic institutions. One by one, the homeopathic medical schools closed and the homeopathic hospitals were converted to standard institutions. Flower Fifth Avenue Hospital and Medical College became New York Medical College; Hahnemann Hospital in San Francisco was recently renamed the Marshall Hale Hospital. With the advent of the "wonder drugs" in the early 1940s homeopathy appeared to be obsolete.

HOMEOPATHY: THE ALTERNATIVE OF THE FUTURE

This dismal prospect is rapidly changing. In an article written in 1970, Harris L Coulter points out that we are witnessing a popular revolt against orthodox medical practices "comparable to the revolt of the 1830s and 1840s which ensconced homeopathy on the American medical scene."

This revolt has gathered steam with the emergence of holistic health, a movement that surfaced in California in the early 1970s. Its practitioners, trained in a variety of disciplines, hold the common belief that medicine has become divorced from natural healing. According to Edward Bauman, coeditor of *The Holistic Health Handbook*, "Holistic Health is a sympathetic response to the distrust and frustration engendered by specialized allopathic medicine." Holistic therapists criticize widespread use of dangerous drugs, the dehumanizing effects of specialization, the failure to cure chronic degenerative disease. The conventional physician prescribes drugs to alleviate the symptoms of arthritis, diabetes, emphysema, but this treatment fails to attack the root of the problem.

Holistic-minded professionals were amazed to stumble upon homeopathy. Here was a "natural" system of medicine that used no toxic drugs, treated the whole person, and, in many instances, cured "hopeless" chronic conditions. Furthermore, the efficacy of homeopathy had been demonstrated by the clinical experience of physicians for over 150 years.

So, with health a national preoccupation, homeopathy is emerging as a vigorous alternative to standard medicine. An increasing number of physicians and nurses are enrolling in the summer course offered by the National Center for Homeopathy. People are investigating homeopathy and incorporating it into their lives. Lay people all over the country are forming homeopathic study groups.

Homeopathy is alive and well in other parts of the world. In Britain, members of the Royal Family have been cared for by homeopathic physicians since the reign of Queen Victoria. There are around 200 homeopathic physicians in Britain; the principal hospitals offering such treatment are in London and Glasgow. France has nearly 800 homeopathic physicians, and the movement is also active in Germany, Austria, and Switzerland.

India is a stronghold of homeopathy, with 124 homeopathic medical schools. Central and Latin America are also important centers. In Mexico there are three homeopathic medical colleges, two of which are state supported. There is a similar school of medicine in Brazil, and the medical school in Santiago, Chile includes a professor of homeopathy. Around 450 Argentine physicians are homeopaths.

Homeopathy is on the rise all over the world, owing to the dissatisfaction of both physician and patient with the medical treatment at their disposal. Both are looking for a safe and effective approach to healing and finding the answer in homeopathy.

APPENDIX B

L-TRYPTOPHAN:
LOST SUPPLEMENT, NECESSARY NUTRIENT

In November, 1989, the U.S. Food and Drug Administration requested that all supplemental, over-the-counter sales of the essential amino acid of L-Tryptophan be stopped. Instead, this amino acid is now only available as a prescription drug, not even manufactured by the large pharmaceutical lab in the U.S.

Leading up to this FDA decision had been the recent outbreak of a rare blood disorder involving 31 people who had taken L-Tryptophan, although this amino acid had been used safely and effectively for more than 30 years. The rare blood disorder, called "eosinophilia myalgia," was characterized by chronic fatigue, muscle pain and elevated counts of eosinophils which are a specific type of white blood cell normally elevated only when a person suffers from allergies or intestinal parasites. During the L-Tryptophan scare period, over 900 cases of the blood disorder emerged. Prior to this event, millions of people had used this nutrient without dangerous side effects, to help with low seratonin levels and the resulting insomnia and sleep disorders.

We discuss this situation for two reasons. First, to encourage you to learn which foods contain L-Tryptophan and to be sure to include them in your diet so you can sleep and be healthy. The list of foods which contain good amounts of L-Tryptophan includes raw milk products, chicken, turkey, eggs, spelt, oats and dried figs.

The other reason for our discussion is to alert you to the control of valuable food-nutrients by drug companies, governmental agencies or medical interests. The removal of L-Tryptophan from the health food stores and from hundreds of natural product companies' formulas was a windfall for the pharmaceutical lab that now provides it through doctors by prescription only. Effectively all the competition was eliminated by the FDA's action, allowing the pharmaceutical company to triple the price of L-Tryptophan.

Another related point is that most medical schools still do not offer nutritional training. Unless they have obtained extra nutritional training, doctors are not likely to recommend nutritional or alternative therapies such as food supplements. Therefore, the general public has no longer easy access to the valuable amino acid L-Tryptophan.

As an important thought in this discussion about L-Tryptophan, I want to state that I never was in favor of using individual, free-form amino acids such as L-Tryptophan. Basic nutritional insights teach us that all the amino acids work together. Thus, a person cannot supplement one amino acid continuously without disturbing the balance of the entire amino acid picture. Nevertheless, the action by the FDA cannot be condoned.

To clarify the events even further, clearly nobody wants a supplement that causes a blood disorder. But, in fact, L-Tryptophan did not cause the rare blood disorder. As the story unfolded, it was discovered that a Japanese manufacturer of L-Tryptophan sold a contaminated batch to other companies and suppliers for the American public. Thus, the real problem with L-Tryptophan was contamination from a single lab, not the nutrient itself.

No American-made L-Tryptophan ever caused blood disorders. Nevertheless, American manufacturers of many effective, natural products were banned from providing L-Tryptophan any longer. Reputable companies, built on the highest standards, such as Tyson in San Diego, had to destroy their perfectly good products or ship them overseas. These companies were no longer allowed to sell in the U.S. market which they had built. Instead, their pharmaceutical competitor was now allowed to supply the nutrient and to call it a drug.

It might interest you that a lot of rumors began to circulate once the nature of the events became clearer. Of course, I cannot verify the validity of these rumors which considered it as quite possible that U.S. vested interests hired the Japanese mafia to deliberately sabotage the Japanese manufacturer's L-Tryptophan supply. The contamination would set up the events which were to occur in the U.S., and competitors of the Japanese manufacturer in Japan would emerge with one less concern when the company was put out of business.

As such rumors of conspiracy were whispered, the deaths of consumers reported, and the undisputable power of the FDA in action, few voices could be raised against the removal of L-Tryptophan from the natural health companies. All but a few companies bowed down to governmental oppression in order to stay in business with other products, but without the nutrient L-Tryptophan. And those companies wishing to reestablish L-Tryptophan as an over-the-counter nutrient will encounter years of court battles and deaf ears in what will most likely be a futile endeavor.

L-Tryptophan, of itself, cannot cause the eosinophil blood disorder. The very thorough investigation by regulatory agencies, U.S. manufacturers and clinicians clearly identified that the L-Tryptophan contamination came from one Japanese source. Rather than taking L-Tryptophan away from the American people, better purity standards on imported L-Tryptophan were needed.

Therefore, it was quite unnecessary for the FDA to persecute American manufacturers of nutritional supplements and to serve the vested and conspiratorial interests of pharmaceutical/medical mega-corporations. The events, however, are a reminder that our health interests and freedoms are being eroded, and that there are many companies, associations and individuals with a mission to take away the public's right to food substances in order to make a larger profit off the public.

You will ask, well what about the people who suffered eosinophil-myalgia syndrome (EMS)? It is of special interest that the cure for them is a new wonder drug, L-Tryptophan, disguised with a trade name. Dr. Russell Jaffe, eminent medical doctor and one of our country's most enlightened nutritional researchers, published a report about a number of cures of people debilitated with EMS in which the only treatment was L-Tryptophan with vitamin C.

Somehow, the whole scenario resembles a shell game. Our nutrient L-Tryptophan is gone; it's now a drug; and it's being used to cure the disease caused by the contaminated batch; except now, the cure comes with expensive medical tests, office visits, and a prescription at three times the original cost of L-Tryptophan. Who are the winners and who are the losers of this shell game?

Keep in mind that L-Tryptophan is only one of many effective nutrients that special interest groups would like to seize for their exclusive control. Flax seed oil and other sources of essential lipids, as well as numerous herbs and other amino acids are also targets for control. If a nutrient works and people need it, someone will try to get control of it. Unfortunately, nutrition companies failed to organize and fight for the preservation of L-Tryptophan as a food supplement.

The American people, also, let this important nutrient fall into the hands of the medical/pharmaceutical monopoly. When we let someone else control our food, our health, our air, our water or our energy, we become weak, vulnerable and ultimately enslaved. Stay alerted to further FDA actions and raids on nutritional supplements as this agency continues to enforce the Nutrition Labeling Education Act. And write to your senators and representatives in Congress about these nutritional issues.

APPENDIX C

THE INFLUENCE OF FOOD COOKING ON THE BLOOD CHEMISTRY OF MAN

by Paul Kouchakoff (Swiss) M.D. Institute of Clinical Chemistry, Lausanne, Switzerland

From *Proceedings: First International Congress of Microbiology, Paris*, 1930. Translation by Lee Foundation for Nutritional Research, Milwaukee, Wisconsin.

The living organism is very sensitive to all harmful influences and reacts against them immediately. We see this when we make an analysis of our blood during simple and infectious illness, when extraneous substances are introduced into our system, etc. In such cases the number of white corpuscles changes and the correlation of percentage between them is disturbed. This is one of the indications of a pathological process going on in our system.

After every dose of food, we also observe a general augmentation of white corpuscles, and a change in the correlation of their percentage. This phenomenon has been considered, until now, a physiological one, and is called a digestive leukocystosis.

We use, for our food, raw foodstuffs which have been altered by means of high temperature, and manufactured foodstuffs. How then does each one of these foodstuffs separately act on our blood formula?

We find that, after taking raw foodstuffs, neither the number of white corpuscles nor the correlation of their percentage has changed. Ordinary unboiled drinking water, mineral water, salt, different green foodstuffs, cereals, nuts, honey, raw eggs, raw meat, raw fish, fresh milk, sour milk, butter—in other words, foodstuffs in the state in which they exist in nature, belong to the group of those which do not call forth any infringement in our blood formula.

After the consumption of the same natural foodstuffs, altered by means of high temperature, we find that the general number of white corpuscles has changed, but the correlation of their percentage has remained the same.

After consumption of manufactured foodstuffs not only has the number of white corpuscles changed but also the correlation of percentage between them. To this group belong sugar, wine, chocolate in tablet form, etc.

All our experiments have shown that it is not the quantity, but the quality of food which plays an important role in the alteration of our blood formula, and that 200 milligrams or even 50 milligrams of foodstuffs produce the same reaction as large doses of them. The experiments also show that the reaction in our blood takes place at the moment the food enters the stomach, while the preliminary mastication of food in the mouth softens the reaction.

We have already said that raw foodstuffs, altered by means of high temperature only call forth an augmentation of the general number of white corpuscles. Does this occur only when such foodstuffs are heated to boiling point, or is the same phenomenon called forth by lower temperatures?

It appears that every raw foodstuff has its own temperature which must not be surpassed in heating, otherwise it loses its original virtues and calls forth a reaction in the system. Ordinary drinking water, heated for half an hour to a temperature of 87 degrees centigrade does not change our blood, but this same water, heated to 88 degrees changes it.

We have given the name "critical temperature" to the highest degree of temperature at which a particular foodstuff can be cooked for half an hour in bain marie [double boiler], and eaten, without changing our blood formula.

This critical temperature is not the same for all raw foodstuffs. It varies within a range of ten degrees. The lowest critical temperature for water is 87 degrees (C); for milk it is 88 degrees; for cereals, tomatoes, cabbage, bananas, 89 degrees; for pears, meat, 90 degrees; for butter, 91 degrees; for apples and oranges, 92; for potatoes, 93; for carrots, strawberries and figs, 97 degrees centigrade. (See last paragraph for conversion to Fahrenheit.)

Our experiments show that it is possible to paralyze the action of a foodstuff, once its critical temperature is surpassed. There exist strictly definite laws for this, and the critical temperature plays the first role here.

If a cooked foodstuff is eaten along with the same product in a raw state there is no reaction.

The raw product has neutralized the action which this same product, with its critical temperature surpassed, would have called forth. In other words, the raw product has, so to say, reestablished the virtues of the product altered by a high temperature. Such a reestablishment is also possible when two different products have been absorbed, but with one condition; their critical temperature must either be the same, or else the critical temperature of the raw product must be higher than the critical temperature of the overheated one.

If the critical temperature of a raw product is lower than that of the overheated one, the reaction is sure to take place; in this case, even the augmentation of the quantity of the raw products does not help.

This law remains the same when the raw product is mixed with several overheated ones of the same critical temperature.

If several cooked foodstuffs are taken, each with a different critical temperature, along with raw food, reaction takes place, even if the raw product has a higher critical temperature than that of any of the cooked foodstuffs.

Now we pass on to the third group of foodstuffs, such as sugar, wine, etc., obtained by complicated manufacturing processes, and producing double reaction in our organism. These products may also be consumed without calling forth any reaction, but only when they are introduced into our organism conjointly with no less than two raw foodstuffs of a different critical temperature. Even one raw product has a beneficial influence on this third group, and deprives them of one of their properties, namely the power of altering the correlation of percentage of the white corpuscles.

As regards the proportions in which raw products must be added to cooked food, there is an irreducible minimum. For water, for example, it is 50 percent.

CONCLUSIONS: After over 300 experiments on ten individuals of different age and sex, we have come to the following conclusions:

1. The augmentation of the number of white corpuscles and the alteration of the correlation of the percentage between them which takes place after every consumption of food, and which was considered until now as a physiological phenomenon, is, in reality, a pathological one, called forth by the introduction into the system of foodstuffs altered by means of high temperature, and by complicated treatments of ordinary products produced by nature.

2. After the consumption of fresh raw foodstuffs, produced by nature, our blood formula does not change in any lapse of time, nor in consequence of any combinations.

3. After the consumption of foodstuffs produced by nature, but altered by means of high temperature, an augmentation of the general number of white corpuscles takes place, but the correlation of percentage between them remains the same.

4. After the consumption of foodstuffs produced by nature, but altered by manufacturing processes, an augmentation of the general number of white corpuscles as well as a change in the correlation of their percentages takes place.

5. It has been proved possible to take, without changing the blood formula, every kind of foodstuff which is habitually eaten now, but only by following this rule, viz: that it must be taken along with raw products, according to a definite formula.

6. In a healthy organism, it is not possible, by the consumption of any food to alter the correlation of percentage between the white corpuscles, without augmenting their general number.

7. Foodstuffs do not seem to have any influence on the transitional and the Polymorphonuclear Eosinophiles and the correlation of percentage between them is not altered.

8. We can change our blood formula in the direction we desire by dieting accordingly.

9. Blood examination can only have significance as a diagnosis if it is made on an empty stomach.

Critical Temperature at Which Food Values are Altered

Food	Critical Temperature
Drinking water	191°F
Milk	191°F
Cereals	192°F
Tomatoes	192°F
Cabbage	192°F
Bananas	192°F
Butter	196°F
Apples	197°F
Oranges	197°F
Potatoes	200°F
Carrots	206°F
Strawberries	206°F
Figs	206°F

APPENDIX   D

PRO-VITA! MEAL PLANNING SHEETS

Pro-Vita! is a custom-designed, flexible way to maximize your nutrition in a way that directly affects your health, energy, attitude, and longevity.

Please use the following sheets to plan your diet.

USUAL DIET(What I normally eat)

Breakfast:

Snack:

Lunch:

Snack:

Supper:

Snack:

PRO-VITA! 5+5

Breakfast:
Protein, cooked:

Proteins, raw:

Vegetable, cooked:

Vegetables, raw:

Other:

Lunch: (PROTEIN)
Protein, cooked:

Proteins, raw:

Vegetable, cooked:

Vegetables, raw:

Other:

 OR Lunch: (CARBOHYDRATE)

Complex carbohydrates:

Vegetable, cooked:

Vegetables, raw:

Other:

Supper:
Complex carbohydrates:

Vegetable, cooked:

Vegetables, raw:

Other:

USUAL DIET (What I normally eat)

Breakfast:

Snack:

Lunch:

Snack:

Supper:

Snack:

PRO-VITA! 5+5

Breakfast:
Protein, cooked:

Proteins, raw:

Vegetable, cooked:

Vegetables, raw:

Other:

Lunch: (PROTEIN)
Protein, cooked:

Proteins, raw:

Vegetable, cooked:

Vegetables, raw:

Other:
OR Lunch: (CARBOHYDRATE)

Complex carbohydrates:

Vegetable, cooked:

Vegetables, raw:

Other:

Supper:
Complex carbohydrates:

Vegetable, cooked:

Vegetables, raw:

Other:

PRO-VITA! PLAN

USUAL DIET (What I normally eat)

Breakfast:

Snack:

Lunch:

Snack:

Supper:

Snack:

PRO-VITA! 5+5

Breakfast:
Protein, cooked:

Proteins, raw:

Vegetable, cooked:

Vegetables, raw:

Other:

Lunch: (PROTEIN)
Protein, cooked:

Proteins, raw:

Vegetable, cooked:

Vegetables, raw:

Other:

OR **Lunch:** (CARBOHYDRATE)

Complex carbohydrates:

Vegetable, cooked:

Vegetables, raw:

Other:

Supper:
Complex carbohydrates:

Vegetable, cooked:

Vegetables, raw:

Other:

USUAL DIET (What I normally eat)

Breakfast:

Snack:

Lunch:

Snack:

Supper:

Snack:

PRO-VITA! 5+5

Breakfast:
Protein, cooked:

Proteins, raw:

Vegetable, cooked:

Vegetables, raw:

Other:

Lunch: (PROTEIN)
Protein, cooked:

Proteins, raw:

Vegetable, cooked:

Vegetables, raw:

Other:
OR Lunch: (CARBOHYDRATE)

Complex carbohydrates:

Vegetable, cooked:

Vegetables, raw:

Other:

Supper:
Complex carbohydrates:

Vegetable, cooked:

Vegetables, raw:

Other:

USUAL DIET (What I normally eat)

Breakfast:

Snack:

Lunch:

Snack:

Supper:

Snack:

PRO-VITA! 5+5

Breakfast:
Protein, cooked:

Proteins, raw:

Vegetable, cooked:

Vegetables, raw:

Other:

Lunch: (PROTEIN)
Protein, cooked:

Proteins, raw:

Vegetable, cooked:

Vegetables, raw:

Other:

OR Lunch: (CARBOHYDRATE)

Complex carbohydrates:

Vegetable, cooked:

Vegetables, raw:

Other:

Supper:
Complex carbohydrates:

Vegetable, cooked:

Vegetables, raw:

Other:

USUAL DIET(What I normally eat)

Breakfast:

Snack:

Lunch:

Snack:

Supper:

Snack:

PRO-VITA! 5+5

Breakfast:
Protein, cooked:

Proteins, raw:

Vegetable, cooked:

Vegetables, raw:

Other:

Lunch: (PROTEIN)
Protein, cooked:

Proteins, raw:

Vegetable, cooked:

Vegetables, raw:

Other:

OR Lunch: (CARBOHYDRATE)

Complex carbohydrates:

Vegetable, cooked:

Vegetables, raw:

Other:

Supper:
Complex carbohydrates:

Vegetable, cooked:

Vegetables, raw:

Other:

BIBLIOGRAPHY

Budwig, Dr. Johanna. 1992. *Flax Oil as a True Aid Against Arthritis, Heart Infarction, Cancer and Other Diseases*. Transl. of Fette als wahre Hilfe gegen Arteriousklerose, Herzinfarkt, Krebs. Vancouver, British Columbia: Apple Publishing Company.

Budwig, Dr. Johanna. 1988. *The Photoelements of Life*. Transl. of *Fotoelemente des Lebens* by Associated Partners West (APW).

Choudhary, Harimohan. 1991. *50 Millesimal Potency in Theory and Practice*. New Delhi: B. Jain Publishers.

Clarke, J. H. 1986. *Dictionary of Materia Medica*, vol 2. New Delhi: B. Jain Publishers, reprint.

Cleave, T. L. 1969. *The Saccharine Disease*. J Wright, Keats Publishing.

Cole, K. C. Human Electricity. 1984. *Discover Magazine*, (February).

Erasmus, Udo. 1986. *Fats and Oils. The Complete Guide to Fats and Oils in Health and Nutrition*. Vancouver, BC: Alive Books.

Erasmus, Udo. 1990. *Healing Fats…Killing Fats* .

Frase, Dr. med. W. 1991. Disturbances of Metabolism and Antihomotoxic Therapy. *Biologische Medizin, Internationale Zeitschrift für Biomedizinische Forschung und Therapie*. Vol. 20 (February).

Grant, Doris & Jean Joice. 1989. *Food Combining for Health.* Rochester, VT: Healing Arts Press.

Hahnemann, Samuel. 1974. *Organon of Medicine.* 6th ed. Transl. by William Boericke. New Delhi: B. Jain Publishers.

Hahnemann, Samuel. 1831. *Regeln der homöopatischen Diät.* (Rules of the Homeopathic Diet.) Dresden: Arnold.

Howell. Dr. Edward. 1985. *Enzyme Nutrition.* Avery Publishing Group.

Jaffe, Russell M. 1989. Eosinophilia-Myalgia Syndrome Caused by Contaminated Tryptophan. *International Journal of Biosocial Medical Research* (December).

Lappe, F. M. 1982. *Diet for a Small Planet.* 2nd ed. New York: Ballantine Books.

Lee, Royal. 1950. The Battlefront for Better Nutrition. *The Interpreter.*

Mead, Nathaniel. 1990. The Champion Diet. *East West Journal,* (September).

Morter, M. T. 1988. A Review of the Potential of Hydrogen (pH). In *Clinical Chemistry and Nutrition Guidebook: A Physician's Desk Reference.* Ed. by Paul Yanick & Russell Jaffe. T & H Publishing.

Panos, Maesimund B. & Jane Heimlich. 1980. *Homeopathic Medicine at Home.* Los Angeles: J. P. Tarcher, Inc.

Pottenger, Francis M. 1983. *Pottengers' Cats: A Study in Nutrition.* San Diego: Price Pottenger Foundation.

Revici, Emanuel, M. D. 1961. *Research in Physio-Pathology as Basis of Guided Chemotherapy.* Van Nostrand Co., 1961.

Robbins, John. 1987. *Diet for a New America.* Walpole, NH: Stillpoint Publishing.

Sampsidis, Nicholas. 1983. *Homogenized!* Glenwood Landing, NY: Sunflower Publishing, Inc.

Simopoulos, Artemis, MD & Norman Salem, PhD. 1989. Fatty Acids in Eggs from Range-Fed Greek Chickens. *The New England Journal of Medicine* (Nov. 16).

Steinberg, David. 1990. *Diet for a Poisoned Planet: How To Chose Safe Foods for You and Your Family.* New York: Harmony Books.

Strehlow, Dr. Wighard. 1989. *The Wonderfood Spelt.* Okemos, MI: Purity Foods, Inc.

Strehlow, Dr. Wighard & Gottfried Hertzka, M.D. 1988. *Hildegard of Bingen's Medicine.* Santa Fe, NM: Bear & Company.

Tips, Jack. 1992. *Osteoporosis: The Preventable Disease.* MS.

Tyler, M. L. 1989. *Homeopathic Drug Pictures.* Saffron Walden, Essex: C. W. Daniel Co.

Walb, Dr. Ludwig & Luise Walb. 1988. *Die Haysche Trennkost.* (The Hay Separation Diet.) 40th ed. Heidelberg: Karl F. Haug Verlag.

Wheelwright. *Lectures.*

ABOUT THE AUTHOR

Jack Tips, ND, PhD, brings the message of dynamic, vital health to thousands of people through lectures, seminars, articles, radio, books, television and clinical practice. *"Health is a dynamic state wherein the body, the emotions, and the mind are bio-energetically in accord with the flow of Life Force, expressing adaptability, vitality, and joy."*

Beginning in 1971, his background includes personal studies with many of the world's renowned health leaders: Dr. Bernard Jensen (iridology, naturopathy), Dr. Wilhelm Langreder (German nosode homeopathy), Dr. A.S. Wheelwright (systemic herbology, bioenergetic nutrition, sclerology), Stanley Burroughs (cleansing, color therapy), Dr. Francisco Eizayaga (clinical homeopathy), Dr. Paul Eck (tissue mineral ratios), Dr. Alan Beardall (kinesiology), Dr. Herbert Shelton (fasting, hygiene), and Dr. Robin Murphy (classical homeopathy). He also studied at the Occidental Institute Research Foundation (electro-acupuncture, vega-test, Mora therapy) in Vancouver, BC.

In 1980, Dr. Tips began consulting in the applications of systemic herbology, homeopathy and clinical nutrition. He earned a PhD in Nutrition Science from Clayton University (The Dr. Roger Williams School of Nutrition Science), and an ND (Doctorate of Naturopathy — a 2 year curriculum) from Clayton University in Clayton, Missouri. His dissertation, published as *Conquer Candida and Restore Your Immune System* has received international recognition as a definitive work on the philosophy of natural cure and the challenges of the immune system. He has also authored *The Next Step to Greater Energy, Your Liver...Your Lifeline,* and *The Art and Science of Sclerology, Blood Chemistry & Clinical Nutrition,* as well as numerous articles on women's health. He holds a Fellowship in the American Council of Applied Clinical Nutrition (FACACN), and is certified as a Nutritional Consultant (CNC) by the American Council of Nutrition Consultants. He serves on the board of directors of the Texas chapter of the International and American Association of Clinical Nutritionists. He is registered as a practicing homeopath with the National Center for Homeopathy, Washington, DC, and is a member of the International Foundation for Homeopathy; the Homeopathic Academy of Naturopathic Physicians, and graduate of and active participant with the Hahnemann Academy of North America (CHom).

In 1993, he became a minister for Life Resources, an integrated auxiliary of Freedom Church of Revelation, and established his ministry through Apple-A-Day. His ministry is dedicated to the healing of the whole person with natural methods.

Currently, he is president of the International Sclerology Foundation, teacher with the Westlake Homeopathic Society, and director of the Apple-A-Day Clinic, Austin, Texas, where he consults with individuals, both in person and by phone. He resides in Austin with his wife, children, and step children. Dr. Tips is dedicated to providing people the knowledge and tools to live genuinely healthy lives.

INDEX

Blood cholesterol, 83

Blood pH, 121, 122

Body: carbohydrate as percentage of dry weight of, 51-52; electrical field of, 22-23; innate wisdom of, for healing, 19; protein as percentage of dry weight of, 51

Body cycles: food processing cycle, 107; and glandular typing, 109-11; and health, 105-107; menstrual cycle, 107; meridian/organ clock, 111-13, 176; pH cycle, 102, 113-14, 174-79; timing for when to eat, 107-109

Bok choy, 81, 157

Borscht (recipe), 305

Bottled water, 259

Boyd, William E., 317

Bread, 287

Breakfast: complex carbohydrates for, 175; 5 + 5 meal for, 181-82, 272-73; fruit for, 101-102, 110; sample menus for, 237, 241-43, 282-85; value of, 173-76, 179

Breast milk, 80, 139

Brewer's yeast, 189

Brown rice, 90, 150

Brown rice vinegar, 212

Budwig, Johanna, 60-61, 84, 166

Butter: balanced butter, 86, 90, 211-12; compared with other oils, 88; substitutes for, 212; toxicity of, 86

C vitamin, 93, 221, 226

Cabbage, 81, 157

Calcarea carbonica, 117

Calcarea fluorata, 117

Calcarea phosphoricum, 117

Calcium: in commercial milk, 79, 80; in vegetables, 81, 167

Calcium citrate, preparation of, 81

Cancer: and abnormal lipids, 82; and chlorinated water, 258-59; colon cancer, 95; and excessive amounts of protein,119-120; and fatty acids, 60, 61; and fiber, 42; and improper use of protein, 55; and oils, 32, 66; and oxygen, 12-13; and pH, 123; prevention of, 32, 42, 98, 157; and refined foods, 94; skin cancer, 64, 219

Candida, 187, 267-68

Canned foods, 210

Canola oil, 65, 86, 87, 88, 287

Carbohydrates: for athletes, 53; for breakfast, 175; for children, 52-53; definition of, 91; energy lines of, 151-52, 154; and energy metabolism, 93-96, 132-33; and fruit, 101-104; high carbohydrate diets, 48, 52-53; importance of, by U.S. Department of Agriculture, 33; inadequacy of, as foundation of diet, 25, 28, 48; list of, 100; not to be eaten with 5 + 5 meal, 235; nutritional function of, 53; optimal time for, 174; percentage of dry weight of body, 51-52; in Pro-Vita! Nutrition Pyramid, 32, 91-104; produced by overcooking certain proteins, 150; reasons for not mixing protein with, 147-50; recipes for, 304-08; refined carbohydrates, 92-94, 133, 151- 52, 220; and release of endorphins, 175, 181; role of complex, simple and refined carbohydrates, 91- 93, 151-52; spelt as example of, 96-99; for supper, 238-39

Cardiovascular disease and enzymes, 159; and nutrition, 68-73; statistics on, 68; symptoms of cardiovascular stress, 72-73

Enzyme supplements, 223
Enzymes: in carbohydrates, 93; and cardiovascular health, 70; foods best suited for, 39, 40; loss of, in pasteurized milk, 79, 80; and pH, 114-15; and protein assimilation, 180; and raw vegetables, 157- 60; in vegetables, 42, 157-60
EPA, 83-84
Erasmus, Udo, 84, 86
Eskimos, 83-84
Essential fatty acids (EFA), 83-87. *See also* Oils
Ether, as element of health, 12, 131, 216, 217-18
Exercise, 30, 262-63
Extra-virgin olive oil, 65, 74, 86, 87, 89, 287

F vitamin, 64-66, 74
Fasting, 263-64
Fats: and cholesterol myth, 75-76; in eggs, 76; and essential fatty acids and mono-unsaturated oils, 83-87; in milk, 77-82; and ratio of lipoproteins, 82-83
Fatty acids. *See* Oils
FDA. *See* Food and Drug Administration (FDA)
Fermenation, of soybeans, 23-24
Fertilizers, chemical, 162, 227
Feta cheese, mixed with flax seed oil, 86
Fiber: in carbohydrates, 93; in fruits, 165; in spelt, 98; in vegetables, 42, 164-65
Fire, as element of health, 12, 13, 60, 131, 216, 217
Fish, 26-27; recipes for, 141, 207, 265, 298, 299-300
Fish Fillet, Sauteed (recipe), 299-300
Fish, Marinated (recipe), 298
Fish oils, 59, 66, 83-84
Fish with Herbs (recipe), 299
5 + 5 meal, 166, 181-82, 235-43, 235-43
Five Element Theory, Chinese, 11-14, 131, 216, 218
Flax seed oil, 60, 61-62, 66, 74, 84-89, 222, 287, 328
Flax seeds, 65, 84
Food. *See* Carbyhydrates; Fats; Fruits; Oils; Proteins; and names of specific foods
Food and Drug Administration (FDA), 44, 67, 98, 188, 325-28
Food combining plans: Pro-Vita! Plan, 103-104
Food groups, revision by U.S. Department of Agriculture, 32-33
Food processing cycle, 107
Foundation of Economic Trends, 44
Frase, Med. W., 148
Free radicals, 66-68, 70, 71
French Dressing (recipe), 311
Fried foods, 59, 60, 62, 66, 67, 90, 210
Frozen vegetables, 292-93
Fruit: acid category of, 103; in afternoon and evening, 110-11, 182; appreciation of taste of, 37; for breakfast, 101-102, 110, 175-76, 179; classification according to food-combining schema, 103-104; consequences of limiting diet to raw fruits and vegetables, 159-60; fiber in, 165; impact of commercial farming and synthetic fertilizers on, 37; melon category of, 104; optimal use of, 101-103; in Pro-Vita! Nutrition Pyramid, 32, 101-103; and production of alkalinity in body, 102, 119; sub-acid category of, 103; sugars in, 92; sweet category of, 104

Homeopathy: as alternative of future, 322-23; and body's innate wisdom for healing, 19; compared with standard medicine, 318-19; and concept of bioenergy, 20; definition of,313; history of, 313- 14; principles of, 19, 315-18; reasons for effectiveness of, 317-18; remedies for pH imbalance, 117, 127; and sleep difficulties, 181; and supplementation, 224-26; suppression of, 320-22

Homogenization, of milk, 81-82

Honey, 203

Howell, Edward, 70

Humanization of proteins, 47, 62, 156, 165-66

Hummus, 289

Humor, 275-77

Hydrochloric acid (HCl), 187-89

Hydrogen peroxide soak, 227, 230, 231

Hydrogenated oils, 59, 60, 90, 211

Hypoglycemia, 93, 263

Iceberg lettuce, 43, 162, 163

Illness. *See* Disease; and names of specific diseases

Immune system: and effective protein consumption, 134; function of, 47; and proteins, 156; and spelt, 97-98

Infants: breast milk for, 80; raw goat milk for, 80; substitute baby milk-formula for, 80-81

Inge's Fruit Salad (recipe), 312

Inge's Miso Soup (recipe), 300

Inge's Red Cabbage (recipe), 307

Inge's Spelt Pasta Salad (recipe), 307-08

Insecticides, 227

Insulin, 116, 119

Intestinal tract, and foods best suited for, 39-40

Intrinsic factor, 26-27

Ionization potential of foods, 129

Irradiated foods, 208-09

Italian Dressing (recipe), 308

Jaffe, Russell, 275

Japan, 24, 68, 188

Johnson, Kirk, 134

Juice, preparation of raw red potato juice, 194-95

Juicer, 289

Kale, 157

Kali remedies, 117, 127

Kellogg, Harvey, 164

Kidneys, and meating eating, 57

Kitchen: managing the Pro-Vita! kitchen, 287-93; six steps to a Pro-Vita! kitchen, 254-56

Kouchakoff, Paul, 161

Kreb's cycle, 132

Mexican Chili Sauce (recipe), 309

Milk: allergy to cow's milk, 148; avoidance of commercial milk, 210-11; avoidance of, with meat, 115; breast milk, 80, 139; commercial milk, 78-80, 81-82, 210-11; digestion time of, 139-40; as high- stress protein, 171; homogenization of, 81-82; for infants, 80-81; pasteurization of, 78-81; raw milk, 77, 78-79, 82; substitute baby milk-formula, 80- 81; substitutions for, 253

MIN formula, 224

Mineral supplements, 222, 224

Minerals: in carbohydrates, 93; loss of, in pasteurized milk, 79; in vegetables, 42

Minimum Dose, in homeopathy, 316-17

Miso, 23, 24, 151

Miso Soup (recipe), 300

Mitochondria, 57

Monosaturated oils, 64-65

Mono-unsaturated oils, 85

Morning sickness, 51

Morris, Robert, 259

Morter, Ted, 119-20, 122

Natrum muriaticum, 117, 118

Natrum phosphoricum, 127

Niacin: conversion to niacinamide, 26, 27

"Niacin flush," 27

Niacinamide, 26, 27

Nitsuke method, 292

Nucleo-proteins. See Proteins

Nut milks, 201

NutraSweet, 46, 47, 211

Nutrition: biochemical aspects of, 21, 23-31; and cardiovascular disease, 68-73; and Chinese five element philosophy, 11-14, 131, 216-18; definition of, 4; diet versus, 4-6; effects of, on health and disease, 8-11, 19-20; importance of nutritional plan, 6-8; and natural body cycles, 105-130; and the Natural Law, 3-4, 7; new Pro-Vita! Plan, 18-20; pathways of, 3- 4; and pH cycle, 174-79; Pro-Vita! Nutrition Pyramid, 31-34, 48; Wheelwright's concept of plant bioenergy, 20-23; Wheelwright's low-stress diet, 15-18. See also Pro-Vita! Plan; and specific foods

Nutritional improvements, instructions for, 211-12

Nuts, 65, 163-64, 171, 201, 211; soaking of, 211

Obesity, 204

Octopus, 141

Octopus, Marinated (recipe), 302-303

Oil and Vinegar Dressing (recipe), 311

Oils: abstinence from, 65-66; balanced butter, 86; biochemical values of, 62; Budwig's research on, 60-61, 66; cold-pressed oil, 73-74, 89-90; for cooking, 89; definition of, 59; detrimental oils, 59, 62, 63, 86-87; and diet, 61-63; energy line of, 153, 154; as energy supplier, 132; enhancing protein assimilation with vegetables and high quality oil, 155-66; essential fatty acids, 83-87; fish oils, 59, 83-84; function of, 60; heated oils, 67; high quality, 62, 287; hydrogenated oils, 59, 60, 90, 211; mono-unsaturated oils, 85; monosaturated oils, 64-65; number of fatty acids, 65; omego-3 oils, 83-87; pan-frying at low temperature, 86; polyunsaturated oils, 65, 67; in

Pro-Vita! Nutrition Pyramid, 32, 59-74; proper use of, 89-90; and protein
  humanization, 62, 165-66; and proteins, 59; rancid oils, 62, 66-68, 85, 87, 203,
  277; recommended amount of, 59, 61-62, 65; as required nutrient, 59-60;
  saturated oils, 64; small amount of high quality oils used with protein and
  vegetables, 62; storage of, 90; symptoms of diet too low in, 64; symptoms of too
  many fats in diet, 63; table comparing dietary oils, 88; and Vitamin F, 64-66.
  See also specific types of oil
Oleic acid, 85, 87, 88
Olive oil, 65, 66, 85, 86, 87, 88, 89, 90, 212, 287
Omego-3 oils, 83-87
Omelet, Spinach (recipe), 304
Organic produce, 206, 218, 231-33, 287
Osteoporosis, 84, 95, 118-20, 123
Out-of-season produce, 233
Oxidation rates, 114-16, 136-37, 265-66
Oxygen, sale of, 219

Palm oil, 83, 87, 88
Pan-frying at low temperature, 86
Pasta Salad, Spelt (recipe), 307-08
Pasteurization of milk, 78-81
Peanut butter, 211
Peanut oil, 65, 86, 88, 89
Peas, 150
Pepsin, 114-15
Pesticides, 139, 162
pH: acid-forming foods for alkaline pH, 126; alkaline- forming foods for acid pH,
  125; analysis of, 121- 23; blood pH, 118-19, 121, 122; charting for analysis,
  123-30; homeopathic remedies for pH imbalance, 127; importance of, in
  health, 114-21; as logarithmic scale, 113; measurement of, 122; optimal range
  of, 124, 130, 174; pH cycle, 102, 113-14, 174-79; salivary pH, 122-23;
  symptoms of acid pH, 125-26; symptoms of alkaline pH, 126-27; techniques to
  acidify pH, 126; techniques to alkalize pH, 124-25; urinary pH, 122, 124
Phosphate of Soda, 127
Phosphorus, 62
Pimiento, 70
Pine nuts, 211
Plant bioenergy, 20-23
Plaque system, in cardiovascular health, 69, 70-71
Platelets, 71
PMS, 106
Poached eggs, 195
Polyunsaturated oils, 65, 67
Pork, 136, 148, 171
Potato, Baked (recipe), 307
Potatoes, preparation of raw red potato juice, 194-95
Potentization, Law of, 316-17
Pottenger, Frances M., 79
Pregnancy: morning sickness during, 51; protein consumption during, 50-51
Pritikin Diet, 66
PRO formula, 169

167- 68; improvement of vegetarian diet, 38-42; and "niacin flush," 27; not for everyone, 207; and nutritional problems, 25-28, 56-57, 138-39, 269-70

Very low density lipoproteins (VLDL), 82-83

Vinegars, 189, 212

Vitality Scale, xxi

Vitamin B, 93

Vitamin B complex, 222

Vitamin B-6, 225-26

Vitamin B-12, 26, 27

Vitamin B-17, 98

Vitamin C, 93, 221, 226

Vitamin D, 79, 80, 217

Vitamin E, 67, 90, 258

Vitamin F, 64-66, 74

Vitamin supplements, 29, 220-24

Vitamins: and enzymes, 159; function of, 221; loss of, in pasteurized milk, 79; in vegetables, 42

VLDL. See Very low density lipoproteins (VLDL)

Water: avoidance of tap water, 212, 218, 257-59; bottled water, 259; chlorinated water, 258-59; distilled water, 259; as element of health, 12, 13, 131, 216, 217; necessary amount of, 260; poor quality of tap water, 257-59; purification system for, 259; timing and amount of, 189-90, 237-40, 264; in vegetables, 42; ways to have pure water, 259; and weight loss, 259 Weight loss, 240, 261-62, 263

Wheat, genetic engineering of, 43

Wheat germ, 90

Wheelwright, Stu: "ACX/CTV/CLNZ Pesticide Detox Program" of, 139; author's work with, xiii-xv; AZV supplement of, 223-24; on carbohydrates, 52; cooking vegetables with wok, 86; on effective protein digestion, 147-54; on enhancing protein assimilation with vegetables and high quality oil, 155-66; on excess carbohydrates, 94-95; on 5 + 5 meal, 166, 181-82, 235-43; and genetic engineering of vegetables, 42-43; on glandular typing, 109-10; guidelines for optimal protein use, 143-44, 190; herbal formulas of, 129; on importance of own garden, 44; on ionization potential of foods, 129; Liver Triad program of, 51, 109, 230; on low- stress diet, 15-18; MIN formula of, 224; on optimal time for proteins, 173-82; on pimiento for healthy arteries, 70; on plant bioenergy, 20- 23; PRO formula of, 169; on protein economy, 167- 72; on shrimp, 141-43; on supplementation, 223-24; on Vitamin E, 67

Wheelwright, Stuart (son), 18

Wild rice, 150

Xanthine oxidase (XO), 81

Yard eggs, 76, 196, 210, 229; cooking of, 195-196

Yeast infections, 120

Yeast overgrowth, 187

Yoghurt, mixed with flax seed oil, 86

Yogurt Salad Dressing (recipe), 310, 312

Yogurt Sauce (recipe), 310

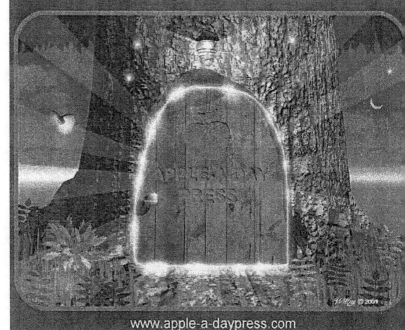

www.apple-a-daypress.com

Apple-A-Day Press

1500 Village West Drive, Suite 77
Austin, TX 78733
Phone: 512-328-3996
Toll Free: 877-442-7753
Fax: 512-263-7787
E-mail: apple-a-day@austin.rr.com

Welcome to Apple-A-Day Press:
Your natural health resource!

Here you'll find some of the most amazing and informative books, courses, and healing programs available in the world today!

Since 1984, Apple-A-Day Press has published insightful books and natural health courses that have helped thousands (even millions) of people with their health. With a primary focus on the research and writings of Dr. Jack Tips, nothing here is like what you've encountered before. At Apple-A-Day, you'll view health and healing from a totally new perspective—one that is deeper, more well-rounded, and watch out—you may catch a dose of dry Texas humor! These books are jam-packed with valuable information that truly brings the gift of health.

You'll find much more information on our web site, www.apple-a-daypress.com including downloads of chapters of our books, other free articles, lab tests, nutritional programs, and health building tools.

It is indeed an honor and a pleasure to share these tools, insights and knowledge with you. It is our foremost desire that this site contribute to your good health, good insight, and good life...Best Wishes in your health endeavors!

Apple-A-Day Press

Natural Healing at Your Fingertips

For more information on your "do it yourself" health improvement system, log on to www.apple-a-daypress.com.

Join the Apple-A-Day Press confidential mailing list and be the first to know about new books, discounts, special offers and seminars. Join on line at www.apple-a-daypress.com.

Toll free order line: 1-877-442-7753
(orders only, 24-hours secure)
Or on-line: www.apple-a-daypress.com

APPLE-A-DAY PRESS

1500 Village West Drive, Suite 77, Austin, Texas, 78733

Phone: 512.328.3996 Fax: 512.263.7787

Website: www.apple-a-daypress.com

Email: apple-a-day@austin.rr.com

Passion Play by Dr. Jack Tips

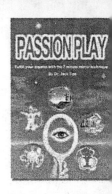

If ever a book could change your life—increase your wealth, improve your relationships, and open your heart—this is it. Absolutely profound and insightful. Believe this—the Mirror Technique is a true shortcut to success in any endeavor. It starts where other self-help books leave off—beyond affirmations, beyond visualization, beyond anything you've ever tried!

Passion Play is the art of combining Sensualization with the Native American Mirror Technique to harness your hidden power of manifestation. Use this technique to awaken your heart, encourage your actions, enliven your dreams, clarify your mission, achieve your goals and discover your true destiny. Passion Play is a new, powerful breakthrough in self-realization and human potential. Wealth, love, romance, success, charity, health, freedom, contentment, joy, exciteme and spiritual adventures await you—within these pages, within your life. Never before has the step-by-step process to recreate yourself, create your future life, and follow your heart's desire based on your core values become so clear, simple, and effective. Now you can discover your passion and begin your play. Passion Play will improve your life—Forever.

333 pages, ISBN 0-929167-20-1 $24.9

The Weight Is Over by Dr. Jack Tips

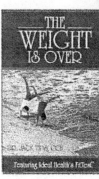

A powerful, health-building book. The last weight-loss book you'll ever need! Much more than how to lose weight, this book teaches how to gain true health! Anyone can benefit from this myth-busting breakthrough!

Get trim now! It's not your fault your weight is up and your energy is down. You've avoided fat, you've increased grains, you've eaten less—just like they told you. But you know what? They told you wrong! Now, for the first time, find out why people have excessive weight and how you can eradicate it. Learn about the perfect, custom-designed eating plan for you as an individual! Take The FitTest—a simple, in-home lab test that reveals how to get trim now. The Weight Is Over is a groundbreaking new program that takes you step by step into a mastery of nutrition—both eating to lose fat and building optimal health simultaneously. Much more than a crash program, this book helps yo build a healthy Pro-Vita! lifestyle that will benefit you for the rest of your life. Learn about:

- So called "bad" foods that are really good for you!
- Super foods that unleash your body's ability to burn fat while you sleep!
- Herbs and nutrients that help you burn fat for energy!
- 'Syndrome X' and how it silently kills people.
- The 12 Optimal Food Factors – never before published insights on everything your diet must provide you to prevent disease and be healthy!

The Weight Is Over is more than guidelines and tips, it is a strategic action plan, based on ove 30-years of research and clinical experience. You'll be taken through the maze of nutrition confusion into a very simple, crystal clear program that brings you success you can keep. It's easy, it's fun, it's effective!

300 pages (limited edition), ISBN 0-929167-21-X $24.9

BOOKS AND TAPES

The Pro-Vita! Plan for Optimal Nutrition by Dr. Jack Tips

A nutrition classic and one of the most important natural health books of the 20th Century! Absolutely a must read for every natural health practitioner and anyone wanting to end the confusion about dietary health.

Here is a simple and comprehensive way to build your health, prevent disease, and increase longevity based on both biochemistry and bio-energy! An extraordinary overview of how to minimize dietary stress and maximize utilization of the highest quality food factors: protein, fat, carbohydrates, minerals, vitamins, enzymes, fiber, nascent water, and bio-energy.

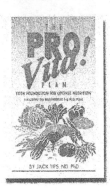

A safe, non-radical nutritional foundation based on 'ancient wisdom' and 'common sense' that can change your life and bring the best of health.

Daily nutrition plans and delicious recipes are included. Learn how to design the optimal nutrition meal and turn your eating experience into a healing experience! You will gain a greater understanding of nutrition and its role in health. A simple approach to more energy, weight loss, improved immunity, and better health!

376 pages, index, ISBN 0-929167-05-8 $22.95

Toll free order line: 1-877-442-7753
Or on-line: www.apple-a-daypress.com

Conquer Candida – Restore Your Immune System by Dr. Jack Tips

Not just another candida book but a natural health milestone. This book goes where others have never dared—a deeper understanding of health and its restoration.

Hailed by readers and natural health practitioners alike as the finest and most easy to understand book about the "canary in the mine shaft" regarding your health. Not just another candida book, here is an in-depth look at the silent, health-undermining pandemic that contributes to allergies, chronic fatigue, PMS, chronic infections, headaches, bloating, memory loss, and immune deficiencies. More importantly, this book explains what to do about these conditions by indicating true causes and offering unique insights based on hundreds of clinical case histories. "Many people blame all their health ailments on candida (yeast fungus), but this is not really the problem! Many people overlook the fact that candida is not only a symptom of impaired immunity, it also predisposes people to further poor health and low energy.

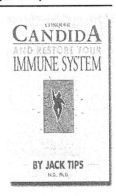

You cannot quickly win the battle against candida by dietary adjustment, but you can with proper natural health therapy." Find out if candida is a factor in your health picture and what to do about it with the Apple-A-Day comprehensive program. This information goes beyond current treatments and offers an understanding of how to truly conquer candida and restore your most optimal health.

163 pages, ISBN 0-929167-00-7 $15.95

BOOKS AND TAPES

Breast Health — A Women's Health Discourse by Dr. Jack Tips

Are you simply waiting and hoping your next mammogram won't steal your life with the dreaded news? Find out what you can do now to not only protect your health but to have overall female hormone balance. Find out why men need to read this material.

From the natural health perspective, there are clear reasons that breast cancer occurs and thus there are clear steps to take to prevent it! In this discourse, you will learn the reasons that the breast tissue is susceptible to disease and learn simple steps to avoid them. Beyond disease concerns, the breasts play an important role in overall female hormonal balance. Breast health is an important part of overcoming PMS, menstrual cramping, endometriosis, and menopausal symptoms. This discourse discusses the role of breast tissue in female endocrine balance and demonstrates how to maintain healthy breast tissue. Features the breast-test and breast massage technique to help prevent breast disease and maintain tissue integrity. Unpublished manuscript.

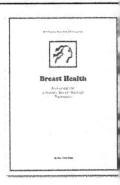

56 pages, illustrations $9.95

The Next Step to Greater Energy: A Unique Perspective on Bioenergy, Addictions and Transformation by Dr. Jack Tips

Are your "little addictions" a clear symptom of a metabolic imbalance? Breaking addictive behaviors is more effective with this information.

Explore the energy systems of the body with emphasis on both the glandular (thyroid and adrenals) and bio-electric energy systems. This book presents a new look at the connection between bio-energy and addictions. Discover energy impostors including substances, activities, and habits. Identify addictions and habits as symptoms of bio-energetic and biochemical imbalances. Discover the true cause of cravings and addictive patterns, and how to correct the underlying imbalances. How to stop smoking is thoroughly discussed. The focus of this practical information is how to obtain freedom and fuller spiritual expression.

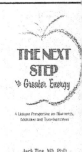

Web download only, www.apple-a-daypress.com, 210 pages, index, ISBN 0-929167-04-X $16.9

Women's Health Discourses by Dr. Jack Tips

Formerly available for sale in this catalog, the discourses on Menopause, PMS, and Osteoporosis among many others are now available for free on the website www.jacktips.com. Enjoy the gift of health-empowering information from Dr. Tips!

BOOKS AND TAPES

Your Liver...Your Lifeline! (The Healing Triad) by Dr. Jack Tips

The liver—the most important organ in your body and a key part of your immune system. Fascinating insights on how to detoxify your entire body by building your inherent liver function. This information changes lives!

Featured at Anthony Robbins' Life Mastery University, here is the key to detoxification and restoration of proper liver function. This is a fascinating look at the liver—your most important organ—its bioforces and the Chinese healing system involving the triad of the liver-stomach-colon. Explains in easy steps how to detoxify your liver, gall bladder and entire body the natural way. Contains provocative insights into how herbs really work to help your body heal. Reveals natural liver treatments and cures. Shows you how to build the very foundation upon which your health rests! Doc Wheelwright discovered seven herbs that he called "miraculous" that support the complex liver systems and created a remarkable breakthrough in liver support. A must read for people with concerns regarding Hepatitis C and anyone wanting to live life in the best of health.

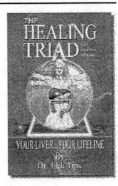

150 pages, illustrations, photos, index, ISBN 0-929167-06-6 $15.95

The Healing Triad (CD's) with Dr. Jack Tips

A candid discussion on the ancient Chinese foundation of healing and the 21st Century applications brought forth by Doc Wheelwright. [Companion discussion that further elaborates on Your Liver...Your Lifeline! (The Healing Triad)]

Master vibrant health in a polluted world! Learn about the ancient healing triad, the truth about parasites, and a simple technique for detecting liver problems. Find out about the liver's role in allergies, PMS, candida, fatigue, and skin problems. In this lively discussion, you'll discover how to improve digestion, detoxification and elimination.

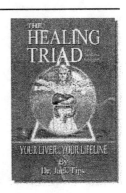

2 CD set in binder, ISBN 0-929167-13-9 $19.95

Save on Healing Triad Set (Book and CDs) $32.95

Toll free order line: 1-877-442-7753
Or on-line: www.apple-a-daypress.com

Cooking with Brooke Recipes by Melane Lohmann

Wonderful, healthful Pro-Vita! Recipes from a wonderful cook.

Delicious Pro-Vita! Recipes served by Brooke Medicine Eagle at the Eagle Song Camp (Blacktail Ranch, Montana). A great companion of simple, tasty recipes based on the Pro-Vita! Plan For Optimal Nutrition.

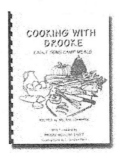

57 pages, spiral bound, illustrated $12.00

A Guidebook to Clinical Nutrition for the Health Professional by Dr. Timothy Kuss

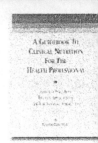

What to do and how to do it. Valuable information on how to help people heal.

A fascinating guide and desk reference through Dr. Wheelwright's work with herbs by one of his leading protégés. Includes a 400-entry Clinician's Manual of herbal protocols, and demonstrates Dr. Wheelwright's bioenergetic research. Full of valuable information on the natural cure of the most common health concerns. Includes more than the Wheelwright herbal system and embraces the full spectrum of natural healing.

Revised in 2001, 275 pages $21.95

Systemic Nutrition/Herbology Training Program (The Training!) by Dr. Jack Tips with Dr. Tim Kuss

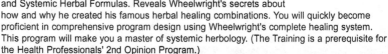

Master the Doc Wheelwright healing formulas and learn his programming secrets with this cassette course that becomes your desk reference book for one of the most advanced healing systems in the world.

For the health professional, this training program features 14 cassette tapes, a discourse on advanced applications of Doc Wheelwright's herbal system, and a 200-page desk reference for thorough training in the applications of Wheelwright's research and Systemic Herbal Formulas. Reveals Wheelwright's secrets about how and why he created his famous herbal healing combinations. You will quickly become proficient in comprehensive program design using Wheelwright's complete healing system. This program will make you a master of systemic herbology. (The Training is a prerequisite for the Health Professionals' 2nd Opinion Program.)

14 cassettes in binder, discourse (protocols), 200-page manual $159.00

For additional health professional offerings, please visit www.jacktips.com

Blood Chemistry & Clinical Nutrition by Dr. Jack Tips

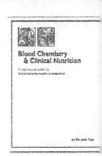

Deep nutritional insights from the ordinary Auto-Chem, SMAC-26/CBC blood test.

For the clinical nutritionist, this manual and desk reference examines each blood test value from the SMAC-26/CBC lab test for its nutritional health implications and provides Systemic Formulas protocols for correcting imbalances. Includes optimal values, pathologies, clinical notes, cross-references, protocols and valuable insights from other clinicians. An absolutely essential tool for the practicing health professional.

123 pages, ISBN 0-929167-07-4 $44.95

Insights in the Eyes: An Introduction to Sclerology by Dr. Jack Tips

Once you know these signs in the whites of the eye, you have insights about the cause of a person's constitution and the chief factors that can limit health.

A brief but thorough introduction to the history, premises, and practice of interpreting the red lines in the white of the eyes for stress patterns and nutritional implications. Features the 30 most common stress lines, commentaries, and excerpts from the ISI Art & Science of Sclerology Certification Course.

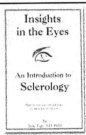

90 pages, illustrations $19.95

The Art & Science of Sclerology Certification Course by Dr. Jack Tips

Red lines in the whites of your eyes—what do they mean? Here's the most accurate, most advanced, most comprehensive, and most simple training in Sclerology—the interpretation of the red lines in the whites of the eyes for their health implications!

You can become a Sclerologist! Here is the most advanced up-to-date information in the world on the interpretation of the red lines in the white of the eyes for their health implications. This course will certify you to interpret what the sclera—the whites of the eyes—is revealing about a person's health.

This is the International Sclerology Institute's (ISI's) distance education certification course and is the definitive and foundational course for

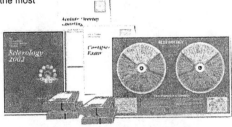

all Sclerologists around the world. Straight from the founder—A.S. Doc Wheelwright—this course teaches you to master the language of the eyes. It contains 7-hours of instructional video (CD-DVD) along with a segment on the adrenal glands taught by Wheelwright; a 300-page manual, a full color laminated wall chart; an acetate overlay system to assist practitioners in charting; and the certification examination. Upon successful completion of the exam requirements, your certificate will be issued by the ISI and you will be certified as a Sclerologist. More information is on the web site www.sclerology-institute.org.

Regular price $699
Limited time special offer price $399

Sclerology Pens

Doc Wheelwright's favorite pen for accurately charting the sclera.

This calligraphic pen delivers red ink via a brush on one end plus a fine-line detail via a nib on the other end. Perfect to capture the prominent veins as well as fine lines and other markings when charting the sclera on paper.

$3.95 each

Toll free order line: 1-877-442-7753 or on-line: www.apple-a-daypress.com

SCLEROLOGY

Sclerology Wall Chart
by the International Sclerology Institute

The worldwide official chart of reflex zones in the white of the eyes.

Sclerology is the art of evaluating the entire body's health stresses from the reflexive red lines in the white of the eyes. This is the official chart, the most accurate and up-to-date one available. Chart outlines zones and lines.

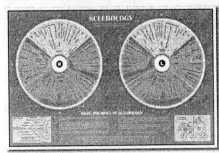

Artfully designed, four color, 11x17   **$19.95**

Sclerology Wall Chart (Organs Depicted)
by the International Sclerology Institute

Attractive, historical Sclerology chart with drawings of organs in the proper zones.

This older version chart, enjoyed by Doc Wheelwright, graphically and artistically depicts the major organ systems in the sclera.

White on Blue, 11X14   **$14.95**

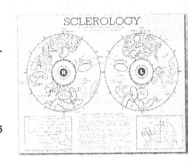

Stories The Eyes Can Tell:
A Sclerology Starter Package by Dr. Jack Tips

Learn the major markings and how to chart the sclera.

Start with the book Insights In the Eyes: An Introduction to Sclerology and then view the Introduction to Sclerology Video (CD-DVD) that presents an overview of Sclerology and a live demonstration of how to chart the eyes while referring to the laminated, color Sclerology Wall Chart. This is a great way to start learning to interpret the secrets of the eyes. A $70 value!

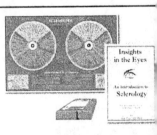

Book, chart, CD-DVD   **$49.95**

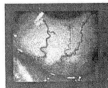

**For more information on Sclerology:
www.sclerology-institute.org**

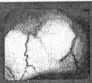

Sclerascope (Sclerology/Iridology) Camera

The ancient science enters the 21st Century! State of the art camera puts sclera (and iris) images on your computer screen for grid analysis and more.

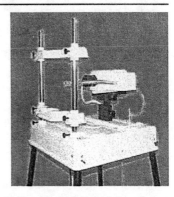

Take advantage of instant photography for immediate analysis with direct input into your own personal computer or laptop. This state of the art instrument has been built to the precise specifications of leading iridologists worldwide and its applications are perfectly applicable for Sclerology.

Unlock and capture the history and all the vital information portrayed in the sclera through the use of the Sclerascope Camera System. It's fast, safe and easy to operate. This complete, turnkey system utilizes the patented, fiber optic, proper spectrum lighting system (180,000 optical fibers) designed for close-up macro enlargements of the sclera (and iris). This unique high intensity, cool lighting system captures the greatest depth of field and the highest resolution, offering the most comfort and protection to the eyes against the dangers of ultra-violet rays that are produced from all photography lighting.

Now you can photograph your patient's sclera (and iris) with this digital camera system and bring it to your computer screen for immediate analysis during the time of visit. This camera system comes with the renowned Iridology Scanning System software included (a $495 value) and a USB connector plug-in—everything you need to operate the camera, to view, enhance and examine the eye's information on the screen.

High Resolution, up to 1.2 million pixels. The image comes directly into your computer. Compatible with Windows 98 for the PC and the Virtual PC program on the Apple/Macintosh.

This 120 volts system is lightweight, yet durable, can be operated on location under any lighting conditions or is completely mobile for easy set-up and use wherever you might travel. (Optional 220V adapters available.)

Features:

- Telescoping legs and supporting platform
- Chin and head rests for customer comfort

Sclerascope Camera Photos

- State of the art digital/video camera. (No previous photography experience necessary)
- Two fiber optical lighting assemblies with macro enlargement lenses
- Travel case
- Complete instruction manual
- One year limited warranty

- Operating System—Iridology Scanning Software. You receive a complete iris scanning grid system to which you will add the independent Sclerology plug in. Features:

Travel Case

  - Patient Database: records patient details, sclera (and iris) signs, suggestions and comments
  - Patient Report Printouts: Includes the option to print out patient sclera and iris images, graphs, suggestions, comments and sclera markings
  - Image Adjustment: through a selection of settings
  - State of the art tools including: Graphic and Text Tools, Image Zooming Tools, Diets, Help files on Constitutions
  - Sclerology Interpretive CD-ROM Software (List: $349. Included.)

Regular price $5950   ISI price $5650.

SCLEROLOGY

The Art & Science of Sclerology Manual CD-ROM

Put the ISI Certification Course Reference Manual in your computer for quick access.

Available only to those enrolled in the Art & Science of Sclerology Certification Course, this CD places the entire Art & Science of Sclerology desk reference manual onto your PC computer or into your "Virtual PC" program on your Apple/Macintosh computer. This program provides a quick search feature that lets you reference any topic in the manual and bring that information into view. Example: if you want to check the pancreas, you can instantly bring all the pancreas line examples to your screen.

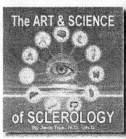

1-CD-ROM   List price $159.95
Special offer, limited time at $99.95

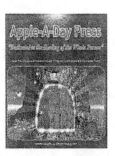

Natural Healing at Your Fingertips

For more information on your "do it yourself" health improvement system, log on to www.apple-a-daypress.com.

Join the Apple-A-Day Press confidential mailing list and be the first to know about new books, discounts, special offers and seminars. Join on line at www.apple-a-daypress.com.

APPLE-A-DAY PRESS

1500 Village West Drive, Suite 77
Austin, Texas, 78733

Phone: 512.328.3996
Fax: 512.263.7787

Website: www.apple-a-daypress.com
Email: apple-a-day@austin.rr.com

Toll free order line: 1-877-442-7753
(orders only, 24-hours secure)
Or on-line: www.apple-a-daypress.com

Apple-A-Day Press
Dedicated to the Healing of the Whole Person

Important News! Our web site www.apple-a-daypress.com offers additional health-enhancing services including Lab Tests, Tried 'N True Nutritional Programs, and Natural Resources (health building products) to bring you more tools for optimal health.

ORDER FORM

Books and Tapes

■ The Weight Is Over* (ISBN 0-929167-21-x)	$24.95 ____	$ _____
■ Passion Play* (ISBN 0-929167-20-1)	$24.95 ____	$ _____
■ The Pro-Vita! Plan for Optimal Nutrition* (ISBN 0-929167-05-8)	$22.95 ____	$ _____
■ Conquer Candida – Restore Your Immune System* (ISBN 0-929167-00-7)	$15.95 ____	$ _____
■ Breast Health – Women's Health Discourse	$9.95 ____	$ _____
■ The Next Step to Greater Energy* (ISBN 9-929167-04-X) (web download)	$16.95 ____	$ _____
■ Your Liver...Your Lifeline! (The Healing Triad)* (ISBN 0-929167-06-6)	$15.95 ____	$ _____
■ The Healing Triad (2 CD set)	$19.95 ____	$ _____
■ The Healing Triad Set (Your Liver...Your Lifeline! book and CDs)	$32.95 ____	$ _____
■ Cooking with Brooke	$12.00 ____	$ _____

For the Health Professional

■ A Guidebook to Clinical Nutrition	$21.95 ____	$ _____
■ Systemic Nutrition/Herbology Training Program (cassettes & manual)	$159.00 ____	$ _____
■ Blood Chemistry & Clinical Nutrition (ISBN 0-929167-07-4)	$44.95 ____	$ _____

Sclerology

■ Insights in the Eyes: An Introduction to Sclerology* (ISBN 9-929167-11-2)	$19.95 ____	$ _____
■ The Art & Science of Sclerology Certification Course (list $699)	$399.00 ____	$ _____
■ Sclerology Pens	$3.95 ____	$ _____
■ Sclerology Wall Chart* (Color)	$19.95 ____	$ _____
■ Sclerology Wall Chart* (Organs Depicted)	$14.95 ____	$ _____
■ Sclerology Starter Package (book, CD, chart)	$49.95 ____	$ _____
■ The Art & Science of Sclerology Manual CD-ROM	$99.95 ____	$ _____

ORDER SUBTOTAL $ _____

* Discount available with purchase of any combination of 12 or more of titles denoted with an asterix. Contact our office for more information.

TAX (if applicable) $ _____

S&H, COD $ _____

TOTAL $ _____

Name _____ Date _____

Address _____

City/State/Zip _____

Phone_____ E-mail _____

Method of Payment ☐ Check ☐ Credit Card

Name on card _____

Card # _____

Exp. Date _____

Signature _____

Order on the Internet at: www.apple-a-daypress.com

Apple-A-Day Press
1500 Village West Drive, Suite 77
Austin, TX 78733

E-mail:
apple-a-day@austin.rr.com

Phone: 512-328-3996
Toll Free: 877-442-7753
Fax: 512-263-7787

ANNOUNCING A PRO-VITA! BREAKTHROUGH

The Pro-Vita! In a Jar

With this reprint of the *Pro-Vita! Plan*, I am very excited to make this announcement. Beginning November 1, 2000, people will be able to have a quick Pro-Vita! meal before rushing off to a busy day. We have just completed the design and manufacture of a powdered beverage nutritional formula called ACCELL that can form the base of a Pro-Vita! meal and meet the 12 Optimal Nutrition Factors taught throughout this book and in its companion book, *The Weight Is Over*.

Two proteges of Dr. Wheelwright—Drs. Timothy Kuss and Jack Tips—joined with Dr. Wheelwright's son, Stu Wheelwright, Jr., and production expert, Dr. Daeyoon Kim, to build a nutritional supplement in the Pro-Vita! tradition.

This supplement, ACCELL, starts with an organic rice protein base, enhanced with the limiting amino acids for a balanced blend of essential proteins. To that is combined an herbal matrix that supports a huge array of natural nutrients. More than just a nutritional drink, ACCELL provides key ingredients for the Healing Triad© (discussed in *Your Liver—Your Lifeline*) of Digestion, Intestines, Liver. Further, it benefits the glucose metabolism; immune anti- inflammatory processes; and is perfect for weight management.

For people who need a quick Pro-Vita! meal without the time of food preparation—great for travel—the basic recipe is: 2 scoops ACCELL in 6–8 oz pure water, plus 2 capsules of an essential fatty acid formula such as BFO, plus 3–5 capsules of pectin fiber (such as Nutri-fiber). For more living enzymes and nascent water, include some crisp raw vegetables such as a stalk of celery or a carrot. These vegetables travel well or can easily be obtained.

So now, a quick drink with some capsules, and a raw vegetable to munch on, a person can be heading down the road with this new breed of "fast food" that genuinely supports the body in countless ways.

This hypo-allergenic, all-natural dietary convenience and approach to supporting the fundamental healing processes of the body took over three years to develop. The result is something that we think will be a wonderful blessing, because now people can easily start their day with super nutrition, even when kitchen facilities are not available.

For more information on this program, please contact your natural health professional. You may contact the publisher for a practitioner near you.

Best wishes in your health endeavors!